Mindfulness-Based Cognitive Therapy

Stuart J. Eisendrath
Editor

Mindfulness-Based Cognitive Therapy

Innovative Applications

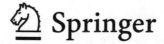 Springer

Editor
Stuart J. Eisendrath
The UCSF Depression Center
Langley Porter Psychiatric Institute
University of California, San Franc
San Francisco, CA, USA

ISBN 978-3-319-80672-3   ISBN 978-3-319-29866-5   (eBook)
DOI 10.1007/978-3-319-29866-5

Printed on acid-free paper

This Springer imprint is published by Springer Nature
The registered company is Springer International Publishing AG Switzerland

I want to thank my wonderful family: Debra, Adam, Allison, Faina, Samson and Mila. They have supported me in my mindfulness explorations.

Contents

Contributors

Marcus Averbeck, Ph.D. Department of Adult Mental Health, Erith Center, Park Crescent, London, UK

Sejal M. Barden, Ph.D. Child, Family and Community Sciences, College of Education, University of Central Florida, Orlando, FL, USA

Michel Bédard, Ph.D. Department of Health Sciences, Lakehead University, Thunder Bay, ON, Canada

Centre for Applied Health Research, St. Jospeh's Care Group, Thunder Bay, ON, Canada

Northern Ontario School of Medicine, Lakehead University, Thunder Bay, ON, Canada

Xavier Borràs, Ph.D. Stress and Health Research Group (GIES), Faculty of Psychology, Universitat Autònoma de Barcelona, Barcelona, Spain

Kate Cavanagh, D.Phil., D.Clin.Psych. Sussex Mindfulness Centre, Sussex Partnership NHS Foundation Trust, Research and Development Department, Sussex Education Centre, Mill View Hospital Site, Neville Avenue, Hove, UK

School of Psychology, University of Sussex, Falmer, East Sussex, UK

Melissa A. Day, M.A. (Clin.), Ph.D. School of Psychology, The University of Queensland, Brisbane, QLD, Australia

Serina Deen, M.D., M.P.H. Department of Psychiatry, University of California, San Francisco, CA, USA

Stuart J. Eisendrath, M.D. The UCSF Depression Center, Langley Porter Psychiatric Institute, University of California, San Francisco, San Francisco, CA, USA

Susan Evans, Ph.D. Weill Cornell Medical College, New York, NY, USA

Todd K. Favorite, Ph.D., A.B.P.P. Department of Psychiatry and University Psychological Clinic, University of Michigan, Ann Arbor, MI, USA

PTSD Clinic, Mental Health Service, VA Ann Arbor Health System, Ann Arbor, MI, USA

Lone Fjorback, M.D., Ph.D. Danish Center for Mindfulness, Aarhus University Hospital, Aarhus, Denmark

Elizabeth Foley, Ph.D. Mind Potential, Caringbah, NSW, Australia

Thomas Forkmann, Ph.D. Institute of Medical Psychology and Medical Sociology, University Hospital of RWTH Aachen University, Aachen, Germany

Carrie Gibbons, M.P.H. Centre for Applied Health Research, St. Joseph's Care Group, Thunder Bay, ON, Canada

Jessica Gonzalez, Ph.D. College of Health and Human Science, School of Education Counseling and Career Development, Colorado State University, Fort Collins, CO, USA

Marian González-García, Ph.D. Department of Psychology, European University of the Atlantic, Santander, Spain

BalanCe Center for Psychology & Mindfulness, Santander, Spain

Kim Griffiths, Ph.D. Department of Adult Mental Health, Erith Center, Park Crescent, London, UK

Katleen Van der Gucht, Ph.D. Faculty of Psychology and Educational Sciences, University of Leuven, Leuven, Belgium

Neil Horn, M.B.Ch.B., UCT., M.R.C.(Psych.) Department of Psychiatry, University of Cape Town, Cape Town, South Africa

Fleur Howells, Ph.D. Department of Psychiatry, University of Cape Town, Cape Town, South Africa

Victoria L. Ives-Deliperi, Ph.D. Department of Neurology, University of Cape Town, Cape Town, South Africa

Fergal W. Jones, Ph.D., Psych.D. Salomons Centre for Applied Psychology, Canterbury Christ Church University, Tunbridge Wells, UK

Sussex Mindfulness Centre, Sussex Partnership NHS Foundation Trust, Research and Development Department, Sussex Education Centre, Mill View Hospital Site, Neville Avenue, Hove, UK

Anthony P. King, Ph.D. Department of Psychiatry and University Psychological Clinic, University of Michigan, Ann Arbor, MI, USA

Research Service, VA Ann Arbor Health System, Ann Arbor, MI, USA

Peter Kuppens, Ph.D. Faculty of Psychology and Educational Sciences, University of Leuven, Leuven, Belgium

Javier González López, M.S. BalanCe Center for Psychology & Mindfulness, Santander, Spain

David Adam Lovas, M.D. Department of Psychiatry, IWK Children's Hospital, Dalhousie University, Halifax, NS, Canada

Department of Psychology and Neuroscience, Dalhousie University, Halifax, NS, Canada

Edel Maex, M.D. ZnA Stresskliniek, St. Elisabeth's Hospital, Antwerp, Belgium

Robin E. McGee, M.P.H. Department of Behavioral Sciences and Health Education, Rollins School of Public Health, Emory University, Atlanta, GA, USA

Kim Griffin McNeil, Ph.D. Department Chair of Translation and Interpretation, European University of the Atlantic, Santander, Spain

Johannes Michalak, Ph.D. Department of Psychology and Psychotherapy, Witten/Herdecke University, Witten/Herdecke, Germany

Lana J. Ozen, Ph.D. Department of Health Sciences, Lakehead University, Thunder Bay, ON, Canada

Centre for Applied Health Research, St. Joseph's Care Group, Thunder Bay, ON, Canada

Filip Raes, Ph.D. Faculty of Psychology and Educational Sciences, University of Leuven, Leuven, Belgium

Hiske van Ravesteijn, M.D., Ph.D. Department of Psychiatry, Radboud University Nijmegen Medical Centre, Nijmegen, The Netherlands

Poppy L.A. Schoenberg, Ph.D. Departments of Psychiatry and Cognitive Neuroscience, Radboud University Medical Center, Nijmegen, The Netherlands

Amanda J. Shallcross, N.D., M.P.H. Department of Medicine and Population Health, New York University, Langone Medical Center, New York, NY, USA

Walter Sipe University of California, San Francisco, CA, USA

Lesley Stafford, Ph.D. Centre for Women's Mental Health, Royal Women's Hospital, Parkville, VIC, Australia

Clara Strauss, D.Phil., Psych.D. Sussex Mindfulness Centre, Sussex Partnership NHS Foundation Trust, Research and Development Department, Sussex Education Centre, Hove, UK

School of Psychology, University of Sussex, Falmer, East Sussex, UK

Tobias Teismann, Ph.D. Department for Clinical Psychology and Psychotherapy, Ruhr-Universität Bochum, Bochum, Germany

Naomi Thomas, Ph.D. Centre for Women's Mental Health, Royal Women's Hospital, Parkville, VIC, Australia

Nancy J. Thompson, Ph.D., M.P.H. Department of Behavioral Sciences and Health Education, Rollins School of Public Health, Emory University, Atlanta, GA, USA

Pallavi D. Visvanathan, Ph.D. Manhattan Mindfulness-Based Cognitive Behavioral Therapy, New York, NY, USA

Elizabeth Reisinger Walker, Ph.D., M.P.H. Department of Health Policy and Management, Rollins School of Public Health, Emory University, Atlanta, GA, USA

Andrew W. Wood, Ph.D. School of Applied Psychology, Counseling, and Family Therapy, Clinical Mental Health Counseling, Antioch University, Seattle, WA, USA

Introduction

Stuart J. Eisendrath

Zindel Segal, John Teasdale, and **Mark Williams** brought Mindfulness-Based Cognitive Therapy (MBCT) into wide exposure with their 2002 treatment book [1]. MBCT was built on the infrastructure of Mindfulness-Based Stress Reduction and it presented a radical departure in the approach to relapse prevention of major depressive disorder. This disorder, with an often chronic and relapsing course, called for a preventive approach in order to decrease the disability and suffering that were so often prevalent. Early studies demonstrated its efficacy in depression relapse prevention [2, 3]. Its utility in preventing relapse in major depressive disorder has demonstrated an efficacy that is not inferior to maintenance antidepressants, the gold standard of prophylactic treatment [4].

MBCT's metacognitive approach indicated that attention to the thought process was important and perhaps even more so than attention to thought content as in traditional cognitive therapy approaches. The metacognitive awareness of thoughts, feelings, and sensations can lead to greater acceptance of mental events and consequent less experiential avoidance. For example, paying attention to thought processes and not

content was one of the important shifts in approach that allowed many patients to engage with the therapeutic process. Previously, they were often firmly attached to a particular thought content that kept them rigidly locked in a specific life stance. MBCT allowed a softer stance, with more self-compassion and flexibility. The mindfulness approach permitted a bigger gap between stimulus and response, with a consequent ability to have a broader range of skillful approaches to situations.

MBCT's applications broadened since its introduction to treatment of a variety of conditions, of which only a limited sampling has been gathered in this book. Ranging from medically unexplained symptoms to social anxiety, and epilepsy to insomnia, the palette of MBCT has covered a wide spectrum. Taking one pass through multiple MBCT applications, as the authors of the chapters in this volume illustrate, MBCT has had a broad international reach. Moreover, the range of chapters indicates MBCT has begun to emerge as a modality with a wide range of utility. MBCT has been drawing substantial investigations that demonstrate transdiagnostic effects. Exactly which component of MBCT produces these effects remains to be elucidated, but the authors raise a number of possibilities. In addition, a number of the authors describe the increased activation of brain areas such as the dorsolateral prefrontal cortex and the anterior cingulate, that are associated with enhanced emotion regulation. At the same time increased

S.J. Eisendrath, M.D. (✉)
The UCSF Depression Center, Langley Porter Psychiatric Institute, University of California, San Francisco, 401 Parnassus Avenue, Office 278, San Francisco, CA 94143-0984, USA
e-mail: stuart.eisendrath@ucsf.edu

© Springer International Publishing Switzerland 2016
S.J. Eisendrath (ed.), *Mindfulness-Based Cognitive Therapy*, DOI 10.1007/978-3-319-29866-5_1

activation of the insula is associated with internal somatic awareness, one of the areas that MBCT helps individuals to focus on.

The book's chapters are divided into primarily focusing on medical problems or psychiatric disorders. Melissa Day begins by describing the application of MBCT to chronic pain. She describes the value of the pain patient changing his/her relationship to such pain catastrophizing thoughts such as "I'm totally useless because of my pain". She lays out the adaptations of MBCT for the pain population that her group has been investigating including psychoeducation regarding pain as well as mindful awareness and acceptance. Day describes her group's work with a headache pain population in finding decreased pain interference and increased acceptance after completing MBCT. She reviews the growing literature on MBCT for other painful conditions as well as Internet-delivered MBCT. She then examines practical issues in the selection of participants and the delivery of MBCT.

Marian González-García, Xavier Borràs, and **Javier González López** bring MBCT into focus as a particularly useful intervention for people living with HIV (PLWH). This population suffers high levels of stress, stigma, anxiety, and depression. Her group's randomized controlled trial of MBCT demonstrated large effect sizes in reducing stress, anxiety, and depression levels. Psychological factors posited to play a role include attention, meta-awareness, and self-regulation. The authors build a strong case for neural mechanisms of change that may involve areas of the brain associated with increased alerting and executive attention including the anterior cingulate cortex (ACC) and dorsolateral prefrontal cortex (DLPFC). The insula may be associated with meta-awareness of experiences of the present moment and bodily states and emotional processing. These issues may be related to self-regulation, including the nonreactivity facet of mindfulness. This, in turn, is also associated with the ACC and its connections to other areas of the brain.

Nancy Thompson, Robin McGee, and **Elizabeth Walker** shine an important light on the potential of distance-delivered MBCT. Their research, including Project Uplift, has examined the impact of MBCT on individuals with chronic medical illnesses such as epilepsy or cystic fibrosis. For such patients, the advantages of telephone or Internet-enabled MBCT have important advantages such as ease of access, low cost, avoidance of transportation problems, and reduced stigma. There are however potential problems with such delivery and the authors address such limitations straightforwardly. They also describe the literature in distance delivery including their own randomized controlled trials. The authors explain the modifications to MBCT that they made and the rationale that went into their decision. In the trials, participants' physical health did not change, but their quality of life improved. This was consistent with the mindfulness facet of improved acceptance as a means of reducing suffering. They call for further research into distance delivery to broaden MBCT's reach.

The problem of traumatic brain injury is being increasingly recognized in a wide-ranging population, from sports participants to military casualties. Depression is one of the most common sequelae of these injuries. **Lana J. Ozen, Carrie Gibbons,** and **Michel Bédard** investigate the impact of MBCT on depression in this population. They point out that often the impact of traumatic injury is amplified by stress, depression, and decreased satisfaction with life. Mindfulness interventions have the potential to impact all of these areas. The authors review the literature examining the utility of mindfulness-based treatment for traumatic brain injury. They then present data from their own groundbreaking work in applying MBCT to this population. Using a pilot study, and randomized controlled trials, the authors found decreased depression, improved quality of life and increased mindfulness and self-compassion in their MBCT cohorts compared to wait list controls. These effects were substantial at levels that were clinically significant. They describe in detail the modifications necessary for working with this population, including patient selection, home practice, and facilitator training. Although future research is necessary, MBCT may represent an important first step in dealing with the emotional after effects of traumatic brain injury.

In describing their work with women suffering breast and gynecological cancer, **Lesley Stafford, Naomi Thomas,** and **Elizabeth Foley** elucidate the central psychological issues with this population. After a thorough review of the literature, they explain how MBCT may be a uniquely suitable modality. They describe the modifications they made to fit their model to the population. They then provide results of their pilot work demonstrating a number of beneficial effects such as improved quality of life and decreased suffering. However, they also found that the logistics and costs of MBCT were challenging to implement. They then developed a second iteration, an abbreviated mindfulness meditation program (MMP) that yielded similar outcomes in a shorter intervention with lower costs and fewer logistical issues.

Andrew Wood, Gonzalez, and **Barden** examine the utility of MBCT in the growing population of caregivers of cancer survivors. They point out that the MBCT program can have beneficial effects for caregivers by providing sharing, support, and a forum for discussing guilt, anger, and sadness. Importantly, MBCT also offers participants the opportunity to learn techniques they can apply at home, even when giving care to loved ones. The authors describe a number of modifications that help target the MBCT sessions to the caregiver population. They lay the groundwork for future empirical investigations.

Hiske van Ravesteijn and **Lone Fjorback** describe their approach of applying MBCT to the challenge of helping individuals with medically unexplained symptoms. They examine the potential sources of such symptoms and the suffering associated with them. They describe MBCT's effects in reducing the experiential avoidance of unpleasant states in such patients. Moreover, many of MBCT's practices are aimed at enhancing authentic awareness of the body and this process may improve the patients' grounding in their bodies. The participants learn that they can tolerate what is present. They can learn to step out of automatic pilot and become more able to observe what is present. They describe specific modifications to facilitate MBCT for this population, and have developed two programs featuring

detailed manuals, one offering more time for psychoeducation about medically unexplained symptoms. Their approach has met with broad acceptance by patients.

The problem of health anxiety, more commonly known as hypochondriasis, can be a challenging condition for patient, family, and physician. **David Lovas** carefully reviews the cognitive behavioral model of health anxiety and identifies the potential mediating features that would be amenable to MBCT as an alternative treatment to CBT. He suggests that MBCT may help individuals regulate their attention to interoceptive and cognitive phenomena. He notes that MBCT may also decrease experiential avoidance, a frequent driver of health anxiety. Given these facets of MBCT, Lovas developed a MBCT program that he describes with session-by-session modifications. The results from open-label, qualitative, and a randomized controlled trial have been promising. They included outcomes such as decreased health anxiety, reassurance seeking, and belief in hypochondriacal cognitions. Taken as a whole, MBCT may be an appealing alternative to CBT for this population.

Amanda Shallcross identifies the cognitive/ affective and increased arousal components that play a significant role in insomnia. She reviews the mindfulness intervention literature including randomized controlled trials and polysomnographic studies. She goes on to develop an integrative cognitive model of insomnia. Building on this, **Shallcross** identifies MBCT features that may be useful in insomnia such as decentering from rumination, attentional control, and acceptance of unpleasant thoughts, feelings, and sensations. She suggests certain modifications for applying MBCT in this population. She concludes by describing the MBCT evidence as being most strong for individuals with depressive disorders who are suffering insomnia.

Major depressive disorder is the number one cause of disability in the developed world. The scope of suffering it brings is extraordinary. **Serina Deen, Walter Sipe,** and **Stuart Eisendrath** investigate the utility of MBCT for this population. They note that many of the cognitive factors found in depressive relapse also play a role in perpetuating the illness in treatment-resistant depression (TRD). This variant causes increased morbidity and mortality and is associated with worse medical illness outcomes. After examining potential mediators of MBCT, the authors describe how these factors may be of benefit in TRD. They use a case example to illustrate the use of a number of modifications of MBCT. These range from shorter sitting meditations to more active meditations such as yoga and walking. They also describe a number of metaphors that help participants understand key elements of MBCT. They describe the current state of the evidence for MBCT for TRD including pilot studies and one large RCT. Future research needs to further examine both the psychological mediators and the neural circuitry of MBCT effects.

Kim Griffiths and **M. Averbeck** report on a very unique approach, applying MBCT for couples. This modality applies to couples (or a participant with a family member or friend) attending a MBCT group. Griffiths and colleagues extensively review the impact of mindfulness on dyadic relationships such as couples, but also other pairs such as teacher and student. They describe the existing literature on the use of MBSR or MBCT to enhance couples relationships. They then trace how MBCT was integrated into their National Health Service clinical operation. They describe modifications to issues such as attendance, in-group discussions, assessment, and suitability. They then give the results of their pilot investigation of MBCT for couples, noting the beneficial effects based on a small sample size. Overall, their work lays the groundwork for future interesting investigations.

Bipolar disorder is one of the most prevalent and costly mental disorders. **Victoria Ives-Deliperi, Fleur Howells**, and **Neil Horn** describe emotional dysregulation and executive dysfunction as the core clinical and psychological features of bipolar disorder. Alterations in neural circuitry, such as between the ventrolateral prefrontal cortex (VLPFC) and amygdala, have been demonstrated in bipolar disorder. In a study by **Ives-Deliperi's group**, MBCT appeared to increase activation in bold signal in the medial prefrontal cortex (MPFC),

similar to pharmacological treatments. EEG findings in bipolar disorder support altered emotional processing that can be reduced with MBCT. Research data suggest that MBCT enhances activation of the MPFC, a region associated with cognitive flexibility. Taken as a whole, MBCT shows promise as a treatment enhancing emotion regulation and executive function.

Thomas Forkmann, Tobias Teismann, and **Johannes Michalak** examine MBCT's utility in one of the most challenging clinical populations, individuals with suicidal risk. They argue that a key element driving this disorder is the individual's attempt to avoid painful emotions, thoughts, sensations, and memories. They note that mindfulness may reduce suicide risk because it targets this experiential avoidance and thereby represents a transdiagnostic therapeutic process in suicidal clients, as well as substance abuse, depression, anxiety, chronic pain, and psychosis.

They also examine MBCT in relation to change in overgeneral memory. Depression has been noted to be associated with decreased specificity of autobiographical memory leading to diminished problem solving ability. This feature has been shown in suicidal patients. As MBCT reverses the finding and enhances the specificity of autobiographical memory, problem solving and suicidality decrease in this population. How MBCT exerts its effects remains an open arena of inquiry, as no formal mediator of these effects has been identified as of yet.

Susan Evans examines the utility of MBCT for generalized anxiety disorder (GAD). A number of treatments are available for this condition but full remission is difficult to achieve. Worry is a prominent symptom often focused on the past or future and not the present moment. Individuals appear to have an emotion regulation deficit with difficulty processing their emotional experiences and managing their emotions. Some of this dysfunction has been associated with hypofunction of the attentional and executive control areas of the prefrontal cortex and anterior cingulate cortex and impaired connectivity to the amygdala. After a thorough review of the literature, **Evans** describes an adaptation of MBCT for GAD. She provides a cogent discussion of specific issues that occur in each session and how they may be approached. She helpfully describes challenges in implementing MBCT in GAD and explains how the group leader can best prepare for leading a group, both technically and via a personal mindfulness practice.

Anthony King and **Todd Favorite** provide a compelling investigation of MBCT for PTSD. Drawing from their extensive experience with PTSD in combat veterans, they have crafted a well-thought out adaptation of MBCT in this population. They carefully review the extant literature on PTSD and its treatments that often feature some form of exposure. They point out that there is a growing literature on therapeutic approaches that do not feature exposure as a focus, including problem solving therapy, acceptance and commitment therapy, interpersonal therapy, and MBCT. They describe modifications of MBCT for PTSD including attention to both process (e.g. shortening meditations) and content (e.g. psychoeducation about PTSD). Their program clearly lays out aspects of MBCT that pose potential pitfalls with PTSD and offer well designed approaches. The authors provide a thorough review of the use of mindfulness intervention in PTSD and include their own work with combat veterans.

Poppy Schoenberg does a masterful job of examining the neuroanatomical, chemical, hormonal, cognitive, and psychological dimensions underpinning attention-deficit hyperactivity disorder (ADHD). She then explains how MBCT can be considered to play a role in both "top down" and "bottom up" regulation of dysregulated processes such as attention and executive control as well as biobehavioral and emotional self-regulatory pathways. She carefully reviews the literature supporting mindfulness effects in enhancing emotion regulation and attention while at the same time identifying the limits of scientific knowledge at this time. Her chapter lays a solid groundwork for future investigations of MBCT for ADHD.

Although MBCT shows promise across a spectrum of conditions, there are problems such as accessibility, availability, and stigma that may limit dissemination. **Fergal W. Jones, Clara Strauss,** and **Kate Cavanagh** examine some

potential solutions to these problems. They describe five approaches for self-help applications of MBCT. These include paper or digital media as well as Internet-delivered multimedia techniques. The five approaches are grounded in traditional MBCT but none require class participation. There is a preliminary but limited evidence base for these self-help approaches. One book-based study found that the intervention lessened depression and anxiety compared to a wait list control. Two open studies of web-based interventions found medium to large effect sizes in outcomes such as reduced depression levels, anxiety symptoms, and perceived stress. These investigations are encouraging and suggest the need for rigorous randomized controlled trials. The interventions hold significant promise of being able to deliver MBCT to a much broader population than currently possible.

Katleen Van der Gucht, Peter Kuppens, Edel Maex, and **Filip Raes** examine the role of mindfulness interventions in the school ages, particularly in adolescence. This population faces changes in emotional, behavioral, and attentional regulation. It is a time when "top down" regulation of emotions may be less available as the adolescent brain continues to develop. The authors note that 50% of European adolescents suffer some level of anxiety and depression. This underlies the need for a widespread, low-level, evidence-based intervention for this population. Schools provide an excellent venue for such interventions. They lay out the evidence for how mindfulness interventions can provide low cost, efficient, widely applicable approaches that are relatively easy to implement. The authors examine the scientific literature for such mindfulness interventions. They then describe practical considerations and guidelines for implementation.

Before closing and allowing you to directly sample some of the innovative applications of MBCT, I would like to thank a number of people. I would like to thank the patients and research participants along with the clinicians and researchers who have expanded our knowledge of MBCT. My core research team of **Erin Gilllung, Maura McLane, Lauren Erickson, Christa Hogan, Dan Mathalon, Mitch Feldman,** and **Kevin Delucchi** have been a pleasure to work with and invaluable in my learning more about the limits of MBCT. I would also like to thank **Zindel Segal** who as one of the original developers of MBCT served to ignite the flame that has spread so widely. Through his encouragement and support, I have been able to help expand the knowledge of MBCT a bit more.

References

 1. Segal Z, Williams JM, Teasdale J. Mindfulness-based cognitive therapy for depression. New York: The Guilford Press; 2002.

 2. Teasdale JD, Segal ZV, Williams JM, Ridgeway VA, Soulsby JM, Lau MA. Prevention of relapse/recurrence in major depression by mindfulness-based cognitive therapy. J Consult Clin Psychol. 2000;68:615–23.

 3. Ma SH, Teasdale JD. Mindfulness-based cognitive therapy for depression: replication and exploration of differential relapse prevention effects. J Consult Clin Psychol. 2004;72:31–40.

 4. Kuyken W, Hayes R, Barrett B, Byng R, Dalgleish T, Kessler D, et al. Effectiveness and cost-effectiveness of mindfulness-based cognitive therapy compared with maintenance antidepressant treatment in the prevention of depressive relapse or recurrence (prevent): a randomised controlled trial. Lancet. 2015;386: 63–73.

Distance Delivery of Mindfulness-Based Cognitive Therapy

Nancy J. Thompson, Robin E. McGee, and Elizabeth Reisinger Walker

Clinical Case Study

M.W. is a 44-year-old divorced African American woman living in rural Georgia. She is unemployed due to epilepsy, and lives in an apartment in her parents' home. She has had two brain surgeries, which reduced but did not eliminate her seizure activity. As a result, she remains unable to drive due to seizures. In addition to seizures, she experiences severe headaches and cognitive problems. The cognitive problems were worsened by her surgeries.

M.W. entered one of our distance-delivered groups to address depression in people with epilepsy. Our program is based upon mindfulness-based cognitive therapy (MBCT) for depression, with modifications for distance delivery and use among people with chronic disease. In the first session, when discussing factors that influence

N.J. Thompson, Ph.D., M.P.H. (✉)
R.E. McGee, M.P.H.
Department of Behavioral Sciences and Health Education, Rollins School of Public Health, Emory University, 1518 Clifton Road, Atlanta, GA 30322, USA
e-mail: nthomps@emory.edu;
robin.mcgee@emory.edu

E.R. Walker, Ph.D., M.P.H.
Department of Health Policy and Management, Rollins School of Public Health, Emory University, 1518 Clifton Road, Atlanta, GA 30322, USA
e-mail: ereisin@emory.edu

mood, M.W. noted that her brain surgeries had affected her word-finding and speech capabilities, which she found embarrassing and difficult. In addition, she reported that she has three sons and a daughter in their late teens and twenties who live with their father and rarely visit. She said she believes he has told the children untruths about her and this, too, affects her mood.

In the second session, when working on identifying thoughts, M.W. identified the thought, "I'm stupid," as one that comes to her mind when she misspeaks or finds the wrong word. She received assistance from the group, and worked on modifying her thought to, "Look how much I can do in spite of what I have been through."

In the third session, which focuses on coping and relaxing, she responded positively to the body scan and reported that it helped her headaches. During the walking meditation in the fourth session, M.W. reported that she enjoys walking and often walks but had never really paid attention to the movement from one foot to the other. She was interested in the fact that it felt odd to be on one foot, a sensation she had never noticed. In the fifth session, M.W. reported that she had continued doing the body scan and it:

…makes the stress go away in my brain. And that means it helps the seizures sometimes…The stress is gone and I've been sleeping better, too…And when you're sleeping better, you know, the whole day can be so much easier to deal with when you're well rested for it. My girl even said, 'Mom, you're actin' different. You're not fussin'.' My mom and dad have also…noticed that, you know, I'm standing up for myself now. I look at them and

I say, 'Look, I'm not a baby. I can do this. It takes me a minute to say words, but I can do it. Even though I can't say it fast enough, I can do it. Watch!' and I show them what I can do.

Session 6, which focuses upon the impermanence of thoughts, occurred just before Thanksgiving. In this session, M.W. reported that she had called her daughter to see if she would visit M.W. Instead of reaching her daughter, M.W.'s ex-husband had gotten on the phone and yelled at M.W., which left her distressed and she ended up having a seizure. During the session's meditation on mindfulness of sounds she found herself relaxing. She shared that she has difficulty with cognitive problem-solving because she gets confused, but she was able to use the mindfulness practice of letting the thoughts go and relax. In the following session she reported,

> It's hard on all holidays because I don't ever get to see my children—they don't call me. But I, uh, this has helped me out on how to just let things go and how to be in this moment right here. It's helped my depression a lot.

Later in the session, when providing guidance to another participant she said, "You gotta put your mind to it…"

In the final session, participants complete a Relapse Action Plan and express thanks. In her Relapse Action Plan, M.W. gave as a reason for keeping up the practice, "It really helps my stress and it helps my seizures stay under control." During the wrap-up, one of the other participants commented, "I'd also like to thank M.W. especially. Just seeing her blossom over the last 2 months has been a wonderful experience," after which another participant chimed in, "and an inspiration." M.W. responded with, "…it comes kinda slow, but it comes. Um, I've been real badly depressed. But now, even after Thanksgiving, I just learned…how to just let things go—don't let it bother you. And I have done really good."

The Problem of Distance Delivery

Reducing Problems Through Distance Delivery

In many respects, distance delivery is not a problem, but rather, a solution to other problems. M.W. exemplifies many of the reasons people may need distance delivery of MBCT. Co-morbid mental and physical health problems are common; research has found that those with mental illness have a higher risk of chronic disease [1]. Furthermore, individuals with chronic physical illness have higher rates of depression, anxiety, and other mental disorders. Like many people with co-morbid mental and physical health problems, it is difficult for M.W. to get out for treatment. Depression alone reduces the motivation to leave home, as do other chronic health problems that leave one feeling unwell. In addition, mobility and transportation difficulties are a fact of life for many people with orthopedic or neurological disorders, including epilepsy. There are specific transportation limitations that M.W. experiences as a result of having active seizures; in all 50 states, people with active seizures are not allowed to drive. M.W.'s transportation and access to care are still further limited by her rural location, as well as economic factors. Like many people with chronic health problems, and particularly people with epilepsy, M.W. is unemployed. In addition, epilepsy is a highly stigmatized disease [2], and having M.W. attend treatment services at a mental health facility could add to the stigma she experiences. Distance delivery of mental health programs like MBCT addresses many of these barriers.

Problems Associated with Distance Delivery

On the other hand, there are also problems associated with the distance delivery of programs like MBCT. General issues include technology concerns, professional practice issues, confidentiality issues, and limitations upon interpersonal communication. In addition, there are issues associated with MBCT, and with co-morbid mental and physical health problems that make distance delivery challenging.

Technology Concerns
Distance delivery requires access to some form of technology such as a telephone, smart phone, or computer with Internet access. This contributes to disparities in access since not all populations have access to telephones, let alone smart phones or computers and the Internet. Furthermore, some

may have access, but be paying by the minute for phone calls or data usage, which can severely limit their use of the technology. Those who do have Internet access may have computers with varied capabilities and processing speeds. This will influence the timing of activities within a session. Also, with Internet delivery, participants must have the computer literacy to be able to navigate the program's platform; therefore, an orientation to the platform and troubleshooting assistance may be necessary. In addition, privacy concerns necessitate being aware of the type of equipment and technology being used by each participant and discussing the limitations with group members. For example, cordless phones are less secure than landlines, and the standard version of Skype is not HIPAA compatible.

With the use of technology comes the potential for technological failures. The Internet can be unavailable or go down, power outages can occur, and phones can run out of battery life before a session is concluded. These failures of technology can influence the timing and flow of the session, creating a late start or an abrupt ending. This, in turn, can impact the effectiveness of the program.

Telephone delivery differs from Internet delivery in that visual materials must be eliminated or provided ahead of time in person or by electronic or paper mail. For Internet delivery, materials must be uploaded in advance, with proper accommodations (e.g., transcripts for audio presentations), and tested to ensure that all elements of the program function properly. In order to provide all the materials a participant will need for an 8-session MBCT program, it may also be necessary to mail some of the materials (e.g., marble, stone, or bead) to those receiving Internet delivery. For either mode of delivery, these steps require a significant degree of advance planning to reduce costs.

Professional Practice Issues

Professional licensing laws and policies also influence distance delivery. Most professionals are licensed at the state level, and when providing treatment, the professional must be licensed in the state in which the participant is receiving the treatment. Thus, if a professional who is licensed to practice in New Hampshire delivers treatment to a participant who is residing across the state line in Vermont or vacationing in Florida, the professional is practicing beyond the scope of his or her license. There are some exceptions, however, where specific conditions are in place, e.g., compacts between states to accept each other's licensure. It is important to know the laws of any state to which you are distance delivering treatment.

Another important consideration is distance delivery within a state when a participant is severely depressed or at risk of suicide. Before distance delivering treatment, a professional should be aware of the available emergency resources within any community to which he or she is delivering care. It is good practice to make contact with these resources ahead of time to let them know you will be delivering care into the area. This will avoid unnecessary delays should you need to contact them in the event of an emergency.

Distance Confidentiality Issues

At the beginning of each session, it is important to determine the location at which the participant is taking part in the session, and whether or not there are other people present in that location. With distance technology, it is possible for a participant to take part in a session in a public location, or with friends or family members in the room. If there are any identifiable limits upon confidentiality, all participants should be made aware of that fact.

Limitations Upon Interpersonal Communication

The degree to which distance delivery is limited with respect to interpersonal communication depends upon the technology being used. Email and discussion boards are solely dependent upon written communication. As a result, there are no voice inflections or tones and facial expressions to assist with interpreting the communication. Telecommunications provide vocal tone and inflection, but still lack facial expressions as an aid to interpreting the communication. Videoconferencing provides the greatest number of cues, allowing more accurate interpretation of comments and statements.

Other Limitations

In addition to the distance delivery concerns raised above, there are some issues related to distance delivery of MBCT, in particular, since the exercises were developed for in-person delivery. There are also issues related to distance delivery to those with co-morbid mental disorders and physical disease, a population that is often in need of distance delivery. These modifications typically relate to the distribution of materials, working around visual cues, and attending to timing. They will be discussed in greater detail below, in the section on modifications.

Theoretical Rationale of MBCT

For Distance Delivery

Cognitive behavioral therapy (CBT) is the most commonly reported distance-delivered form of psychotherapy [3, 4]. Early research found that computer-delivered CBT did not differ from therapist-delivered CBT and the effect was maintained at 2-month follow-up [5]. Furthermore, computerized CBT can improve evidence-based therapy access, while reducing the costs and lack of availability of face-to-face therapists [6]. It also has benefits for treating mood disorders among groups who may avoid face-to-face therapy due to stigma, but programs targeting these groups are rare [7]. Additional research has found no difference in the effect of face-to-face, video-delivered, or audio-delivered CBT upon process and outcome variables, and all modes of delivery were superior to an untreated control group [8]. Thus, CBT is a promising alternative when moving from face-to-face to distance delivery.

Considered part of the third wave of CBT, MBCT is particularly well-suited to distance delivery. One reason for this is that many of the exercises are derived from mindfulness-based stress reduction (MBSR) [9], which is taught as a course. As a result, the facilitator can easily lead many of the activities, and much of the participants' work is going on internally as they are led in these activities. This allows delivery via a relatively basic level of technology. Furthermore, in terms of visual requirements, handouts are already created and available for MBCT and can be provided in hard copy or electronically ahead of time.

For Co-morbid Mental and Physical Disease

MBCT is also well-suited for people with co-morbid mental and physical illness, since MBSR was designed to address stress in people with medical illness [10]. In addition to stress, people with chronic physical illness are at high risk of other mental disorders such as anxiety and depression [11]. In turn, these common mental disorders impact cognitive capabilities. Cognitive performance has been shown to have an inverse linear relationship with depression, while its relationship with anxiety is in the form of an inverted u; mild anxiety increases cognitive performance and severe anxiety impairs it [12, 13]. As already entioned, an advantage of MBCT is that it may carry a lower cognitive burden than other CBT programs. In several of our studies of people with co-morbid depression and chronic disease, participants reported that the cognitive burden associated with challenging and changing thoughts through CBT was taxing. These participants found relief once we shifted toward MBCT. Thus, our experience suggests that "letting go" of a thought as taught in MBCT, although not simple, may be less cognitively demanding than holding and challenging a thought.

Modifications of MBCT

Although patterned after MBCT, our program, Project UPLIFT, is structured somewhat differently. In part, this is because it was first designed in response to a call for a home-based depression treatment program for people with epilepsy. We designed our program for delivery by telephone conference call or asynchronously via the Web. At the time we developed the program, MBCT had not yet been studied as a first-line treatment program, but only as a program to prevent depression relapse after successful treatment. We were interested in using MBCT as a foundation for our program because cognitive difficulties are common among people with epilepsy and, as noted above, the cognitive burden associated with challenging and changing thoughts through CBT can be great. Having previously worked with mindfulness, we considered it possible that the mindfulness practice of "letting go" of a thought might prove to be a less cognitively demanding task. In the interest of ensuring adequate treatment, however, we began the eight-session Project UPLIFT program with an emphasis on CBT skills, which were already demonstrated to be effective for first-line treatment. In fact, UPLIFT is an acronym for Using Practice (referring to the practice of mindfulness) and Learning to Increase Favorable Thoughts (referring to CBT).

Table 2.1 presents a comparison of the eight sessions in our Project UPLIFT program with the eight sessions of MBCT. We devoted the first session to identifying thoughts, the second session to challenging and changing thoughts, and the third session to coping and relaxing. We introduced the Body Scan in the third session, as we shifted from CBT to MBCT. Sessions 4 through 7 were focused on different mindfulness techniques and the program wrapped up with relapse action planning.

Table 2.1 Comparison of MBCT and UPLIFT sessions

MBCT session	UPLIFT sessions
1. Automatic pilot	1. Monitoring thoughts[a]
2. Dealing with barriers	2. Challenging and changing thoughts[a]
3. Mindfulness of the breath	3. Coping and relaxing
4. Staying present	4. Attention and mindfulness
5. Allowing/letting be	5. The present as a calm place
6. Thoughts are not facts	6. Thoughts as changeable and impermanent
7. How can I best take care of myself?	7. Pleasure and reinforcement[a]
8. Using what has been learned in the future	8. Relapse action plans

[a]Presentation of CBT skills

Modifications for Distance Delivery

As noted previously, the modifications to MBCT that were required for distance delivery typically centered around the distribution of materials, working around visual cues, and the length of the exercises. For example, the raisin exercise presents an issue regarding distribution of materials. This exercise begins by having the facilitator go around the class to give each participant several "objects" (raisins) for use in the exercise. To conduct this exercise at a distance would require that we either mail each participant several raisins before the session in which the exercise took place, or ask that he or she purchase raisins for use in the session. In either case, participants need to have some raisins on hand for the session. Neither of these alternatives is satisfactory, especially when dealing with people with mobility, transportation, cognitive, or financial limitations. To address this issue, we modified the exercise to use gardening pebbles that looked similar to one another. These were sealed in a zip-lock bag and included in the notebooks that were mailed to the participants before the program began. They were instructed to have these notebooks with them during each session. We also moved this activity from the first session to a later session, to ensure that participants would be accustomed to having their materials with them.

The telephone version of Project UPLIFT necessitated that we work around visual material. For many activities, we provided handouts that were included in a notebook. Because of the visual limitation, however, we did not include activities like the presentation and discussion of the video *Healing from Within*.

The guided walking meditation also presented some challenges for distance delivery. The in-person version included in MBCT requires that the participant be able to hear the guided instructions while walking. This is easily done in a classroom setting, or by playing a digital audio file on the computer, but it becomes more difficult when using a telephone without a speaker option, especially when it is a landline with a short cord. We modified our instructions to incorporate the possibility of holding a tele-phone and to allow pacing an area with a length of two to three strides.

In addition, the mindful walking and some of the other MBCT exercises also recommend con-tinuing the exercise for 10–15 min. This duration of quiet in a distance-delivered session can lead to difficulties. While less problematic when meeting face-to-face, prolonged "dead air" dur-ing a videoconference or telephone call can cause some phones or computers to go into a "locked" or "hibernation" mode, or cause participants who are in a private location to become particularly drowsy or fall asleep. To address this issue, we shortened the duration of several activities and inserted periodic guiding statements by the facili-tator. Participants were then encouraged to prac-tice on their own for longer periods of time between sessions.

For Co-morbid Depression and Chronic Disease

It is critical to understand the culture of the popu-lation to whom you are delivering MBCT, and whether or not specific MBCT activities are appropriate to this culture. Particular attention should be paid to the nature of the population's disease. For example, raisins are dehydrated and, thus, more sugar-dense than their whole-grape counterparts. Consequently, consuming raisins may be unacceptable to people with diabetes. Similarly, for people with pulmonary diseases such as asthma, chronic obstructive pulmonary disease, or cystic fibrosis, a focus on the breath can be highly anxiety-provoking. In our work with cystic fibrosis, we found a focus on the skin to be acceptable. This point of focus was personal and ever-present, like the breath, but avoided a focus on disease-affected organ systems.

Also, as already noted, cognitive difficulties are associated with anxiety and depression and can be exacerbated in the presence of co-morbid chronic diseases, particularly those affecting the nervous system. Participants with these difficulties may need shortened, repetitive, and/or rephrased instructions. Especially during the early sessions,

before their mindfulness skills have been enhanced, when left without prompting, participants may lose track of the activity under way. This, too, argues against prolonged periods of silence in the course of distance delivery of MBCT to this population.

Evidence of Using MBCT for Distance Delivery

Review of Studies

Most research on distance delivery of psychologi-cal interventions has focused on CBT [3, 4]. Internet-based CBT interventions are efficacious and effective and, as mentioned above, may be particularly useful for reaching individuals who cannot receive treatment through traditional methods [4, 14, 15]. Meta-analyses suggest these interventions are effective for depression and anxiety [15, 16], as well as for a number of other mental health conditions [16]. Similarly, inter-ventions delivered by computer are as effective as face-to-face interventions while reducing thera-pist time [15, 16]. The mechanisms through which distance-delivered CBT interventions influence outcomes are similar to those of face-to-face CBT, which likely contributes to the equivalence between modes of delivery [16]. Telephone deliv-ery appears to have similar results to face-to-face delivery for individuals with less severe disorders [17]. However, one study reported that at 6-month follow-up, treatment outcomes may be better for face-to-face delivery [18].

Distance-delivered interventions may be delivered to a wide variety of client groups and settings [4]. On the other hand, Web-based inter-ventions may exclude subgroups with reduced Web access and literacy [3]. Participants who receive distance-delivered interventions report similar levels of satisfaction for computer and face-to-face treatments [15]. Receiving CBT over the computer offers convenience, provides participants the opportunity to proceed at their preferred pace, is low cost, and allows for pri-vacy [15]. Data from eight studies that included cost-effective analyses suggested that Internet-delivered CBT is a cost-effective intervention when compared with no treatment [16]. Similar conclusions about cost-effectiveness have been suggested for telephone delivery [17].

One challenge of distance delivery of CBT is the high dropout rate. A meta-analysis of 40 studies identified a dropout rate of 57 % [4]. However, interventions that are supported by therapists (28 %) or administrators (38 %), rather than no support (74 %), had lower dropout levels. Additionally, Internet-based CBT interventions that are supported by therapists or administrators are more effective in treating depression than self-directed interventions [4, 14].

Few studies have evaluated distance delivery of MBCT programs. In addition to Project UPLIFT [19, 20], two other distance delivery of MBCT interventions have been evaluated [21–23]. The first study combined elements of MBSR and MBCT through an 8-week, online, mindfulness course. The interactive sessions were led by two mindfulness instructors, and participants completed the course at their own pace [23]. Immediately after and at 1-month follow-up, participants reported reduced levels of stress, anxiety, and depression. The effect sizes were similar to other interventions, such as face-to-face mindfulness courses and CBT for stress. The authors evaluated the amount of meditation that participants reported and found that increased meditation was related to greater improvements in stress, anxiety, and depression [23].

The second study, Mindful Mood Balance, evaluated web-based delivery of a mindfulness intervention that incorporated the core elements of MBCT for delivery over the Web, to reduce residual depressive symptoms [21, 22]. The eight-session intervention started by focusing on the principles of mindfulness for the first four sessions, followed by CBT principles for the last four sessions. The sessions were guided by online group leaders and lasted for 60–90 min. Participants were assigned home practice at the end of each session. The intervention was designed to have individuals work through the material on their own time. They could interact with other participants by posting anonymous questions. Through exit interviews and qualitative methods, the authors concluded that the benefits of the web-based format included flexibility and comfortability of doing the program from home [21]. Compared with an in-person group, the web-based format lacked interactivity between the group leaders and participants. Participants indicated that they would have preferred adding a community component, such as participating in a Web-based group, and having the opportunity to receive feedback from a professional therapist [21]. The effectiveness of the intervention was assessed through an open trial of 100 participants and participants were matched to 100 participants receiving usual depression care [22]. Participants in the Mindful Mood Balance reported significantly reduced depressive severity that was sustained over 6 months. These studies have concluded that delivering MBCT over the Internet is feasible and promising for preventing depression relapse [21, 22].

A search of PsychInfo, Medline, and Google Scholar suggests that Project UPLIFT is the only distance-delivered MBCT program that has been assessed through randomized, controlled trials [3, 24]. To date, we have conducted two randomized, controlled trials of the program. The Centers for Disease Control and Prevention (CDC) funded the first study, which included development and initial testing of Project UPLIFT as a home-based depression treatment program for people with epilepsy [20, 25]. As previously mentioned, we designed the program for delivery by telephone conference call, or asynchronously via the Web. Using a crossover design, forty participants with epilepsy from Georgia were randomly assigned to one of four strata: Project UPLIFT via telephone, Project UPLIFT via Web, treatment-as-usual (TAU) followed by Project UPLIFT by telephone, or TAU followed by Project UPLIFT by Web. All groups were assessed at baseline, after intervening in the UPLIFT conditions but not in the TAU conditions (~8–12 weeks), and after intervening in the TAU conditions (~16–20 weeks). At the interim assessment (i.e., 8–12 weeks), knowledge and skills had increased significantly more and depressive symptoms had decreased significantly more in the UPLIFT condition than in TAU. Telephone and Web groups did not differ. The decrease in depressive symptoms persisted for the additional 8 weeks of follow-up. On the basis of this study, CDC listed Project UPLIFT among evidence-based epilepsy self-management programs and the program was highlighted in the 2012 Institute of Medicine (IOM) report entitled *Epilepsy Across the Spectrum* [26].

The second, larger randomized, controlled trial of Project UPLIFT was funded by the National Institute for Minority Health and Health Disparities [NIMHD; 19]. This study was designed to determine whether Project UPLIFT could be used to *prevent*, rather than *treat*, depression among people with epilepsy. This study included 128 participants with epilepsy and mild/moderate depressive symptoms from Georgia, Michigan, Texas, and Washington. The design matched that of the first study with one exception: participants were randomized to UPLIFT or TAU and, within the conditions, they were allowed to self-select their mode of delivery since the modes had been shown not to differ in the prior study. About two-thirds of the participants did not have a preference for mode of delivery. The incidence of onset of major depressive disorder was significantly lower in the UPLIFT condition (0.0%) than in the TAU condition (10.7%). As in the first study, the program significantly increased knowledge and skills and reduced depressive symptoms when compared with TAU. In addition, the program significantly increased satisfaction with life and reduced reported number of seizures when compared with TAU [19].

In addition to the trials above, we have also completed a pilot study of Project UPLIFT for adults with cystic fibrosis. This study demonstrated that the program reduced both symptoms of depression and symptoms of anxiety (publication in preparation). Two other pilot studies of Project UPLIFT are currently in progress: one to reduce stress in women with heart disease and one for caregivers of people with epilepsy. At present, studies of the cultural appropriateness of our epilepsy version of UPLIFT for African Americans and for Hispanics are also in progress, funded by the CDC.

Mechanisms of Change

As a part of the first study of Project UPLIFT, we developed an instrument to assess knowledge and skills. The knowledge instrument assessed knowledge about depression, its relationship to thoughts, and factors that can influence mood. The skills we assessed were directly linked to those included in our program and included: *cognitive skills* such as monitoring thoughts, remembering that thoughts are not facts, and letting thoughts pass; *mindful awareness skills* such as paying attention during everyday activities, focusing on the present moment, and attending to the breath; and *behavioral skills* such as practicing seeing and hearing meditations, performing pleasurable activities, and activating behavior. Using structural equation modeling, we assessed the path from participation in our program, to score on the knowledge and skills assessment, to score on a standardized depression assessment. In doing so, we found that participation in our program influenced change in depression score indirectly, through a change in knowledge and skills [19]. Thus, the change in depression resulting from our distance-delivered program was a result of a change in the knowledge and skills of our participants.

It appears that mindfulness, in particular, may have been an important element of our program. In addition to reducing their depression, Project UPLIFT also produced a significant increase in participants' satisfaction with life [19]; the satisfaction of those receiving our program increased significantly compared to those receiving TAU. This is particularly noteworthy because, during the course of the study, the physical health of those participating in Project UPLIFT did not change and, if anything, declined. The physical health of the TAU group did not change, either. Thus, our finding that the life satisfaction increased for those who took part in Project UPLIFT is consistent with the premises of mindfulness. Through attention, we can see the ways in which we attach thoughts to suffering that exacerbate it; by letting go of these thoughts, we reduce suffering [9].

Practical Considerations of MBCT for Distance Delivery

Participant Selection and Number

There are some participant selection criteria that are important considerations when using distance delivery. First and foremost, we want to ensure the safety of participants. Thus, distance delivery should not be considered for those with active suicidal ideation or a suicide plan, unless there are no in-person services available locally. In the case where no local services are available, the facilitator must to ensure that back-up safety services are available in close proximity to the participant, and that visual contact with the participant is part of the delivery in order to monitor safety and affect. For distance delivery, we also want to ensure that participants are not so depressed that they cannot actively take part in the group activities. We found distance delivery to be effective for people who scored in the severe range of depression on baseline screening tests, but the degree of effectiveness of the program appeared to decline somewhat at very high levels of depression.

Our program was co-facilitated by a trainee and a person with the same chronic disease as the participants and our groups were restricted to seven or fewer participants. With two facilitators, seven participants were almost too many for everyone to participate in the activities of the telephone groups; four to six appeared to be the ideal size to allow people sufficient time to participate. In contrast, seven participants was too small a number for our asynchronous Web-based groups. Having groups in the size range of 14–15 would have reduced the time participants had to wait until someone other than a facilitator responded to their posts. The longer participants had to wait for responses, the more disappointed they became.

Facilitator Training

Project UPLIFT is a manualized program. When we train facilitators, we provide them with facilitator manuals, participant manuals, and CDs containing the recordings of our meditations and exercises. The telephone facilitator's manual includes a script that can be followed, and the same script is provided through the text and recordings in the Web version. The part of the manual that cannot be scripted is the response to participant discussion. During our training, each trainee is responsible for co-facilitating at least one UPLIFT session and is provided with feedback regarding his or her responses.

An important aspect of the training of our facilitators and co-facilitators is in mindfulness. It is important that they understand what mindfulness is and is not, and how to respond to participants in such a way as to teach them this distinction, as well. Without care in this area, mindfulness can be misinterpreted as "positive thinking" or "thinking a happy thought," rather than becoming aware of our thinking and of our ability to remove our attention from thoughts, or to let them go. While the professionals-in-training who facilitated for us were selected for their prior exposure to the study of mindfulness, mindfulness training was an especially important component of the training of our co-facilitators, i.e., the peers with the chronic disease being addressed. As Project UPLIFT has been disseminated to professionals in additional states, we have also had to ensure this understanding of mindfulness among the professionals, as well.

For both facilitators, it has also been important to provide training in distance delivery. This includes concerns regarding safety. For example, it was important to obtain the name of a designated contact person for each person with epilepsy in our phone groups, in case someone experienced a seizure during a conference call. If this were to happen, one of the facilitators would drop off the conference call to make contact with the designated person while the other facilitator continued on the call. In addition to safety, training about distance delivery included how to encourage participation and group cohesion. This was more difficult for asynchronous Web groups; in these, the facilitators had to have a strong presence throughout the discussion and assist the participants in seeing the commonality among their comments. For the phone groups, the skills required of the facilitator included drawing similar parallels, but also assisting people who got spoken over, since there are no visual cues about who is speaking via telephone. Moreover, training in the timing of pauses during meditations and other activities has been key. As previously discussed, long lapses can be problematic with distance delivery.

The third important area of training is with regard to the disease being addressed. Some disease-specific concerns affect both modes of delivery, Web and telephone. Since some of the particular diseases may have their particular mental health effects, it is important that the facilitators have a sense of these issues, to reduce the number of surprises during a session. There are additional disease-related concerns that seem to be more important for the training of phone facilitators who are working in "real time." For example, in working with people with epilepsy, it was important that facilitators understand some of the cognitive struggles the participants might encounter. It was also important that they know that an absence seizure can take the form of an interruption or pause as a person is speaking. With cystic fibrosis, it was important that the facilitators be aware of the participants' need for coughing, although it might be disruptive during some exercises. The co-facilitators were very helpful in contributing to this portion of the training.

Home Practice

We did not stress home practice in our groups because the feedback from our focus groups was that it felt daunting. We made assignments from session to session, for what we termed "on-your-own" practice. We also asked people to report on their past week's on-your-own practice during our check-ins, but we did not track the amount of practice or put other emphasis on it. Instead, we encouraged people in the small ways they could practice, and emphasized that any practice is better than none. The longest practice we suggested during our program was 20 min. We also provided guided CDs to assist participants between sessions.

Web-Specific Issues

There are some particular practical issues related to delivery via the Web. In the section on technology concerns, we mentioned that different types of equipment have differing capabilities. This may mean that a page does not display as it was designed, or that some participants are not seeing what others are seeing. It is important to pilot test your Websites with a wide range of participants like those you wish to reach. One of the biggest practical issues for Web-based delivery is the significant cost of developing an interactive Website. Frequently, by the time the materials are developed, uploaded, and beta tested, technology has changed sufficiently to necessitate a new version. Furthermore, it can be difficult to find a permanent home for a site, and the resources to keep it up to date. A feasible solution may be to employ Web-based videoconference delivery, with a simple site from which participants can download program materials. Videoconferencing may help to overcome some of the drawbacks of asynchronous Web delivery by enabling greater interaction among the participants.

Summary/Conclusions

Overall, distance-delivered MBCT provides the opportunity to bring this evidence-based form of therapy to people whose physical and/or mental health would not allow them to attend it in person. Distance delivery can overcome barriers related to distance, transportation, mobility, high risk of infection, and stigma. It can also reduce the costs associated with delivery of MBCT. For many of these reasons, distance delivery offers particular benefits to those with co-morbid chronic disease.

Evidence has found distance-delivered MBCT to be effective in reducing symptoms of depression and anxiety, preventing relapse, and improving physical symptoms and satisfaction with life [19, 22]. Furthermore, the qualitative responses from participants have been positive across authors and studies, including words like "functional," "practical," and "flexible" [21, 25]. In the words of one Project UPLIFT participant, "Thank you for helping me because I have been depressed and now I can cope" [25].

While these results are promising, offering the potential to provide service to populations that might otherwise be neglected, there are a variety of issues to be considered before undertaking distance delivery. While interpersonal communication can be difficult under the best of circumstances, it is further complicated with distance delivery in the absence of visual and auditory cues. Moreover, there are technology-related concerns related to access, cost, and privacy, as well as failure of the technology. There are also professional practice issues related to state-level licensing, client safety at a distance, and the need for back-up services in areas from which one is distant. In addition, there are confidentiality issues related to both the technology in use and the inability to determine from a distance exactly who is present. These are important issues to tackle as we move forward with the promising practice of providing MBCT at a distance.

References

1. De Hert M, Correll CU, Bobes J, Cetkovich-Bakmas MA, Cohen DA, Asai I, Detraux J, Gautam S, Moller HJ, Ndetei DM, Newcomer JW. Physical illness in patients with severe mental disorders. I. Prevalence, impact of medications and disparities in health care. World Psychiatry. 2011 Feb 1;10(1):52–77.
2. de Boer HM, Mula M, Sander JW. The global burden and stigma of epilepsy. Epilepsy Behav. 2008;12(4):540–6.
3. Charova E, Dorstyn D, Tully P, Mittag O. Web-based interventions for comorbid depression and chronic illness: a systematic review. J Telemed Telecare. 2015;21(4):189–201.
4. Richards D, Richardson T. Computer-based psychological treatments for depression: a systematic review and meta-analysis. Clin Psychol Rev. 2012;32(4):329–42.
5. Selmi PM, Klein MH, Greist JH, Sorrell SP, Erdman HP. Computer-administered cognitive-behavioral therapy for depression. Am J Psychiatry. 1990;147(1):51–6.
6. Marks IM, Mataix-Cols D, Kenwright M, Cameron R, Hirsch S, Gega L. Pragmatic evaluation of computer-aided self-help for anxiety and depression. Br J Psychiatry. 2003;183:57–65.
7. Rozbroj T, Lyons A, Pitts M, Mitchell A, Christensen H. Assessing the applicability of e-therapies for depression, anxiety, and other mood disorders among lesbians and gay men: analysis of 24 web- and mobile phone-based self-help interventions. J Med Internet Res. 2014;16(7):e166.
8. Day SX, Schneider PL. Psychotherapy using distance technology: a comparison of face-to-face, video, and audio treatment. J Counsel Psychol. 2002;49(4):499–503.
9. Segal ZV, Williams JMG, Teasdale JD. Mindfulness-based cognitive therapy for depression: a new approach to preventing relapse. New York: Guilford; 2002.
10. Kabat-Zinn J. Full catastrophe living: using the wisdom of your body and mind to face stress, pain, and illness. New York: Dell Publishing; 1990.
11. Chou SP, Huang B, Goldstein R, Grant BF. Temporal associations between physical illnesses and mental disorders--results from the Wave 2 National Epidemiologic Survey on Alcohol and Related Conditions (NESARC). Compr Psychiatry. 2013;54(6):627–38.
12. Bierman EJ, Comijs HC, Jonker C, Beekman AT. Effects of anxiety versus depression on cognition in later life. Am J Geriatr Psychiatry. 2005;13(8):686–93.
13. Salthouse TA. How general are the effects of trait anxiety and depressive symptoms on cognitive functioning? Emotion. 2012;12(5):1075–84.
14. Spek V, Cuijpers P, Nyklicek I, Riper H, Keyzer J, Pop V. Internet-based cognitive behaviour therapy for symptoms of depression and anxiety: a meta-analysis. Psychol Med. 2007;37(3):319–28.
15. Andrews G, Cuijpers P, Craske MG, McEvoy P, Titov N. Computer therapy for the anxiety and depressive disorders is effective, acceptable and practical health care: a meta-analysis. PLoS One. 2010;5(10):e13196.
16. Hedman E, Ljotsson B, Lindefors N. Cognitive behavior therapy via the Internet: a systematic review of applications, clinical efficacy and cost-effectiveness. Expert Rev Pharmacoecon Outcomes Res. 2012;12(6):745–64.
17. Hammond GC, Croudace TJ, Radhakrishnan M, Lafortune L, Watson A, McMillan-Shields F, et al. Comparative effectiveness of cognitive therapies delivered face-to-face or over the telephone: an observational study using propensity methods. PLoS One. 2012;7(9):e42916.
18. Mohr DC, Ho J, Duffecy J, Reifler D, Sokol L, Burns MN, et al. Effect of telephone-administered vs face-to-face cognitive behavioral therapy on adherence to therapy and depression outcomes among primary care patients: a randomized trial. J Am Med Assoc. 2012;307(21):2278–85.
19. Thompson NJ, Patel AH, Selwa LM, Stoll SC, Begley CE, Johnson EK, et al. Expanding the efficacy of Project UPLIFT: distance delivery of mindfulness-based depression prevention to people with epilepsy. J Consult Clin Psychol. 2015;83(2):304–13.
20. Thompson NJ, Walker ER, Obolensky N, Winning A, Barmon C, Diiorio C, et al. Distance delivery of mindfulness-based cognitive therapy for depression: Project UPLIFT. Epilepsy Behav. 2010;19(3):247–54.
21. Boggs JM, Beck A, Felder JN, Dimidjian S, Metcalf CA, Segal ZV. Web-based intervention in mindfulness meditation for reducing residual depressive symptoms and relapse prophylaxis: a qualitative study. J Med Internet Res. 2014;16(3):e87.

22. Dimidjian S, Beck A, Felder JN, Boggs JM, Gallop R, Segal ZV. Web-based mindfulness-based cognitive therapy for reducing residual depressive symptoms: an open trial and quasi-experimental comparison to propensity score matched controls. Behav Res Ther. 2014;63C:83–9.

23. Krusche A, Cyhlarova E, Williams JM. Mindfulness online: an evaluation of the feasibility of a web-based mindfulness course for stress, anxiety and depression. BMJ Open. 2013;3(11):e003498.

24. van Beugen S, Ferwerda M, Hoeve D, Rovers MM, Spillekom-van Koulil S, van Middendorp H, et al. Internet-based cognitive behavioral therapy for patients with chronic somatic conditions: a meta-analytic review. J Med Internet Res. 2014;16(3):e88.

25. Walker ER, Obolensky N, Dini S, Thompson NJ. Formative and process evaluations of a cognitive-behavioral therapy and mindfulness intervention for people with epilepsy and depression. Epilepsy Behav. 2010;19(3):239–46.

26. England MJ, Liverman CT, Schultz AM, Strawbridge LM. Epilepsy across the spectrum: promoting health and understanding. Institute of Medicine (IOM), editor. Washington, D.C.: The National Academies Press; 2012.

Mindfulness-Based Cognitive Therapy for Insomnia

Amanda J. Shallcross and Pallavi D. Visvanathan

Clinical Case Study

Patient Presentation

Manu is a 51-year-old married man with multiple lifetime depressive episodes seeking mindfulness-based treatment for depression relapse prevention. At intake his depressive symptoms reflected partial remission from depression (Beck Depression Inventory score of 18). Manu reported being in good health overall with no chronic medical conditions apart from depression. Manu's primary goal for treatment was to "learn ways to prevent another [depressive] episode"; however, initial interviews revealed that sleep difficulties were a source of considerable distress and were inter-related with mood issues (e.g., patient reported low mood on days following poor sleep which resulted in heightened anxiety about getting enough sleep in order to avoid depressed mood).

A.J. Shallcross, N.D., M.P.H. (✉)
Department of Medicine and Population Health, New York University, Langone Medical Center, 227 E. 30th Street, 6th Floor, New York, NY 10026, USA
e-mail: Amanda.shallcross@nyumc.org

P.D. Visvanathan, Ph.D.
Manhattan Mindfulness-Based Cognitive Behavioral Therapy, 276 Fifth Avenue, Suite 905, New York, NY 10001, USA
e-mail: visvanathan@mindfultherapynyc.com

Manu reported difficulty with sleep initiation (average sleep onset latency of 90 min) and sleep maintenance (woke 2–3 times each night). Average total sleep time was roughly 5 h but average time in bed was 9 h (consistent sleep schedule of 9:30 pm to 6:30 am). His sleep efficiency was 56 %. Manu denied use of nicotine, caffeine, and alcohol. Manu indicated that over the past several months he had reduced his overall activity levels (socializing with friends, engaging in activities with wife and children) in favor of "resting" in his bed as a response to daytime fatigue and to make up for the sleep he was not getting at night.

Treatment Course

Manu participated in the 8-week mindfulness-based cognitive therapy (MBCT) group intervention for depression relapse prevention [1]. Weekly 2.5 h sessions focused on mindfulness skills (increasing awareness of thoughts, emotions, and physical sensations, and the tendency to react with attachment or aversion to these internal experiences; and developing a nonjudgmental and accepting stance toward internal experiences) and psychoeducation about depression and relapse (e.g., the cognitive model of depression, links between sad mood, negative automatic thoughts, and maintenance of low mood). A detailed description of session content and homework assignments is available in the MBCT manual [1].

Manu had expressed an interest in mindful-ness and remained engaged throughout treat-ment. After the first several sessions, he noted a tendency to frequently scan for signs of low mood and would engage in maladaptive second-ary appraisals if any emerged—"why am I feeling down again—I'm going to be depressed—I will never get better". Manu found that these thoughts were typically associated with increased auto-nomic arousal—"tightness and fluttering" in his chest and stomach and noted that, at bedtime, he experienced many negative thoughts and beliefs ("I have to get 8 h to make up for last night" "I can't function on less than 8 h") and feelings (frustration, anxiety, hopelessness).

Manu struggled with the concept of letting go of the effort to control thoughts rather than the thoughts themselves. Like many other individu-als new to mindfulness meditation, Manu held the idea that he must rid his mind of distressing thoughts and described attempts to "just cut it off". In session 6 however, Manu reported sitting with his worry thoughts and his physical sensa-tions of anxiety and using his breath to bring his attention back whenever he "ended up down-stream". Manu noted that he did not fall asleep but felt less tense and overwhelmed by needing to get to sleep. During one inquiry session, Manu expressed frustration with not falling asleep despite "doing all the right things" like abstaining from coffee and alcohol and giving himself plenty of time to sleep. The facilitator inquired about Manu's experience of sleepiness and noted that he may be confusing fatigue with sleepiness. Manu was encouraged to observe the difference between these sensations.

Treatment Outcome

Post-MBCT training, Manu reported an average total sleep time of 6.5 h with sleep efficiency >90 %. He had adjusted his time in bed to approximately 7 h after realizing that he did not need as much sleep as he had previously believed. He reported satisfac-tion with the amount and quality of sleep and ability to function effectively in the daytime. His BDI score was reduced to a score of 7.

Pathway for Clinical Improvement

Manu's skill development in the three key domains influenced by MBCT likely contributed to resolution of sleep difficulties. First, Manu's *awareness* of ruminative thought cycles led him to practice *attentional control* thereby supporting "decentering" from worry thoughts and distorted beliefs and resulting in reductions in negative primary and secondary (metacognitive) apprais-als and physiological arousal. Practicing mindful awareness also decreased time spent on sleep-interfering behaviors like calculating time left to sleep. Finally, increased *acceptance* of difficult thoughts, emotions, and physical sensations allowed Manu to let go of his desire (and desper-ate behaviors) to make sleep happen. Each of these skills likely contributed to Manu's overall diminished worry about the consequences of poor sleep and increased confidence in his ability to function well in the daytime with fewer hours of sleep than previously believed.

The Problem of Insomnia

Insomnia is a complex disorder of varied etiol-ogy that is characterized by the presence of an individual's report of difficulty with sleep [2]. The complexity of insomnia is due, in part, to a lack of universally defined diagnostic criteria. Hallmark symptoms common to the three differ-ent classification systems used to diagnose insomnia include difficulties in initiating sleep or in maintaining sleep [3–5]. The term "insomnia" has different meanings based on an individual's clinical presentation. Ohayon and Reynolds [6] compare "insomnia" to "pain" whereby it can be considered a complaint (related to sleep duration or quality), a symptom (part of a sleep or other organic disorder), or a diagnosis (e.g., primary insomnia or secondary insomnia, a consequence of a primary diagnosis such as substance abuse or medical or mental illness). Prevalence rates of insomnia vary based on the degree of distinction between these domains and also the diagnostic classification system used. Results from a recent epidemiological study that differentiated the various presentations of insomnia indicate that 37 % of individuals reported sleep complaints (e.g., light or short sleep and sleep dissatisfaction), 35 % reported at least one symptom of insomnia (difficulty initiating or maintaining sleep and nonrestorative sleep at least 3 nights per week), and 7 % met diagnostic criteria for insomnia based on the DSM-IV classification [6].

Insomnia is associated with a range of debilitating outcomes including increased psychosocial and physical morbidities, financial consequences, and mortality. Decades of population-based studies demonstrate that individuals with insomnia experience significantly impaired quality of life on nearly all domains including mental, emotional, physical, and social functioning (for review, see [7]). Individuals with sleep disturbance also experience significant daytime impairment, which frequently leads to poor work performance, higher rates of absenteeism, and economic loss [8]. Finally, insomnia is causally linked with higher mortality including increased suicide [9] and preventable accidental deaths (e.g., motor vehicle accidents) [10].

Identification of the causal determinants of insomnia is difficult not only because of nonstandard diagnostic and classification systems but also because the symptom profile of insomnia overlaps considerably with other psychological and physical health conditions. Indeed, insomnia is more frequently associated with psychiatric disorders, most commonly depression, than any other disorder [11]. Consensus regarding whether insomnia is antecedent to or a result of psychiatric disorders has not been reached; however, at least one large-scale epidemiological study demonstrated that insomnia more often preceded rather than followed incident cases of a mood disorder [12]. Still, it is widely agreed that there may be bidirectional relationships between insomnia and psychiatric disorders and that these conditions share pathophysiological pathways that make individuals vulnerable to both conditions [2].

Several models have been proposed to explain the pathophysiology of insomnia (Psychobiological

Inhibition Model [13]; Hyperarousal Model [14]; Cognitive Model [15]; Neurocognitive Model [16]). Common to each of these is that cognitive/affective processes play a primary role in activating the clinical complaint of insomnia [13] and that mental hyperarousal [15] or deficits in achieving mental de-arousal [13] contribute to the maintenance and chronicity of this disorder. In Fig. 3.1, we present a model of insomnia that integrates core cognitive and behavioral processes from several extant theoretical frameworks (e.g., [17, 18]). In general, insomnia is thought to be initiated and perpetuated by the following sequential cognitive and behavioral processes: (1) Excessive daytime and nighttime rumination [19]; (2) Primary arousal (i.e., initial negative appraisal about daytime consequences of poor sleep that results in distress and physiological activation)—"If I don't sleep tonight, I'm going to fail at my job tomorrow and be fired" [15]; (3) Secondary arousal (i.e., the negative secondary or metacognitive evaluation or judgment of initial (primary) arousal, which leads to continuing distress and physiological activation)—"I hate how I'm feeling and shouldn't be feeling this way." [18]; (4) Excessive monitoring of and selective attention to internal (e.g., bodily sensations) and/or external (e.g., clock) sleep cues that are either consistent or inconsistent with falling asleep [15]. Hand in hand with selective attention is a dysfunctional perceived need for control and engagement in sleep effort (e.g., actively trying to sleep or increasing sleep opportunity) [20]; (5) Distorted perceptions about sleep impairment (i.e., regularly overestimating sleep loss). Misperceptions of sleep deficit frequently lead to excessive negative cognitions about sleep thus fortifying a vicious cycle of chronic insomnia.

On the basis of this integrative cognitive model of insomnia, the most successful interventions for sleep disturbance are those that target each of the key predisposing vulnerabilities, namely negative cognitions, dysfunctional cognitive and affective and behavioral regulatory strategies (e.g., suppression, selective attention, monitoring, sleep effort) and distorted perceptions about sleep.

Fig. 3.1 A model for
MBCT's effects on
cognitive and metacognitive
risk processes for the
development and
maintenance of insomnia

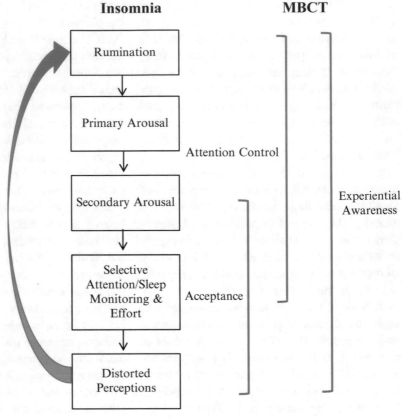

Theoretical Rationale of MBCT for Insomnia

Cognitive behavior therapy for insomnia (CBT-I) is one of the most widely researched psychobehavioral interventions for insomnia. CBT-I has evolved as a multicomponent treatment approach and combines: (1) cognitive strategies such as thought restructuring to change dysfunctional beliefs and attitudes about sleep; and (2) behavioral techniques such as sleep restriction and stimulus control to promote healthy sleep habits [21]. Although CBT-I is considered to be an effective and first-line treatment (for review and meta-analysis, see [22, 23]), a significant proportion (19–26 %) of individuals do not benefit from CBT-I, and the average overall improvement among those who do respond is only 50–60 % [24]. This change, while statistically significant, does not represent enough clinical improvement to classify those who do respond to CBT-I as

"good sleepers" [15]. Thus, additional and/or complementary treatment approaches are needed for the substantial number of CBT-I "nonresponders" and for those who have experienced only partial symptomatic relief from CBT-I.

One particularly promising treatment approach for insomnia is MBCT. MBCT was developed as a treatment to prevent depression relapse in individuals with recurrent major depressive disorder. It is based on the Mindfulness-Based Stress Reduction (MBSR) program and combines mindfulness meditation practices with cognitive therapy to help reduce depressogenic and ruminative thinking, common antecedents to major depression relapse. Several RCTs have demonstrated MBCT is effective for reducing depression relapse and depressive symptoms [25–27]. Three theoretical considerations indicate that MBCT may be a promising treatment for insomnia.

First, MBCT is believed to target experiential awareness, attentional control, and acceptance; deficits in each of these domains have been linked to poor sleep [18, 28, 29]. For instance, mindfulness-based practices, such as breath-focused meditation, body scanning, and mindful stretching, promote experiential awareness of a range of experiences including internal (e.g., thoughts, emotions, physiological sensations) and external stimuli (e.g., sights, sounds) [30]. During these exercises, participants acquire skills in attentional control by focusing attention on the breath (sustained attention) and redirecting attention to this anchor whenever one's thoughts wander (attention inhibition) [31]. Finally, participants learn to change their relationship to their experiences by learning to accept, rather than avoid or control negatively perceived thoughts, emotions, and physical sensations. Skills in acceptance are learned by nonjudgmentally observing one's thoughts, feelings, and physical sensations and by viewing such experiences as passing mental events, rather than facts [32].

Experiential awareness, attentional control, and acceptance, the three domains putatively improved by MBCT, collectively target each of the cognitive and behavioral vulnerabilities associated with poor sleep (see Fig. 3.1). First, increased awareness of internal and external experiences (e.g., thoughts and behaviors) should target each of the processes that contribute to the maintenance of insomnia: (1) rumination; (2) primary arousal; (3) secondary arousal; (4) sleep monitoring/selective attention and effort; and (5) distorted perceptions. Second, attentional control should enable individuals to disengage from negative thoughts and/or beliefs about sleeplessness by disrupting selective attention toward internal/external sleep-related threat cues. Thus, skills in attentional control should target processes (1)–(4) above. Finally, skills in acceptance should foster a less contentious and more flexible relationship to one's thoughts, emotions, and sensations by promoting the ability to approach, rather than avoid, and to engage with such experiences with equanimity instead of with judgment. Therefore, acceptance should target the following processes: (3) secondary arousal; (4) sleep monitoring/selective attention and effort; and (5) distorted perceptions.

A second consideration that indicates that MBCT may be a helpful treatment for insomnia is that insomnia is frequently comorbid with mood disorders like depression [33], and extensive studies have shown MBCT is effective for preventing depression and reducing depressive symptoms [26, 27, 34]. Thus, although the relationship between depression and insomnia is likely bidirectional [35], one would expect that MBCT-related reductions in depression relapse and depressive symptoms may also lead to improvements in sleep.

Finally, the mindfulness skills imparted through MBCT have broad implications for well-being and may additionally have long-term effects that are sustained over time. For example, mindfulness can be applied to a range of daily psychological and behavioral phenomena (e.g., healthy decision making) that may either directly (i.e., via processes discussed above) or indirectly (e.g., via improvements in chronic disease symptomology) reduce insomnia. Relatedly, MBCT may have cumulative benefits that are sustained over the long term [36]. Collectively, these features of MBCT suggest that it may be a particularly promising intervention for individuals who suffer from insomnia.

Evidence of MBCT for Insomnia and Mechanisms of Change

The majority of the evidence for mindfulness-based interventions (MBIs) for insomnia comes from studies that have tested the MBSR intervention or a tailored derivative of this protocol for insomnia (e.g., mindfulness-based therapy for insomnia or MBTI: [27, 37]). A thorough review of such studies is beyond the scope of this chapter. However, compelling evidence from three recent studies demonstrates especially promising effects of MBTI on objective and subjective assessments of insomnia. MBTI combines mindfulness meditation exercises modeled after the MBSR protocol with CBT-I. In a single-arm study with participants who met diagnostic criteria for psychophysiological insomnia (a subtype of primary insomnia characterized by heightened arousal in bed) [38], MBTI was associated with improvements in self-reported total wake time (TWT), number of awakenings, time in bed, sleep efficiency, insomnia symptom severity, and pre-sleep somatic and cognitive arousal [37]. These improvements were maintained over a 12-month follow-up period [39]. Building on the limitations of single-arm trial, Ong and colleagues [40] conducted a three-arm RCT comparing MBTI versus MBSR versus a self-monitoring control condition (SM). Compared to SM, MBTI and MBSR demonstrated superior effects on self-reported TWT, pre-sleep arousal, insomnia severity, and objective measures of TWT and total sleep time (TST) using wrist actigraphy. Effects of MBTI and MBSR were maintained at a 6-month follow-up and the highest rates of improvement on the Insomnia Severity Index (ISI:[41]) and insomnia remission were found in the MBTI group.

Results from these studies demonstrate that features of MBSR can be combined with elements from the CBT-I protocol to yield a viable treatment for chronic insomnia. Effect sizes for MBTI are comparable to those found for other behavioral interventions for insomnia [42, 43], and MBTI appears to be superior to MBSR for reducing self-reported severity of insomnia symptoms over the long term. One advantage to adding a mindfulness component to the CBT-I intervention may be that MBTI presents an additional treatment option for patients who relate more to acceptance-based approaches than to cognitive restructuring. Also, the benefits of mindfulness may generalize across greater domains of healthy functioning (e.g., reductions in somatic complaints associated with other comorbid conditions) that may directly or indirectly improve sleep. Given the especially high comorbidity between insomnia and certain chronic diseases and mood disorders, developing and testing MBIs that target multiple risk factors for insomnia is critical. For example, MBCT's effects on emotion regulation [44, 45] and reductions in rumination and mood disorder symptoms [46], which are each linked to sleep disturbance [19, 47], suggest it may be an additional treatment option for insomnia.

To date, five studies have examined the effects of the standard MBCT intervention or a modified version of the protocol for insomnia (for review, see [48]). Initial pilot testing of MBCT's effects on reducing symptoms of primary insomnia was conducted by Heidenreich and colleagues [49]. The standardized 8-week MBCT protocol was modified with "cognitive elements tailored to patients with primary insomnia rather than a depressive disorder." Results indicated pre–post improvements in self-reported total sleep time and several domains of thought control as well as reductions in sleep-related monitoring and worry. Ree and colleagues [50] conducted an additional single arm study in a heterogeneous group of adult outpatients with psychiatric presentations. Immediately following the MBCT intervention, self-reported insomnia severity symptom scores decreased from subthreshold insomnia to values within the normal range. Post-treatment improvements were maintained at 3-month follow-up with a large effect size. A more recent study that similarly employed a pre–post design examined the effects of MBCT on self-reported sleep disturbance among older adults with history of depression or anxiety in partial or full remission [51]. The MBCT protocol was modified slightly for the aging sample (e.g., length of seated meditations and duration of each weekly session were slightly shorter to accommodate the aging sample). Results indicated that participants experienced a 14.5 % improvement in self-reported sleep problems.

Although promising, conclusions about the efficacy of MBCT for insomnia are difficult to draw based on these studies due to the lack of a control group and objective and comprehensive subjective (e.g., sleep diaries) measures of sleep and limited reported information regarding modifications made to the MBCT protocol (i.e., [49]).

The strongest evidence for the effects of MBCT for insomnia comes from two sets of results from a randomized controlled trial conducted by Britton and colleagues [52, 53]. Individuals with recurrent depression in full or partial remission and with residual sleep complaints were randomized to either MBCT or a waitlist control condition (WLC). Objective assessments of sleep were measured via polysomnography (PSG), and comprehensive assessments of self-reported sleep were measured with sleep diaries at baseline and over the course of the intervention.

Their first investigation included a medication-free sample [52]; the second included individuals who were taking ADM [53]. Polysomnography data from the initial study indicated that, contrary to hypotheses, MBCT participants experienced significantly more awakenings during the initial or "light" sleep stage (Stage 1) and decreased "deep sleep" or slow wave sleep (Stages 3 and 4) relative to controls. Subjective reports from sleep diaries indicated that sleep was improved in the MBCT group but not over and above improvements in the control condition. Participants in the MBCT group experienced greater improvements in depressive symptoms compared to the control condition and these reductions were associated with improvements in both objective and subjective assessments of sleep.

Results from the second study in individuals currently taking ADM indicated that MBCT participants spent less time awake in bed (TWT: total wake time) and had higher sleep efficiency relative to controls, according to both objective (PSG) and subjective measures (sleep diaries). However, when "wake after sleep onset" (WASO) and "sleep onset latency" (SOL) were analyzed separately (the two indices of TWT), no differences were found using objective PSG and only SOL approached statistical significance using subjective sleep diaries. Also, no changes were found in the total amount of sleep or the amount of "deep" (Stages 3 and 4) or "light" (Stage 1) sleep as a result of MBCT. Finally, improvements in self-reported sleep continuity (e.g., sleep efficiency and WASO), but not objective measures of sleep were correlated with reductions in depression symptoms.

What can be concluded about the effects of MBCT on insomnia from these studies? First, both studies suggest that MBCT is effective for improving self-reported sleep. Further, the magnitude of the effect of MBCT on TWT is comparable to MBTI [40]. Second, objective improvements in sleep as a result of MBCT were found only in the sample taking ADM. The medication-free sample experienced increased sleep disturbance according to objective assessments. The beneficial effect in individuals currently taking ADM may represent an additive advantage of MBCT

plus medication on objective sleep outcomes. Also, complete depression remission rates in the MBCT group among the medication-free sample were lower (35%) than the sample taking ADM (50%), which may indicate that individuals in full remission are more likely to experience objective sleep benefits from MBCT. This interpretation is consistent with theoretical considerations that endorse the use of MBCT as a depression prevention intervention that may be most effective for individuals with minimal depressive symptoms [54]. Further work is needed to identify which types of patients with insomnia complaints are most likely to benefit from MBCT.

Two notable limitations of these investigations should guide future scientific inquiry into the benefits of MBCT for insomnia. First, the long-term effects of MBCT for sleep complaints are largely unknown. Among the five MBCT studies to date, only Ree and colleagues [50] examined the effects of MBCT beyond an immediate post-intervention assessment. Second, the clinical profile of participants across these studies was heterogeneous, which limits conclusions about generalizability. For example, only three MBCT studies included patients who met specified insomnia symptom criteria [49, 52, 53]. Also, with the exception of the study conducted by Heidenrich and colleagues [49], each study examined the effects of MBCT for comorbid mood disorders and insomnia symptoms. Therefore, minimally, results may generalize only to the 40% of individuals with comorbid psychopathology and insomnia.

Mechanisms

The authors are unaware of any study that has formally tested mechanisms underlying the effects of MBCT for insomnia. Two studies demonstrated the effects of MBCT for thought control and rumination. It is unclear, however, whether these improvements correlated with changes insomnia [49, 51]. In the two RCTs of MBCT for insomnia, reductions in depressive symptoms were related to improvements in sleep disturbance, which suggests that improvements in mood may be one possible mechanism underlying the effects of MBCT for sleep disturbance [52, 53]. One additional hypothesis put forward by Britton and colleagues is that, similar to ADM, MBCT may increase neurotransmitters (e.g., norepinephrine, serotonin, and dopamine) [52]. This idea may explain their paradoxical finding whereby improved mood and subjective sleep quality was experienced with a concomitant increase in objectively measured sleep arousal [52].

The wider literature on MBIs for insomnia offers additional insight into candidate mechanisms. Evidence for MBTI-related reductions in pre-sleep arousal [37, 39, 40] suggests this may be a mechanism of MBIs that is consistent with conceptual models [15, 18] and preliminary evidence which indicated that cognitive and somatic arousal predict sleep disturbance [55]. Given the bidirectional link between mood disorders and sleep, additional mechanisms worthy of consideration are those that explain MBCT's effects on depressive disorder outcomes (e.g., self-compassion, improved attentional control, emotion regulation) (for a review, see [56]).

The collective literature on MBIs for insomnia and MBCT for depression provides insight into several plausible mechanisms by which MBCT reduces insomnia. Future investigations are needed to understand the specificity of the effects of MBIs for insomnia (e.g., benefits due to mindfulness rather than nonspecific therapeutic elements such as alliance with instructor or group members) as well as the mechanisms underlying MBIs. A definitive test of each of these would require several assessments of the hypothesized mediator (i.e., pre-intervention, during, and post-intervention) in order to detect the time-course of intervention-related changes, and a demonstration that the mechanisms of MBCT differ from the mechanisms underlying the effects of attention control conditions [27]. Prior to this, however, additional work may be required to first develop a clear conceptual model to guide the testing of treatment mechanisms [18]. Ong and colleagues' "two-level model of sleep-related arousal" [18] has laid the necessary initial groundwork by integrating extant theory from cognitive and behavioral models with mindfulness-based concepts and

processes (e.g., metacognition and secondary arousal) that are associated with sleep disturbance and that are targeted by MBIs.

Modifications of MBCT for Insomnia

The strongest evidence for the effects of MBCT is for individuals with comorbid insomnia complaints and elevated depressive or anxiety symptoms or recurrent major depressive disorder [50–53]. It appears that MBCT may be effective for this patient population, in part, because it targets cognitive and physiological vulnerabilities that underlie both disorders. We provide a few additional considerations for the delivery of MBCT to this population. We recommend that providers be familiar with the diagnosis of insomnia and be able to rule out other sleep disorders (e.g., circadian rhythm sleep–wake disorders, obstructive sleep apnea hypopnea, restless legs syndrome, nightmare disorder) that may contribute to, or complicate, patients' symptoms, and that may necessitate a referral to a sleep specialist. We also recommend that providers screen for substance use, including caffeine, nicotine, and alcohol, as these can have deleterious effects on sleep and mood, and because patients may need additional information and/or substance use treatment prior to engaging in MBCT.

With regard to modification of group session content, we recommend the dissemination of basic information on sleep processes. For example, information on sleep drive and guided discussion to help participants distinguish sleepiness from fatigue may support important behavioral changes (e.g., reducing sleep effort) [18, 57]. Also, to prevent the use of mindfulness practice as a form of sleep effort, providers may want to discourage the use of formal mindfulness practice at bedtime for the first several sessions [37]. Finally, daytime sleepiness and fatigue may affect patients' ability to learn and retain session information. Thus, providers will want to consider timing of group sessions and may schedule session times only after a discussion with participants about when they experience the lowest levels of sleepiness and/or fatigue over the course of the day.

Summary and Conclusions

Nearly 40 % of individuals suffer from symptoms of insomnia. Despite being common and a risk factor for a range of morbidities and mortality, a significant portion of individuals with insomnia go untreated [58] or do not experience benefit from prevailing nonpharmacological interventions [59]. Theoretical considerations from widely accepted models of insomnia and from conceptual frameworks of the cognitive processes targeted by mindfulness-based practices suggest that MBCT may be a promising intervention for insomnia. Another reason MBCT may be a favorable treatment for insomnia is because it reduces depression, which is experienced by over 1 in 3 individuals with insomnia. Because these two disorders are thought to share common pathophysiological pathways, improvements in depression should also reduce symptoms of insomnia. Indeed, compelling preliminary empirical evidence indicates that MBCT reduces symptoms of insomnia in individuals with depressive symptoms and a history of recurrent major depression [52, 53]. Further, the magnitude of MBCT-related improvements in self-reported sleep is similar to those observed in another trial of mindfulness-based therapy for insomnia (MBTI), a newly developed intervention that combines mindfulness exercises from MBSR with CBT-I [40]. Collectively, these studies demonstrate that interventions featuring mindfulness meditation have positive patient-reported benefits and may be viable options for individuals with insomnia seeking treatments that are not based strictly on cognitive behavioral techniques. Additional research is needed to determine the varying degrees of efficacy among mindfulness-based approaches for insomnia (e.g., MBSR, MBCT, and MBTI) and how each of these compares to standard psychobehavioral treatments such as CBT-I.

Also, further work is needed to understand the mechanisms underlying each of these interventions and also which treatments will confer the greatest benefit for which types of patients. Based on the strongest evidence to date, it appears that MBCT may be ideally suited to treat insomnia in individuals with comorbid depression symptoms. Some early evidence suggests that a tailored MBCT protocol that includes information on sleep education may be effective for improving self-reported sleep in individuals with primary insomnia [49]. Treatment development studies and RCTs are needed to test whether the effects of such modifications are stronger than those for extant mindfulness-based treatments that reduce symptoms of insomnia (e.g., MBTI and the standardized MBCT and MBSR protocols).

In sum, MBCT appears to be a promising intervention for reducing symptoms of insomnia, particularly individuals with depressive symptoms and a history of depression.

References

1. Segal Z, Williams MG, Teasdale JD. Mindfulness-based cognitive therapy for depression. New York, NY: The Guilford Press; 2013.
2. Roth T. Insomnia: definition, prevalence, etiology, and consequences. J Clin Sleep Med. 2007;3(5 Suppl):S7–10.
3. American Psychiatric Association. Diagnostic and statistical manual of mental disorders: DSM-5 2013. Available from: http://dsm.psychiatryonline.org/book.aspx?bookid=556.
4. World Health Organization. International classification of diseases 10th Revision 2015. Accessed 24 July 2015. Available from: http://www.who.int/classifications/icd/en/.
5. American Academy of Sleep Medicine. International classification of sleep disorders: diagnostic and coding manual 2. Westchester; 2005.
6. Ohayon MM, Reynolds 3rd CF. Epidemiological and clinical relevance of insomnia diagnosis algorithms according to the DSM-IV and the International Classification of Sleep Disorders (ICSD). Sleep Med. 2009;10(9):952–60. doi:10.1016/j.sleep.2009.07.008.
7. Ishak WW, Bagot K, Thomas S, Magakian N, Bedwani D, Larson D, et al. Quality of life in patients suffering from insomnia. Innov Clin Neurosci. 2012;9(10):13–26.
8. Kessler RC, Berglund PA, Coulouvrat C, Hajak G, Roth T, Shahly V, et al. Insomnia and the performance of US workers: results from the America insomnia survey. Sleep. 2011;34(9):1161–71. doi:10.5665/sleep.1230.
9. Turvey CL, Conwell Y, Jones MP, Phillips C, Simonsick E, Pearson JL, et al. Risk factors for late-life suicide: a prospective, community-based study. Am J Geriatr Psychiatry. 2002;10(4):398–406.
10. Leger D, Bayon V, Ohayon MM, Philip P, Ement P, Metlaine A, et al. Insomnia and accidents: cross-sectional study (EQUINOX) on sleep-related home, work and car accidents in 5293 subjects with insomnia

from 10 countries. J Sleep Res. 2014;23(2):143–52. doi:10.1111/jsr.12104.

11. Benca RM. Consequences of insomnia and its therapies. J Clin Psychiatry. 2001;62 Suppl 10:33–8.

12. Ohayon MM, Roth T. Place of chronic insomnia in the course of depressive and anxiety disorders. J Psychiatr Res. 2003;37(1):9–15.

13. Espie CA. Insomnia: conceptual issues in the development, persistence, and treatment of sleep disorder in adults. Annu Rev Psychol. 2002;53:215–43. doi:10.1146/annurev.psych.53.100901.135243.

14. Riemann D, Spiegelhalder K, Feige B, Voderholzer U, Berger M, Perlis M, et al. The hyperarousal model of insomnia: a review of the concept and its evidence. Sleep Med Rev. 2010;14(1):19–31. doi:10.1016/j.smrv.2009.04.002.

15. Harvey AG. A cognitive model of insomnia. Behav Res Ther. 2002;40(8):869–93.

16. Perlis ML, Giles DE, Mendelson WB, Bootzin RR, Wyatt JK. Psychophysiological insomnia: the behavioural model and a neurocognitive perspective. J Sleep Res. 1997;6(3):179–88.

17. Harvey AG, Tang NK. (Mis)perception of sleep in insomnia: a puzzle and a resolution. Psychol Bull. 2012;138(1):77–101. doi:10.1037/a0025730.

18. Ong JC, Ulmer CS, Manber R. Improving sleep with mindfulness and acceptance: a metacognitive model of insomnia. Behav Res Ther. 2012;50(11):651–60. doi:10.1016/j.brat.2012.08.001.

19. Carney CE, Harris AL, Moss TG, Edinger JD. Distinguishing rumination from worry in clinical insomnia. Behav Res Ther. 2010;48(6):540–6. doi:10.1016/j.brat.2010.03.004.

20. Espie CA, Broomfield NM, MacMahon KM, Macphee LM, Taylor LM. The attention-intention-effort pathway in the development of psychophysiologic insomnia: a theoretical review. Sleep Med Rev. 2006;10(4):215–45. doi:10.1016/j.smrv.2006.03.002.

21. Morin CM. Cognitive-behavioral therapy of insomnia. Sleep Med Clin. 2006;1(3):375–86. doi:10.1016/j.jsmc.2006.06.008.

22. Trauer JM, Qian MY, Doyle JS, Rajaratnam SM, Cunnington D. Cognitive behavioral therapy for chronic insomnia: a systematic review and meta-analysis. Ann Intern Med. 2015;163(3):191–204. doi:10.7326/m14-2841.

23. Taylor DJ, Pruiksma KE. Cognitive and behavioural therapy for insomnia (CBT-I) in psychiatric populations: a systematic review. Int Rev Psychiatry. 2014;26(2):205–13. doi:10.3109/09540261.2014.902808.

24. Morin CM, Culbert JP, Schwartz SM. Nonpharmacological interventions for insomnia: a meta-analysis of treatment efficacy. Am J Psychiatry. 1994;151(8):1172–80.

25. Kuyken W, Hayes R, Barrett B, Byng R, Dalgleish T, Kessler D, et al. Effectiveness and cost-effectiveness of mindfulness-based cognitive therapy compared with maintenance antidepressant treatment in the prevention of depressive relapse or recurrence (PREVENT): a randomised controlled trial. Lancet. 2015;386(9988):63–73. doi:10.1016/s0140-6736(14)62222-4.

26. Williams JM, Crane C, Barnhofer T, Brennan K, Duggan DS, Fennell MJ, et al. Mindfulness-based cognitive therapy for preventing relapse in recurrent depression: a randomized dismantling trial. J Consult Clin Psychol. 2014;82(2):275–86. doi:10.1037/a0035036.

27. Shallcross AJ, Gross JJ, Visvanathan PD, Kumar N, Palfrey A, Ford BQ, et al. Relapse prevention in major depressive disorder: mindfulness-based cognitive therapy versus an active control condition. J Consult Clin Psychol. 2015;83(5):964–75. doi:10.1037/ccp0000050.

28. Woods H, Marchetti LM, Biello SM, Espie CA. The clock as a focus of selective attention in those with primary insomnia: an experimental study using a modified Posner paradigm. Behav Res Ther. 2009;47(3):231–6. doi:10.1016/j.brat.2008.12.009.

29. Harvey A. The attempted suppression of presleep cognitive activity in insomnia. Cogn Ther Res. 2003;27(6):593–602. doi:10.1023/A:1026322310019.

30. Jha AP, Krompinger J, Baime MJ. Mindfulness training modifies subsystems of attention. Cogn Affect Behav Neurosci. 2007;7(2):109–19.

31. Tang YY, Ma Y, Wang J, Fan Y, Feng S, Lu Q, et al. Short-term meditation training improves attention and self-regulation. Proc Natl Acad Sci U S A. 2007;104(43):17152–6. doi:10.1073/pnas.0707678104.

32. Shallcross AJ, Troy A, Mauss IB. Regulation of emotions under stress. Emerging trends in the social and behavioral sciences. John Wiley & Sons, Inc.; Hoboken, New Jersey. 2015.

33. Staner L. Comorbidity of insomnia and depression. Sleep Med Rev. 2010;14(1):35–46. doi:10.1016/j.smrv.2009.09.003.

34. Ma SH, Teasdale JD. Mindfulness-based cognitive therapy for depression: replication and exploration of differential relapse prevention effects. J Consult Clin Psychol. 2004;72(1):31–40. doi:10.1037/0022-006x.72.1.31.

35. Talbot LS, Stone S, Gruber J, Hairston IS, Eidelman P, Harvey AG. A test of the bidirectional association between sleep and mood in bipolar disorder and insomnia. J Abnorm Psychol. 2012;121(1):39–50. doi:10.1037/a0024946.

36. Mathew KL, Whitford HS, Kenny MA, Denson LA. The long-term effects of mindfulness-based cognitive therapy as a relapse prevention treatment for major depressive disorder. Behav Cogn Psychother. 2010;38(5):561–76. doi:10.1017/s135246581000010x.

37. Ong JC, Shapiro SL, Manber R. Combining mindfulness meditation with cognitive-behavior therapy for insomnia: a treatment-development study. Behav Ther. 2008;39(2):171–82. doi:10.1016/j.beth.2007.07.002.

38. Edinger JD, Bonnet MH, Bootzin RR, Doghramji K, Dorsey CM, Espie CA, et al. Derivation of research diagnostic criteria for insomnia: report of an American Academy of Sleep Medicine Work Group. Sleep. 2004;27(8):1567–96.

39. Ong JC, Shapiro SL, Manber R. Mindfulness meditation and cognitive behavioral therapy for insomnia: a naturalistic 12-month follow-up. Explore (NY). 2009;5(1):30–6. doi:10.1016/j.explore.2008.10.004.

40. Ong JC, Manber R, Segal Z, Xia Y, Shapiro S, Wyatt JK. A randomized controlled trial of mindfulness

meditation for chronic insomnia. Sleep. 2014;37(9):1553–63. doi:10.5665/sleep.4010.

41. Morin CM, Belleville G, Bélanger L, Ivers H. The insomnia severity index: psychometric indicators to detect insomnia cases and evaluate treatment response. Sleep. 2011;34(5):601–8.

42. Edinger JD, Wohlgemuth WK, Radtke RA, Marsh GR, Quillian RE. Cognitive behavioral therapy for treatment of chronic primary insomnia: a randomized controlled trial. JAMA. 2001;285(14):1856–64.

43. Buysse DJ, Germain A, Moul DE, Franzen PL, Brar LK, Fletcher ME, et al. Efficacy of brief behavioral treatment for chronic insomnia in older adults. Arch Intern Med. 2011;171(10):887–95. doi:10.1001/archinternmed.2010.535.

44. Britton WB, Shahar B, Szepsenwol O, Jacobs WJ. Mindfulness-based cognitive therapy improves emotional reactivity to social stress: results from a randomized controlled trial. Behav Ther. 2012;43(2):365–80. doi:10.1016/j.beth.2011.08.006.

45. Troy A, Shallcross AJ, Davis TS, Mauss IB. History of mindfulness-based cognitive therapy is associated with increased cognitive reappraisal ability. Mindfulness. 2013;4(3):213–22. doi:10.1007/s12671-012-0114-5.

46. Keune PM, Bostanov V, Hautzinger M, Kotchoubey B. Mindfulness-based cognitive therapy (MBCT), cognitive style, and the temporal dynamics of frontal EEG alpha asymmetry in recurrently depressed patients. Biol Psychol. 2011;88(2–3):243–52. doi:10.1016/j.biopsycho.2011.08.008.

47. Baglioni C, Spiegelhalder K, Lombardo C, Riemann D. Sleep and emotions: a focus on insomnia. Sleep Med Rev. 2010;14(4):227–38. doi:10.1016/j.smrv.2009.10.007.

48. Larouche M, Cote G, Belisle D, Lorrain D. Kind attention and non-judgment in mindfulness-based cognitive therapy applied to the treatment of insomnia: state of knowledge. Pathol Biol (Paris). 2014;62(5):284–91. doi:10.1016/j.patbio.2014.07.002.

49. Heidenreich T, Tuin I, Pflug B, Michal M, Michalak J. Mindfulness-based cognitive therapy for persistent insomnia: a pilot study. Psychother Psychosom. 2006;75(3):188–9. doi:10.1159/000091778.

50. Ree MJ, Craigie MA. Outcomes following mindfulness-based cognitive therapy in a heterogeneous sample of adult outpatients. Behav Chang. 2007;24(02):70–86. doi:10.1375/bech.24.2.70.

51. Foulk MA, Ingersoll-Dayton B, Kavanagh J, Robinson E, Kales HC. Mindfulness-based cognitive therapy with older adults: an exploratory study. J Gerontol Soc Work. 2013;57(5):498–520. doi:10.10 80/01634372.2013.869787.

52. Britton WB, Haynes PL, Fridel KW, Bootzin RR. Polysomnographic and subjective profiles of sleep continuity before and after mindfulness-based cognitive therapy in partially remitted depression. Psychosom Med. 2010;72(6):539–48. doi:10.1097/PSY.0b013e3181dc1bad.

53. Britton WB, Haynes PL, Fridel KW, Bootzin RR. Mindfulness-based cognitive therapy improves polysomnographic and subjective sleep profiles in antidepressant users with sleep complaints. Psychother Psychosom. 2012;81(5):296–304. doi:10.1159/000332755000332755.

54. Segal ZV, Teasdale JD, Williams JMG. Mindfulness-based cognitive therapy: theoretical rationale and empirical status. In: Hayes SC, Follette VM, Linehan MM, editors. Mindfulness and acceptance: expanding the cognitive-behavioral tradition. New York: Guilford Press; 2004. p. 45–65.

55. Wicklow A, Espie CA. Intrusive thoughts and their relationship to actigraphic measurement of sleep: towards a cognitive model of insomnia. Behav Res Ther. 2000;38(7):679–93.

56. van der Velden AM, Kuyken W, Wattar U, Crane C, Pallesen KJ, Dahlgaard J, et al. A systematic review of mechanisms of change in mindfulness-based cognitive therapy in the treatment of recurrent major depressive disorder. Clin Psychol Rev. 2015;37:26–39. doi:10.1016/j.cpr.2015.02.001.

57. Ong J, Sholtes D. A mindfulness-based approach to the treatment of insomnia. J Clin Psychol. 2010;66(11):1175–84. doi:10.1002/jclp.20736.

58. Ozminkowski RJ, Wang S, Walsh JK. The direct and indirect costs of untreated insomnia in adults in the United States. Sleep. 2007;30(3):263–73.

59. Murtagh DR, Greenwood KM. Identifying effective psychological treatments for insomnia: a meta-analysis. J Consult Clin Psychol. 1995;63(1):79–89.

Mindfulness-Based Cognitive Therapy Improves Depression Symptoms After Traumatic Brain Injury

Lana J. Ozen, Carrie Gibbons, and Michel Bédard

The Case of Mary

Mary, a 60-year-old woman, was heading into work on a brisk winter's morning. It had snowed overnight and she was admiring the freshly covered white trees. As she left her house, hurrying to work, Mary stepped off her front porch and suddenly slipped on a patch of black ice hidden beneath the fluffy, light snow. As she fell, her brief case flung out of her hand and she landed flat on her face, hitting the front of her head on the ice-covered concrete path. When Mary opened her eyes, her neighbour was gazing down at her and said she had been unconscious for a couple of minutes. Mary remembered falling and knew where she was, but felt confused and a bit dizzy. Her neighbour told her she had seen her fall from her window and quickly ran to her.

Mary had lost consciousness for a couple of minutes, in which time her neighbour panicked and called 911.

Shortly after, Mary was lying in a computed tomography (CT) scanner, her head pounding. The doctor told her that the results were unremarkable and that she could go home. He recommended to see her family doctor if she continued experiencing symptoms. Mary made an appointment as soon as she got home. The next day, her friend had to drive her to the appointment as she was still a bit dizzy and had a terrible headache. Her doctor told her that she probably sustained a mild traumatic brain injury (TBI) and would need a few days of rest. Those few days turned into months.

For the first week after the injury, Mary was extremely tired and had difficulty concentrating. Light and loud noise irritated her and intensified

L.J. Ozen, Ph.D. (✉)
Department of Health Sciences, Lakehead University, 955 Oliver Rd, Thunder Bay, ON, Canada P7B 5E1

Centre for Applied Health Research, St. Joseph's Care Group, 580 Algoma St. N, Thunder Bay, ON, Canada P7B 5G4
e-mail: ozenl@tbh.net

C. Gibbons, M.P.H.
Centre for Applied Health Research, St. Joseph's Care Group, 580 Algoma St. N, Thunder Bay, ON, Canada P7B 5G4
e-mail: gibbonsc@tbh.net

M. Bédard, Ph.D.
Department of Health Sciences, Lakehead University, 955 Oliver Rd, Thunder Bay, ON, Canada P7B 5E1

Centre for Applied Health Research, St. Joseph's Care Group, 580 Algoma St. N, Thunder Bay, ON, Canada P7B 5G4

Northern Ontario School of Medicine, Lakehead University, 955 Oliver Rd, Thunder Bay, ON, Canada P7B 5E1
e-mail: mbedard@lakeheadu.ca

her persistent headache. She noticed that she was also more forgetful and distracted, frequently losing track of what she was doing as soon as she stepped into another room. After a few weeks, she also noticed that she was feeling quite sad, and it was difficult to shake off. Mary was typically an enthusiastic up-beat person and this underlying sadness was new to her.

Mary tried to go back to work the second week after her injury and realized it was hopeless. She found it extremely difficult to concentrate, felt continually fatigued and was too distracted by ongoing headaches. She ended up taking a month off work. Her sadness seemed to increase during this 'free time', as she found it difficult to complete simple daily tasks (e.g. bills, grocery shopping, reading the newspaper). She did not even feel like socializing, one of her favourite past times before her fall. Mary went back to work on reduced hours after a month. She could not believe how mentally fatigued she felt and how hard it was to get through the day without napping several times. She started noticing a lot of negative self-talk – 'what's wrong with me?', 'why can't I get better', 'I'm worthless', 'I'm a failure'. After 3 months, Mary's physical and cognitive symptoms had almost completely diminished and she was back fulltime at work. However, the sadness persisted and she felt exhausted and unmotivated to do anything after a day's work. She worried that she was depressed. Mary's symptoms are common after mild TBI, and worse after moderate to severe, which is unfortunate considering the high prevalence of TBI.

The Problem of Traumatic Brain Injury (TBI)

TBI presents a significant public health concern with considerable impact on rates of disability and traumatic death [1–3]. The annual incidence rate of TBI in the United States has been calculated at 506.4 per 100,000 [4]. The Centers for Disease Control and Prevention [5] estimates that in 2010 there were 2.5 million emergency department visits, hospitalizations, and deaths attributed to TBI. A recent study looking at premature

mortality due to neurological conditions in hospitals in the United States found that TBIs accounted for the highest number of years of potential life lost [6]. Based on the Canadian Community Health Survey, Statistics Canada data indicate that in 2009–2010 there were 98,440 Canadians, or just over 2 % of the population over age 12, who experienced a brain injury [7]. In Europe, estimates have found an incident rate of 235 per 100,000 with an estimated 775,500 new injuries each year [8].

TBI is defined as 'an alteration in brain function, or other evidence of brain pathology, caused by external force' [9]. Injuries of this nature may comprise loss of consciousness, memory loss of events leading up to the injury or immediately after, neurological deficits, disorientation and/or mental confusion. The epidemiology of TBI is challenging to fully assess for a variety of reasons including varying definitions of TBI and severity, and dissimilar data collection methods and practices in different jurisdictions [4]. In addition, a large number of injuries go unreported or are not treated in a hospital setting. This is particularly true of mild TBIs comprising 70–90 % of all TBIs [1]. It is estimated that mild TBI may impact more than 600 out of every 100,000 people if cases not treated in hospital are taken into account [1].

There are millions of individuals who live with residual issues post-TBI. It is estimated that 3.2–5.3 million Americans are living with TBI-related disability [5] and in Europe this number tops 6.2 million [8]. Residual symptoms comprise a host of cognitive, physical and/or psychological problems that may continue over an extended period. Deficits in cognitive abilities, such as executive dysfunction and memory and learning problems, are often documented after TBI [10,11]. Memory loss, attention problems, decline in organizational thinking skills and learning are symptomatic of TBI and these deficits lead to significant debilitating effects [12,13]. Many individuals experience significant issues with sleep and fatigue [14–16]. Another challenging concern for individuals living with TBI is chronic pain, most often experienced in the form of headaches [17–19].

People with TBI are also at an increased risk for developing long-term psychiatric disorders, including depression, generalized anxiety disorder and posttraumatic stress disorder [20,21]. A study of over 1500 individuals with TBI found that 26% experienced major depression and 22% experienced minor depression 1 year post-injury [22]. These findings were independent of injury severity. Of those who did not express depression symptoms 1 year post-injury, 26% were found to have depression at the 2-year mark [23]. Similarly, a recent review examining data from 99 studies reported that 27% of people with TBI were diagnosed with major depressive disorder or dysthymia and 38% reported symptoms of depression that reached clinically significant levels [24]. Not surprisingly, the cognitive, physical and psychological changes may further exacerbate one's risk for developing depression or at the very least, depression symptoms. The continued prevalence of depression post-injury is worrisome because it is possibly the best predictor of psychosocial adjustment [25], even 10 years after the TBI [26]. Also, the risk of death by suicide after TBI is 3–4 times greater than the general population [27].

Several Reasons May Explain Why Depression Symptoms Remain Many Years Post-Injury

The psychological and emotional issues arising from TBI may simply go untreated because the physical, behavioural and cognitive issues are the primary focus [28–30]. The presence of depression may also not be recognized, especially in the mild TBI group [30,31]. Another important contributor to the presence of depression post-injury may be the lack of intervention studies relying on the best research designs available. There is a paucity of randomized controlled trials (RCTs) for treatment options for depression after TBI [27–29] and research conducted to support pharmacological treatment lacks the rigor required to establish best practices [32,33]. One recent meta-analysis did find some support for medications to treat depression after mild TBI, but this did not

extend to the results from controlled trials [27]. Additionally, in a review of treatment of depression post-TBI [34], it was concluded that there is insufficient evidence to make recommendations to clinicians about psychosocial interventions that may be of benefit.

Theoretical Rationale of MBCT for Traumatic Brain Injury

Why some individuals have better outcomes than others remains to be fully investigated. It is possible that individuals who adjust better emotionally to the injury and have higher resilience develop more adaptive coping styles [35,36], which strongly suggests that interventions aimed at dealing with the emotional adjustment may result in better outcomes. Despite the emergence of such possibilities, the emotional consequences of TBI, and what some individuals report as a loss of 'self' [37] or change in self-concept [38], are often not addressed by conventional rehabilitation approaches. In fact, TBI may result in a constellation of emotional difficulties and their interactions may directly hamper recovery.

In particular, Strom and Kosciulek [39] outlined some of the complex inter-relationships between perceived stress, depression, hope and life satisfaction after a TBI. They point out that as individuals adjust to their 'new' lives after injury, the higher stress some experience is predictive of greater depression symptoms and this depression, in turn, is predictive of lower hope. Moreover, those individuals who focus on their impairments as a result of a TBI are at greater risk of experiencing depression symptoms regardless of injury severity [40]. New approaches that would allow individuals with a TBI to adjust emotionally to the situation created by the injury may positively affect mood and other outcomes. Thus, there is a great need for rehabilitation efforts to address the emotional consequences post-TBI [41].

Kangas and McDonald [42] argue that mindfulness approaches may help individuals with TBI 'reclaim' their lives as they accept limitations as a result of their injuries. This assertion is supported by accumulating evidence in the 1980s and 1990s for the benefits of mindfulness meditation training on physical and psychological outcomes in other clinical populations. For example, patients with chronic pain reported improved pain and psychological symptoms, including anxiety and depression, after partaking in an 8-week Mindfulness-Based Stress Reduction program (MBSR; [43]); these improvements were still present 7- [43] and 15-months later [44]. The authors suggest that, through meditation training, participants learned to uncouple the sensory experience of pain from the automatic affective/evaluative reaction, ultimately reducing suffering through cognitive reappraisal. MBSR had also shown to be successful at reducing anxiety, panic and depression symptoms for people with anxiety disorders, benefits that persisted at a 3-month [45] and 3-year follow-up [46]. The authors attributed the symptom reductions to the ability to identify anxious thoughts as thoughts rather than reality, allowing for a range of responses to a particular thought. Also, participants learned to view anxiety-related symptoms as opportunities to engage in mindful coping strategies, rather than habitual patterns of emotional reactivity.

Similarly, with the goal of improving depression and quality of life for people with TBI, our research group conducted a pilot study [47] using techniques adapted from MBSR [43] and Kolb's Experiential Learning Cycle [48]. The group comprised of 12 weekly sessions, which focused on well-being, empowerment and quality of life through the utilization of meditation, breathing exercises, group discussion and practicing present moment awareness. Participants were recruited through various local sources, were at least 18 years of age, were required to speak and read English, and had already completed standard treatments for their injury. Participants were also required to have insight into their condition and were excluded if they had a major concurrent mental illness, substance abuse or suicide ideation.

Ten individuals with TBI completed the mindfulness intervention and three dropouts acted as controls. The time since injury for participants ranged from 3 to 10 years. Compared to the control group, participants in the intervention group had a significant improvement in quality of life

$(F(1, 11)=5.70, p=.036)$, as observed on the mental health component of the Short-Form Health Survey-36 (SF-36, [49])). Participants' scores on this scale post-intervention were aligned with Canadian norms and indicated clinically significant change (Cohen's $d=0.34$). A significant reduction in depression symptoms $(F(1, 10)=6.48, p=.029)$, was captured on the cognitive-affective subscale of the Beck Depression Inventory–II (BDI-II, [50]) and the total BDI-II score nearly achieved statistical significance $(p=.059)$. We were able to assess seven participants 1 year after the end of the intervention [51] and found that the significant improvements in mental health and depression symptoms observed post-intervention were maintained at follow-up.

A decade after our initial pilot study, further evidence started to accumulate for the benefits of mindfulness training for people with TBI. In particular, Azulay and colleagues [52] developed a 10-week MBSR-based program for individuals with mild TBI and conducted it with 22 people enrolled over a 2-year period. From pre- to post-intervention, they found statistically significant increases in self-efficacy and quality of life, and noted that these changes fell in the clinically meaningful range (Cohen's $d=.50$ and .43 respectively). Smaller, but still statistically significant, improvements on measures of executive functioning and attentional regulation were also reported. Moreover, Johansson and colleagues [53] delivered an RCT of MBSR to individuals with TBI $(n=11)$ and stroke $(n=18)$ who were experiencing mental fatigue as a result of their injuries. Scores on the Mental Fatigue Scale (MFS) statistically improved in participants in the treatment $(n=15)$ compared to the control group $(n=14)$. Pre- to post-intervention changes in measures of depression and anxiety symptoms were not statistically significant when the treatment and control groups were compared (values not reported). The authors conducted a follow-up study with an 8-month advanced modified MBSR program comprising monthly meetings based on Buddhist virtues and meditation practices known for cultivating compassion, loving-kindness, appreciative joy and equanimity [54]. Fourteen participants from the original study completed the enhanced program and results from the MFS indicated continued reduced mental fatigue, as well as significant and sustained positive effects on information processing and attention. While this MBSR research provides some evidence for benefits of mindfulness training on outcomes after TBI, the interventions were not targeted at reducing depression.

Encouraged by the preliminary results showing that MBSR adapted for TBI improved depression on the cognitive subscale of the BDI-II [47], we were interested in continuing to investigate mindfulness for depression after TBI. Coincidentally, during this same time period, Segal and colleagues [55] were tasked with finding a maintenance version of cognitive therapy to reduce the risk of relapse in recurrent depression. It was well-known that cognitive therapy worked for depression in the acute phase by explicitly teaching patients to change the content of depressive thinking. However, their early work on developing a maintenance therapy [56] suggested that it could be equally true that patients were also changing their relationship to their negative thoughts and feelings, not merely the content. Somewhat familiar with the work of Jon Kabat-Zinn, the authors read *Full Catastrophe Living* [57]. They were struck by the similarities in which MBSR and cognitive therapy were thought to be benefiting patients— through the process of 'decentering' (i.e. seeing thoughts simply as thoughts, rather than reflecting reality). Ultimately, this overlap is what led the authors to create a successful group program, MBCT, to prevent relapse in recurrent depression.

The core skill taught in MBCT is the ability 'to recognize and disengage from mind states characterized by self-perpetuating patterns of ruminative, negative thought' (p. 74; [55]). In MBCT, through the practice of mindfulness meditation, cognitive therapy exercises and group discussion, participants learn to become aware of and respond skilfully, instead of reacting automatically, to unpleasant thoughts and feelings related to their depression. Teasdale and colleagues [58] published their first article reporting that MBCT did, in fact, significantly reduce the risk of depressive relapse. Since the original publication, MBCT has been effective in preventing relapse in recurrently

depressed individuals compared to those who continue with treatment as usual [59,60], waitlist controls [61,62] and placebo [63,64]. MBCT is also a recommended therapy for prevention of depressive relapse in the UK [65].

Research was showing that it was the mindfulness component that was helping participants relate differently to their negative thoughts and feelings, ultimately reducing the risk of depression [66]. We were interested in further investigating the treatment of depression symptoms after TBI. With the strong evidence of MBCT for recurrent depression and MBSR for anxiety and depression symptoms in various populations, we sought to adapt MBCT for TBI. In 2008, our research group received funding from the Ontario Neurotrauma Foundation to pilot MBCT for depression after TBI for a future multi-site RCT.

Modifications of MBCT for Traumatic Brain Injury

The MBCT intervention [55] was customized to address issues associated with TBI (e.g. problems with attention, concentration, memory, fatigue). The duration of the intervention was increased from the original 8-week program to 10 weeks. Each weekly session was shortened from the standard 2-2½ h to 1½-h and recommended daily meditation home practice was reduced from 45 min to 1 h per day to 20–30 min. The length of the in-class meditation sessions was shortened and included frequent reviews. Further adaptations included simplified language, the use of repetition and visual aids to help reinforce concepts. More attention was paid to fostering learning conditions to encourage an environment of trust and non-judgment. Connections between learning activities were made more explicit. For example, participants recorded their observations and questions on 'new learning' forms to encourage deeper reflection on usual modes of behaviour and habits of mind in day-to-day activities. The facilitator posed questions regarding the 'new learning' forms throughout the sessions, such as 'Are you committing yourself to the practice in the ways that you would like?' and 'What do you need to do to commit more to the practice?'

Participants were supplied with handouts from each session and received the book *The Mindful Way through Depression: Freeing Yourself from Chronic Unhappiness* [67]. Participants were not required to read the book, but were instructed to use the accompanying CD to guide meditations. Some sessions included additional handouts adapted from MBSR (e.g. 'The Attitudinal Foundation of Mindfulness Practice'). Other handouts were created to supplement course material and assist with home practice, including a 'Mindful Movement Exercises' instruction page and 'Standing Mindful Movement Ideas' handout. A handout was also created to adapt the 'defining the territory of depression' material to be specific to TBI. In particular, the 'Recovering from Depression after a Traumatic Brain Injury' handout included information on the prevalence of depression after TBI, followed by the diagnostic criteria for depression and a discussion about automatic negative thoughts and the symptoms of depression.

Evidence of MBCT for TBI Including Mechanisms of Change

MBCT Pilot Study

The first intervention of MBCT for depression after TBI was a pilot study consisting of 20 participants who expressed symptoms of depression as measured on the BDI-II [68]. All participants experienced their TBI at least 1 year prior to the study. A significant reduction in depression symptoms was found on all measures used to assess this variable, including the BDI-II ($p=.001$), Patient Health Questionnaire-9 (PHQ-9; $p=.003$; [69,70]), the depression subscale of the Hospital Anxiety and Depression Scale ($p=.023$) [71] and the depression subscale of the Symptom Checklist–90 ($p=.023$) [72]. There was also a significant reduction in the number of participants who were classified with major depressive disorder pre- to post-intervention on both the BDI-II ($p=.03$) and PHQ-9 ($p=.01$). These robust results provided strong rationale for a large-scale randomized controlled trial (RCT).

MBCT Randomized Controlled Trial

The development of the facilitators' capacity to provide the MBCT intervention was the first phase of the multi-site RCT. Thus, the first year was devoted to training 10 clinicians to become facilitators of the intervention (see training protocol below, [73]). As part of training, facilitators at three different sites led a trial of non-clinical healthy participant groups to practice their newly learned skills. After training facilitators to deliver the intervention, participants with TBI were recruited and assessed for the RCT at all sites. To be included in the study, participants had to show evidence of depression symptoms, indicated by a score of 16 or higher on the BDI-II. The time since injury for participants was an average of 4 years [74]. In a parallel group analysis, a greater reduction in the total score on the BDI-II was found for the MBCT intervention group compared to the waitlist control group ($F=4.99$, $p=.029$) with a medium effect size (Cohen's $d=0.56$). When we examined data from participants 3 months after the end of the intervention (data were also collected from controls after they crossed over and received the intervention), a reduction in depression symptoms on all measures was observed ($ps<.001$), including the BDI-II, PHQ-9 and the depression subscale of the SCL-90. Both the Philadelphia Mindfulness Scale (PHLMS) and the Toronto Mindfulness Scale (TMS) were used to examine change in mindfulness. While changes were in the expected direction, none achieved statistical significance ($p>.05$).

To return to the case example, Mary was hopeful when she came across a recruitment advertisement in her local newspaper looking for people with TBI-related depression symptoms to participate in a program called Mindfulness-Based Cognitive Therapy. It had been 6 months since the injury and she was still experiencing sadness and negativity, so she thought she would give it a try. Some of the questions on the initial questionnaires that the researchers asked her to complete surprised Mary as she could relate to many of them (e.g. 'I can't get pleasure from the things I used to enjoy'). Mary was encouraged during the first part of the program as she was instructed to merely see her thoughts as thoughts (negative or positive) and let them pass by. She was also amazed that other people in the group had also been having similar negative thoughts, and more so, that these thoughts are common after TBI.

Mary committed to completing each week's meditation practices and found the 10-min sitting meditation and mindful stretching particularly helpful. As the course went on, she found that it was easier to observe when she started ruminating about a negative thought or feeling she was having and come back to what she was doing (e.g. focusing on the breath or completing a task at work). Not being so caught up with trying to figure out her sadness allowed her to be present throughout her day, and gradually Mary realized that the thoughts had less influence on how she was feeling. Close to the completion of the course, she noticed she had more motivation to partake in activities after work and that she was enjoying them as she used to before her brain injury. The researchers contacted Mary 3 months after she completed the course to have her fill out more questionnaires. She had kept up with her 10-min meditation practice 3–4 times a week and was feeling grateful for the positive effects the mindfulness practices were having on her mood, wellbeing and quality of life.

Clinical Significance of Mindfulness for Depression after TBI

The significant findings from our three studies [47,68,74] provide strong support for the use of mindfulness interventions to improve depression symptoms after TBI. Statistically significant differences based on group data, however, do not always translate into meaningful differences in clinical applications, nor do they provide information about treatment response variability within the sample [75,76]. Accordingly, we developed a three-criterion standard based on well-established measures (reliable change, severity change and five-point change) to assess clinically significant change in BDI-II scores for each individual who completed a mindfulness intervention in our three previous studies (including participants in the

waitlist control group in the RCT who later crossed-over and partook in the intervention) [77]. Reliable change is calculated using a standard formula to determine whether the extent of change in each individual's pre-to-post intervention score is more than fluctuations of an imprecise measuring tool [75]. Five-point change, or minimally important clinical difference, determines if pre- to post-treatment scores changed by at least five points [78,79]. Severity change indicates whether each individual's pre- to post-treatment scores differ according to BDI-II severity cut-offs along a depression symptom continuum [50,80]. We predicted that the majority of the total participants with TBI (N=90) who partook in a mindfulness intervention in one of our three studies would have BDI-II scores that improved according to the three-criterion standard for clinical significance.

Results indicated that 50% of participants (45/90) met all three criteria: BDI-II scores reliably improved by at least five points into a lesser severe symptom category post-intervention [77]. Importantly, none of the participants had BDI-II scores that deteriorated and the remaining 50% had scores that did not change. Future research could benefit from exploring individual characteristics in people with TBI to help determine factors related to treatment response (e.g. age, sex, time since injury, cognitive ability). These results, however, do not rule out that the clinically significant improvement was due to factors unrelated to the mindfulness intervention (i.e. results are based on pre- to post-treatment data). Thus, separate analyses were conducted on participant data from the RCT only. Results revealed that the majority of participants had BDI-II scores that improved in the treatment group, 20/38 (53%), compared to a minority in the waitlist control group, 13/38 (34%). Notably, none of the participants in the treatment group had BDI-II scores that deteriorated compared to 5/38 (13%) participants in the control group. That 34% of participants in the control group experienced an improvement in depression indicates that factors unrelated to the mindfulness interventions may also positively affect depression symptoms, although not to the same extent as observed in the treatment group, and attests to the importance of conducting controlled trials.

Combined data from the three studies show, as would be expected, that each determinant of clinical significance used individually was less conservative than the three-criterion standard. Starting with reliable change, 71% (64/90) of participants had BDI-II scores that improved, indicating that almost three-fourth of participants had change that was above and beyond variations of an imprecise measuring tool [75]. This proportion is similar to previous reports of group interventions for people with depression in non-TBI samples. For example, reliable improvement in depression symptoms was reported after cognitive therapy in 64% of participants [81] and after acceptance and commitment therapy in 58% of participants (treatment as usual, [82]). In this study, 54% of participants (49/90) had scores that improved by at least five points and 58% (52/90) of participants had BDI-II scores that improved by at least one symptom severity category. A recent study reported similar results using both of these criteria in a non-TBI population: 54% of participants with depression showed improved symptoms by at least five points into a lesser severe category on the PHQ-9 after cognitive behavioural therapy ([83]). These findings suggest that mindfulness interventions for depression may benefit a similar proportion of people with TBI as cognitive therapy does for depression in non-TBI populations.

Mechanisms for Change after MBCT

Results from the non-clinical participant sample who completed the MBCT intervention during the facilitator training phase of our RCT [73] provided some insight into mechanisms underlying MBCT-related change [84]. Self-reported state (Toronto Mindfulness Scale; TMS; [85]) and trait mindfulness (Philadelphia Mindfulness Scale; PHLMS; [86]) measures were compared with self-reported psychological symptoms (Global Severity Index and the Positive Symptom Total of the Symptom Checklist-90-Revised; SLC-90-R; [72]). Pre- to post-intervention symptom reductions on the Global Severity Index of the SLC-90-R were significantly associated with higher baseline scores on the curiosity subscale

of the TMS (state mindfulness), $r (26) = -.49$, $p = .008$, and an increased pre- to post-intervention scores on the acceptance subscale of the PHLMS (trait mindfulness), $r (26) = -.46$, $p = .015$ [84]. These results suggest that the higher the individuals' ability to reflect on their immediate experiences with mindful curiosity prior to MBCT, the greater the reduction in overall psychological distress reported after MBCT. Also, as individuals' increase their ability to accept mental events without ruminating or suppressing them (acceptance subscale of PHLMS) pre- to post-MBCT, they report a corresponding reduction in overall psychological distress.

These associations found in our research with healthy individuals are in line with previous research examining state and trait mindfulness qualities. For example, scores on the acceptance subscale of the PHLMS were negatively related to anxiety and depression symptoms and positively associated with happiness and quality of life in student samples [86]. Also, increased state mindfulness (as measured by the Mindfulness Awareness Attention Scale) after MBSR was negatively related to self-reported medical symptoms, depression and anxiety [87]. Thus, higher levels of both state (e.g. curiosity) and trait mindfulness (e.g. acceptance) may be important contributors to the improvement in psychological symptoms reported after mindfulness interventions. Similar findings have also been reported in people with recurrent depression after MBCT. Individuals with higher levels of mindfulness (e.g. accepting without judgment and acting with awareness) or capacity for self-compassion after MBCT had lower rates of depression over a year later [88] and reduced depression scores at 6-month follow-up [89]. Further research supported these findings and added that the ability to acknowledge negative affect without becoming overwhelmed by it is a skill learned after MBCT that may protect patients from future depression [90,91].

The improvement in depression symptoms after MBCT in people with TBI may also be related to increases in mindfulness and self-compassion, but to our knowledge, this possibility has yet to be empirically investigated. We did not find an improvement in mindfulness pre- to post-intervention in our RCT using the TMS or PHLMS

[74], which may be a result of the scales not capturing the true facets of mindfulness, or perhaps not being as responsive to change as the BDI-II. Still, we are interested in further examining the potential association between improvements in mindfulness and depression pre- to post-intervention. Future research could also examine such mechanisms of change after MBCT, as well as examine neural changes in this population. For example, research shows that increases in the size of brain areas responsible for attentional and sensory processing (i.e. prefrontal cortex and right anterior insula) are significantly thicker in meditators than non-meditators, especially in those who practiced regularly and those with greater experience [92]. Evidence also indicates that brain areas responsible for emotional learning, memory and self-related processing are thicker in participants after MBSR compared to a waitlist control group ([93] from MBCT manual).

In addition to these structural changes, functional neural changes have also been documented. For instance, using functional magnetic resonance imaging (fMRI) during a mental task, two distinct forms of self-awareness (narrative and experiential modes) have been found to uncouple through mindfulness training. In particular, the neural activity in brain areas responsible for maintaining attention on body experience was found to increase (experiential mode), while the areas responsible for automatically activating 'stories' about the self decreased (narrative mode; [94]). Also, after MBSR training, participants had less neural reactivity to sadness provocation than participants who had not undergone the training [95]. That similar neural mechanisms underlie the improvement in depression symptoms after MBCT for people with TBI has yet to be elucidated.

Practical Considerations of MBCT for Traumatic Brain Injury

Patient Selection

For both our MBCT pilot study [68] and multi-site RCT [74], participants were recruited through local outpatient programs/clinics for individuals with neurological injury and rehabilitation, media coverage, and through family physicians, psychologists, chiropractors and nurses. Participants were all 18 years of age or older, were required to speak and read English, and had completed standard treatments for their injury. Participants on antidepressants and other medications (e.g. pain- and anxiety-related medication) were permitted to participate in the study. Participants were excluded if they had a major concurrent mental illness, substance abuse, or suicide ideation. Participants' data were included in the analyses if they completed the MBCT intervention, as well as the pre- and post-treatment assessment sessions (to provide a realistic estimate of the actual effect of the intervention, if it were offered in a typical clinical setting, all participants who provided outcome data were included regardless of their attendance to the weekly sessions). In order to be included in the study, participants must have undergone standard treatments for the injury. Time since injury was not included in the inclusion/exclusion criteria, which is a factor that could be controlled for in future research (e.g. is there an optimal time post-TBI to receive MBCT?) Also, future research could document TBI severity and determine if it is related to treatment response.

Home Practice

While an essential element of mindfulness interventions, to our knowledge, the effect of home practice on treatment-related outcomes has not yet been empirically investigated for people with TBI after partaking in MBCT. In general, documenting adherence to home practice has been minimal in the mindfulness literature. For example, one review examined 98 articles that studied the effects of mindfulness-focused group interventions on various outcome measures [96]. Of these articles, 24 articles related amount of home practice to study outcomes and the methods by which practice amounts were measured and reported varied greatly. For example, daily between-session practice amounts were reported for 11 articles (mean=31.8 min per day; range=5–58 min), weekly amounts of practice for two articles (55.9 and 84 min, respectively), and mean total practice of whole program for three articles (5.3, 15.8, and 30.3 h, respectively). Of the 24 articles, 13 demonstrated at least partial support for the predicted relationship between home practice and clinical outcomes, and 11 did not find the expected associations. Of those that did find some support, the amount of home practice was positively related to improved mood, mindfulness, wellbeing, happiness and coping; and negatively related to stress, anxiety, depression and rumination [96].

A recent study provided evidence for the importance of the quality of home practice on clinical outcomes for participants enrolled in MBSR (i.e. how participants attend to the present moment, along with their degree of openness to whatever arises). Using a newly created measure, Practice Quality-Mindfulness, Del Re et al. [97] suggested that higher practice quality during MBSR may lead to greater improvements in psychological symptoms after the intervention (overall score on the Depression, Anxiety and Stress Scale; DASS). Also, Snippe et al. [98] reported that, over the course of an MBSR program, daily mindfulness home practice during the day predicted increases in mindfulness, which was followed by improvements in both positive (liveliness and cheerfulness) and negative (anger, fatigue or tension) affect for at least one day. These studies provide some support for the benefits that practicing meditation at home can have on mood while participating in a mindfulness program.

Although we did not formally record participants' home practice, its importance was recognized in our research group's adaptation of MBCT for TBI. In particular, all participants were provided with supplementary handouts to assist with home practice (e.g., Standing Mindful Movement Ideas). Also, 'new learning' forms were provided and discussed each session to address potential issues with home practice (e.g. 'Are you committing yourself to the practice in the ways that you would like?' and 'What do you need to do to commit more to the practice?'). Future mindfulness research would benefit by having participants with TBI record the type, frequency, duration and/or quality of home practice during MBCT to assess if practice is related to the extent of depression symptom reduction.

Facilitator Training

Crane and colleagues [99] outlined training stages for MBCT instructors beginning with foundational training and progressing to basic and advanced teacher training. Basic teacher training contains similar components to the first year of our RCT (e.g. relevant clinical background, participating in MBCT teacher training). These guidelines include participation in a mindfulness program and teacher training, professional training in mental or physical healthcare, knowledge and experience with the population that the course will be delivered to, as well as ongoing commitment to continued development (e.g. personal meditation practice, regular supervision by an experienced mindfulness teacher, further training).

The first year of our RCT [74] was devoted to training clinicians [73]. The training began with a 2-day retreat to introduce mindfulness. This was then followed up with bi-weekly teleconferences and mentorship from an experienced instructor and support from other facilitators within the group. During this period, the facilitators were supported in the development of their own personal mindfulness practice. All facilitators attended a 5-day MBCT teacher training program run by the University of California San Diego Centre for Mindfulness. Next, the RCT culminated with trialling the intervention with 'healthy' participants (e.g. friends, family and colleagues). Sessions from this trial were recorded and assessed by an external reviewer experienced in the delivery of MBCT. The reviewer provided written qualitative feedback as well as conducting teleconferences with the each of the facilitators. Written comments from the reviewer were integrated into on-going, bi-weekly meetings to maximize support provided to the facilitators. These meetings continued for the duration of the RCT to support the facilitators.

Summary/Conclusions

The research conducted by our team over the past decade has led to results that are promising for people experiencing symptoms of depression after TBI. The strongest evidence to date is that MBCT adapted for individuals with TBI resulted in significant improvements in depression symptoms to an extent that was clinically meaningful for half of those who took the interventions. For those who did not show clinical improvement, it is possible that MBCT may have delayed or prevented depression symptoms from deteriorating overtime if left untreated.

Future research could benefit from exploring individual characteristics in people with TBI to help determine factors related to treatment response (e.g. age, sex, time since injury, severity of TBI, cognitive ability).

Treatment adherence is another important factor that would help to understand individual symptom changes during and after MBCT. For example, participants could record the type, frequency, duration and/or quality of home practice during MBCT to assess if it is related to the extent of depression symptom reduction. Further investigations could also examine mechanisms of change after MBCT (e.g. mindfulness and self-compassion), as well as the neural changes in this population. That similar neural mechanisms underlie the improvement in depression observed in people with recurrent depression after MBCT has yet to be elucidated for people with TBI.

Targeting depression after TBI using gold standard RCT methodology is crucial as depression may be the best predictor of psychosocial adjustment long after injury. Also, death by suicide is much higher after TBI compared to the general population. Improving depression symptoms through MBCT may be the first step at targeting the complex emotional sequela after TBI. MBCT may also enhance overall quality of life after TBI and improve the ability to partake in activities of daily living. Determining if mindfulness training could boost the gains achieved with other forms of interventions typically used after TBI may be the next logical step.

Acknowledgments We would like to acknowledge the following funding agencies and organizations that supported this research: Ontario Neurotrauma Foundation, St. Joseph's Care Group, Canada Research Chair program, and the Technology Evaluation in the Elderly Network. Our thanks are also extended to Melissa Felteau, MAdEd, for adapting the MBCT curriculum for depression symptoms after TBI, for training and mentoring the MBCT facilitators and for facilitating some of the mindfulness interventions. In addition, we would like to recognize all of the clinicians who underwent extensive MBCT teacher training, cultivated their own personal meditation practice and facilitated MBCT for the RCT. We also appreciate the contributions of all of the co-authors who helped with the MBCT for TBI projects over the past decade (see original papers).

References

1. Cassidy JD, Carroll LJ, Peloso PM, Borg J, von Holst H, Holm L, et al. Incidence, risk factors and prevention of mild traumatic brain injury: results of the WHO collaborating centre task force on mild traumatic brain injury. J Rehabil Med. 2004;43:28–60.
2. Coronado VG, Xu L, Basavaraju SV, McGuire LC, Wald MM, Faul MD, et al. Surveillance for traumatic brain injury-related deaths--United States, 1997–2007. MMWR Surveill Summ. 2011;60(5):1–32.
3. World Health Organization. Neurological disorders: public health challenges. Geneva, Switzerland: WHO Press; 2006.
4. Corrigan JD, Selassie AW, Orman JA. The epidemiology of traumatic brain injury. J Head Trauma Rehabil. 2010;25(2):72–80.doi:10.1097/HTR.0b013e3181ccc8b4.
5. Centers for Disease Control and Prevention. Report to congress on traumatic brain injury in the United States: epidemiology and rehabilitation. Atlanta, GA: National Center for Injury Prevention and Control; 2014. Division of Unintentional Injury.
6. Rosenbaum BP, Kelly ML, Kshettry VR, Weil RJ. Neurologic disorders, in-hospital deaths, and years of potential life lost in the USA, 1988–2011. J Clin Neurosci. 2014;21(11):1874–80. doi:10.1016/j.jocn.2014.05.006.
7. Billette JM and Janz T. Injuries in Canada: Insights from the Canadian community health survey. (No. 82-624-X). Statistics Canada; 2011.
8. Tagliaferri F, Compagnone C, Korsic M, Servadei F, Kraus J. A systematic review of brain injury epidemiology in Europe. Acta Neurochir. 2006;148(3):255–68. doi:10.1007/s00701-005-0651-y. discussion 268.
9. Menon DK, Schwab K, Wright DW, Maas AI, Demographics and Clinical Assessment Working Group of the International and Interagency Initiative toward Common Data Elements for Research on Traumatic Brain Injury and Psychological Health. Position statement: definition of traumatic brain

injury. Arch Phys Med Rehabil. 2010;91(11):1637–40. doi:10.1016/j.apmr.2010.05.017.

10. Clune-Ryberg M, Blanco-Campal A, Carton S, Pender N, O'Brien D, Phillips J, et al. The contribution of retrospective memory, attention and executive functions to the prospective and retrospective components of prospective memory following TBI. Brain Inj. 2011;25(9):819–31. doi:10.3109/02699052.2011.589790.

11. Ponsford JL, Downing MG, Olver J, Ponsford M, Acher R, Carty M, et al. Longitudinal follow-up of patients with traumatic brain injury: outcome at two, five, and ten years post-injury. J Neurotrauma. 2014;31(1):64–77. doi:10.1089/neu.2013.2997.

12. Chamelian L, Feinstein A. The effect of major depression on subjective and objective cognitive deficits in mild to moderate traumatic brain injury. J Neuropsychiatry Clin Neurosci. 2006;18(1):33–8.

13. Ziino C, Ponsford J. Selective attention deficits and subjective fatigue following traumatic brain injury. Neuropsychology. 2006;20(3):383–90.

14. Castriotta RJ, Murthy JN. Sleep disorders in patients with traumatic brain injury: a review. CNS Drugs. 2011;25(3):175–85. doi:10.2165/11584870-000000000-00000.

15. Mollayeva T, Kendzerska T, Mollayeva S, Shapiro CM, Colantonio A, Cassidy JD. A systematic review of fatigue in patients with traumatic brain injury: the course, predictors and consequences. Neurosci Biobehav Rev. 2014;47:684–716. doi:10.1016/j.neubiorev.2014.10.024.

16. Ouellet MC, Beaulieu-Bonneau S, Morin CM. Insomnia in patients with traumatic brain injury: frequency, characteristics, and risk factors. J Head Trauma Rehabil. 2006;21(3):199–212.

17. Lew HL, Lin PH, Fuh JL, Wang SJ, Clark DJ, Walker WC. Characteristics and treatment of headache after traumatic brain injury: a focused review. Am J Phys Med Rehabil. 2006;85(7):619–27.

18. Lucas S, Hoffman JM, Bell KR, Dikmen S. A prospective study of prevalence and characterization of headache following mild traumatic brain injury. Cephalalgia. 2014;34(2):93–102. doi:10.1177/033310241349964.

19. Ryan LM, Warden DL. Post concussion syndrome. Int Rev Psychiatry. 2003;15(4):310–6. doi:10.1080/0954 0260310001606692.

20. Bryant RA, O'Donnell ML, Creamer M, McFarlane AC, Clark CR, Silove D. The psychiatric sequelae of traumatic injury. Am J Psychiatry. 2010;167(3):312–20. doi:10.1176/appi.ajp.2009.09050617.

21. Rogers JM, Read CA. Psychiatric comorbidity following traumatic brain injury. Brain Inj. 2007;21(13–14):1321–33. doi:10.1080/02699050701765700.

22. Hart T, Brenner L, Clark AN, Bogner JA, Novack TA, Chervoneva I, et al. Major and minor depression after traumatic brain injury. Arch Phys Med Rehabil. 2011;92(8):1211–9. doi:10.1016/j.apmr.2011.03.005.

23. Hart T, Hoffman JM, Pretz C, Kennedy R, Clark AN, Brenner LA. A longitudinal study of major and minor depression following traumatic brain injury. Arch Phys Med Rehabil. 2012;93(8):1343–9. doi:10.1016/j.apmr.2012.03.036.

24. Osborn AJ, Mathias JL, Fairweather-Schmidt AK. Depression following adult, non-penetrating traumatic brain injury: a meta-analysis examining methodological variables and sample characteristics. Neurosci Biobehav Rev. 2014;47:1–15. doi:10.1016/j.neubiorev.2014.07.007.

25. Ownsworth T, Fleming J. The relative importance of metacognitive skills, emotional status, and executive function in psychosocial adjustment following acquired brain injury. J Head Trauma Rehabil. 2005;20(4):315–32.

26. Draper K, Ponsford J, Schonberger M. Psychosocial and emotional outcomes 10 years following traumatic brain injury. J Head Trauma Rehabil. 2007;22(5):278–87.

27. Simon G, Tate R. Suicidality in people surviving a traumatic brain injury: prevalence, risk factors and implications for clinical management. Brain Injury 2007;21:1335–51.

28. Barker-Collo S, Starkey N, Theadom A. Treatment for depression following mild traumatic brain injury in adults: a meta-analysis. Brain Inj. 2013;27(10):1124–33. doi:10.3109/02699052.2013.801513.

29. Jorge RE. Neuropsychiatric consequences of traumatic brain injury: a review of recent findings. Curr Opin Psychiatry. 2005;18(3):289–99.

30. Nygren-de Boussard C, Holm LW, Cancelliere C, Godbolt AK, Boyle E, Stalnacke BM, et al. Nonsurgical interventions after mild traumatic brain injury: a systematic review. Results of the international collaboration on mild traumatic brain injury prognosis. Arch Phys Med Rehabil. 2014;95(3 Suppl):S257–64. doi:10.1016/j.apmr.2013.10.009.

31. Carroll LJ, Cassidy JD, Peloso PM, Borg J, von Holst H, Holm L, et al. Prognosis for mild traumatic brain injury: results of the WHO collaborating centre task force on mild traumatic brain injury. J Rehabil Med. 2004;43:84–105.

32. Gracey F. Mood and affective problems after traumatic brain injury. Adv Clin Neurosci Rehabil. 2002;2(3):18–20.

33. Lee HB, Lyketsos CG, Rao V. Pharmacological management of the psychiatric aspects of traumatic brain injury. Int Rev Psychiatry. 2003;15(4):359–70.

34. Warden DL, Gordon B, McAllister TW, Silver JM, Barth JT, Bruns J, et al. Guidelines for the pharmacologic treatment of neurobehavioral sequelae of traumatic brain injury. J Neurotrauma. 2006;23(10):1468–501.

35. Fann JR, Hart T, Schomer KG. Treatment for depression after traumatic brain injury: a systematic review. J Neurotrauma. 2009;26(12):2383–402. doi:10.1089/neu.2009.1091.

36. Anson K, Ponsford J. Who benefits? Outcome following a coping skills group intervention for traumatically brain injured individuals. Brain Inj. 2006;20(1):1–13.

37. Losoi H, Silverberg N, Waljas M, Turunen S, Rosti-Otajarvi E, Helminen M, et al. Resilience is associated with outcome from mild traumatic brain injury. J Neurotrauma. 2015;32(13):942–9. doi:10.1089/neu.2014.3799.

38. Nochi M. "Loss of self" in the narratives of people with traumatic brain injury: a qualitative analysis. Soc Sci Med. 1998;46(7):869–78.

39. Ponsford J, Kelly A, Couchman G. Self-concept and self-esteem after acquired brain injury: a control group comparison. Brain Inj. 2014;28(2):146–54. doi:10.3109/02699052.2013.859733.

40. Strom TQ, Kosciulek J. Stress, appraisal and coping following mild traumatic brain injury. Brain Inj. 2007;21(11):1137–45.

41. Malec JF, Testa JA, Rush BK, Brown AW, Moessner AM. Self-assessment of impairment, impaired self-awareness, and depression after traumatic brain injury. J Head Trauma Rehabil. 2007;22(3):156–66.

42. Ownsworth T, Haslam C. Impact of rehabilitation on self-concept following traumatic brain injury: an exploratory systematic review of intervention methodology and efficacy. Neuropsychol Rehabil. 2014;26:1–35. doi:10.1080/09602011.2014.977924.

43. Kangas M, McDonald S. Is it time to act? the potential of acceptance and commitment therapy for psychological problems following acquired brain injury. Neuropsychol Rehabil. 2011;21(2):250–76. doi:10.1080/09602011.2010.540920.

44. Kabat-Zinn J. An outpatient program in behavioral medicine for chronic pain patients based on the practice of mindfulness meditation: theoretical considerations and preliminary results. Gen Hosp Psychiatry. 1982;4(1):33–47.

45. Kabat-Zinn J, Lipworth L, Burney R. The clinical use of mindfulness meditation for the self-regulation of chronic pain. J Behav Med. 1985;8(2):163–90.

46. Kabat-Zinn J, Massion AO, Kristeller J, Peterson LG, Fletcher KE, Pbert L, et al. Effectiveness of a meditation-based stress reduction program in the treatment of anxiety disorders. Am J Psychiatry. 1992;149(7):936–43.

47. Miller JJ, Fletcher K, Kabat-Zinn J. Three-year follow-up and clinical implications of a mindfulness meditation-based stress reduction intervention in the treatment of anxiety disorders. Gen Hosp Psychiatry. 1995;17(3):192–200.

48. Bédard M, Felteau M, Mazmanian D, Fedyk K, Klein R, Richardson J, et al. Pilot evaluation of a mindfulness-based intervention to improve quality of life among individuals who sustained traumatic brain injuries. Disabil Rehabil. 2003;25(13):722–31.

49. Kolb DA. Experiential learning: experience as the source of learning and development. Englewood Cliffs, NJ: Prentice-Hall; 1984.

50. Ware JE, Kosinski M. SF-36 physical and mental health summary: a manual for users of version 1. Lincoln, RI: QualityMetric; 2001.

51. Beck AT, Steer RA, Brown GK. Beck depression inventory-II (BDI-II). Toronto: The Psychological Corporation, Harcourt Brace; 1996.

52. Bédard M, Felteau M, Gibbons C, Klein R, Mazmanian D, Fedyk K, and Mack G. A mindfulness-based intervention to improve quality of life among individuals who sustained traumatic brain injuries: one-year follow-up. *The Journal of Cognitive Rehabilitation, Spring.* 2005; p. 2–7.

53. Azulay J, Smart CM, Mott T, Cicerone KD. A pilot study examining the effect of mindfulness-based stress reduction on symptoms of chronic mild traumatic brain injury/postconcussive syndrome. J Head Trauma Rehabil. 2012;28(4):323–31. doi:10.1097/HTR.0b013e318250ebda.

54. Johansson B, Bjuhr H, Ronnback L. Mindfulness-based stress reduction (MBSR) improves long-term mental fatigue after stroke or traumatic brain injury. Brain Inj. 2012;26(13–14):1621–8. doi:10.3109/02699052.2012.700082.

55. Johansson B, Bjuhr H, Rönnbäck L. Evaluation of an advanced mindfulness program following a mindfulness-based stress reduction program for participants suffering from mental fatigue after acquired brain injury. Mindfulness. 2015;6:227–33. doi:10.1007/s12671-013-0249-z.

56. Segal ZV, Williams JMG, Teasdale JD. Mindfulness-based cognitive therapy for depression. A new approach to preventing relapse. New York: The Guilford Press; 2002.

57. Teasdale JD, Segal Z, Williams MG. How does cognitive therapy prevent depressive relapse and why should attentional control (mindfulness) training help? Behav Res Ther. 1995;33:25–39.

58. Kabat-Zinn J. Full catastrophe living: using the wisdom of your body and mind to face stress, pain, and illness. 15th ed. New York: Random House, Inc.; 2009.

59. Teasdale JD, Williams JMG, Soulsby JM, Segal ZV, Ridgeway VA, Lau MA. Prevention of relapse/recurrence in major depression by mindfulness-based cognitive therapy. J Consult Clin Psychol. 2000;68:615–23.

60. Bondolfi G, Jermann F, der Linden MV, Gex-Fabry M, Bizzini L, Rouget BW, et al. Depression relapse prophylaxis with mindfulness-based cognitive therapy: replication and extension in the Swiss health care system. J Affect Disord. 2010;122(3):224–31. doi:10.1016/j.jad.2009.07.007.

61. Godfrin KA, van Heeringen C. The effects of mindfulness-based cognitive therapy on recurrence of depressive episodes, mental health and quality of life: a randomized controlled study. Behav Res Ther. 2010;48(8):738–46. doi:10.1016/j.brat.2010.04.006.

62. Britton WB, Haynes PL, Fridel KW, Bootzin RR. Polysomnographic and subjective profiles of sleep continuity before and after mindfulness-based cognitive therapy in partially remitted depression. Psychosom Med. 2010;72(6):539–48. doi:10.1097/PSY.0b013e3181dc1bad.

63. Keune PM, Bostanov V, Hautzinger M, Kotchoubey B. Mindfulness-based cognitive therapy (MBCT), cognitive style, and the temporal dynamics of frontal EEG alpha asymmetry in recurrently depressed patients. Biol Psychol. 2011;88(2–3):243–52. doi:10.1016/j.biopsycho.2011.08.008.

64. Meeting F, Whiting S, and Williams CM. An Exploratory Study of Group Mindfulness-Based Cognitive Therapy for Older People with Depression. Mindfulness. 2015;6(3):467–74.

65. Segal ZV, Bieling P, Young T, MacQueen G, Cooke R, Martin L, et al. Antidepressant monotherapy vs sequential pharmacotherapy and mindfulness-based cognitive therapy, or placebo, for relapse prophylaxis in recurrent depression. Arch Gen Psychiatry. 2010;67(12):1256–64. doi:10.1001/archgenpsychiatry.2010.168.

66. National Collaborating Centre for Mental Health; NICE clinical guideline 90: depression: the treatment and management of depression in adults (partial update of NICE clinical guideline 23). London: National Institute for Health and Clinical Excellence; 2009.

67. Segal ZV, Williams JMG, Teasdale JD. Mindfulness-based cognitive therapy for depression. New York: Guilford Press; 2013.

68. Williams M, Teasdale J, Segal Z, Kabat-Zinn J. The mindful way through depression: freeing yourself from chronic unhappiness. New York, NY: The Guilford Press; 2007.

69. Bédard M, Felteau M, Marshall S, Dubois S, Gibbons C, Klein R, et al. Mindfulness based cognitive therapy: benefits in reducing depression following a traumatic brain injury. Adv Mind Body Med. 2012;26(1):14–20.

70. Kroenke K, Spitzer RL, Williams JB. The PHQ-9: validity of a brief depression severity measure. J Gen Intern Med. 2001;16(9):606–13.

71. Kroenke K, Spitzer RL. The PHQ-9: a new depression diagnostic and severity measure. Psychiatr Ann. 2002;32(9):509–15.

72. Zigmond A, Snaith R. The hospital anxiety and depression scale. Acta Psychiatr Scand. 1982;67:361–70.

73. Derogatis LR. SCL-90-R administration, scoring, and procedures manual. Minneapolis: National Computer Systems; 1994.

74. Gibbons C, Felteau M, Cullen N, Marshall S, Dubois S, Maxwell H, et al. Training clinicians to deliver a mindfulness intervention. Mindfulness. 2014;5(3):232–7. doi:10.1007/s12671-012-0170-x.

75. Bédard M, Felteau M, Marshall S, Cullen N, Gibbons C, Dubois S, et al. Mindfulness-based cognitive therapy reduces depression symptoms in people with a traumatic brain injury: results from a randomized controlled trial. J Head Trauma Rehabil. 2014;29(4):13–22. doi:10.1097/HTR.0b013e3182a615a0.

76. Jacobson NS, Truax P. Clinical significance: a statistical approach to defining meaningful change in psychotherapy research. J Consult Clin Psychol. 1991;59(1):12–9.

77. Ogles BM, Lunnen KM, Bonesteel K. Clinical significance: history, application, and current practice. Clin Psychol Rev. 2001;21(3):421–46.

78. Ozen LJ, Dubois S, Gibbons C, Short MM, Bédard M. (2015). Mindfulness interventions improve depression symptoms after traumatic brain injury: are individual changes clinically significant? Manuscript submitted for publication.

79. Hiroe T, Kojima M, Yamamoto I, Nojima S, Kinoshita Y, Hashimoto N, et al. Gradations of clinical severity and sensitivity to change assessed with the beck depression inventory-II in Japanese patients with depression. Psychiatry Res. 2005;135(3):229–35. doi:10.1016/j.psychres.2004.03.014.

80. Lowe B, Unutzer J, Callahan CM, Perkins AJ, Kroenke K. Monitoring depression treatment outcomes with the patient health questionnaire-9. Med Care. 2004;42(12):1194–201.

81. Tingey RC, Lambert MJ, Burlingame GM, Hansen NB. Assessing clinical significance: proposed exten-sions to method. Psychother Res. 1996;6(2):109–23. doi:10.1080/10503309612331331638.

82. Strauss C, Hayward M, Chadwick P. Group person-based cognitive therapy for chronic depression: a pilot randomized controlled trial. Br J Clin Psychol. 2012;51(3):345–50. doi:10.1111/j.2044-8260.2012.02036.x.

83. Hayes L, Boyd CP, Sewell J. Acceptance and commitment therapy for the treatment of adolescent depression: a pilot study in a psychiatric outpatient setting. Mindfulness. 2011;2(2):86–94. doi:10.1007/s12671-011-0046-5.

84. Williams AD, Andrews G. The effectiveness of internet cognitive behavioural therapy (iCBT) for depression in primary care: a quality assurance study. PLoS One. 2013;8(2), e57447. doi:10.1371/journal.pone.0057447.

85. Klein R, Dubois S, Gibbons C, Ozen LJ, Marshall S, Cullen N, et al. The Toronto and Philadelphia mindfulness scales: associations with satisfaction with life and health-related symptoms. Int J Psychol Psychol Ther. 2015;15(1):133–42.

86. Lau MA, Bishop SR, Segal ZV, Buis T, Anderson ND, Carlson L, et al. The Toronto mindfulness scale: development and validation. J Clin Psychol. 2006;62(12):1445–67.

87. Cardaciotto L, Herbert JD, Forman EM, Moitra E, Farrow V. The assessment of present-moment awareness and acceptance: the Philadelphia mindfulness scale. Assessment. 2008;15(2):204–23.

88. Carmody J, Reed G, Kristeller J, Merriam P. Mindfulness, spirituality, and health-related symptoms. J Psychosom Res. 2008;64(4):393–403. doi:10.1016/j.jpsychores.2007.06.015.

89. Kuyken W, Watkins E, Holden E, White K, Taylor RS, Byford S, et al. How does mindfulness-based cognitive therapy work? Behav Res Ther. 2010;48(11):1105–12. doi:10.1016/j.brat.2010.08.003.

90. Bieling PJ, Hawley LL, Bloch RT, Corcoran KM, Levitan RD, Young LT, et al. Treatment-specific changes in decentering following mindfulness-based cognitive therapy versus antidepressant medication or placebo for prevention of depressive relapse. J Consult Clin Psychol. 2012;80(3):365–72. doi:10.1037/a0027483.

91. Leary MR, Tate EB, Adams CE, Allen AB, Hancock J. Self-compassion and reactions to unpleasant self-relevant events: the implications of treating oneself kindly. J Pers Soc Psychol. 2007;92(5):887–904. doi:10.1037/0022-3514.92.5.887.

92. Raes F, Dewulf D, Van Heeringen C, Williams JM. Mindfulness and reduced cognitive reactivity to sad mood: evidence from a correlational study and a non-randomized waiting list controlled study. Behav Res Ther. 2009;47(7):623–7. doi:10.1016/j.brat.2009.03.007.

93. Lazar SW, Kerr CE, Wasserman RH, Gray JR, Greve DN, Treadway MT, et al. Meditation experience is associated with increased cortical thickness. Neuroreport. 2005;16(17):1893–7.

94. Holzel BK, Carmody J, Vangel M, Congleton C, Yerramsetti SM, Gard T, et al. Mindfulness practice leads to increases in regional brain gray matter density. Psychiatry Res. 2011;191(1):36–43. doi:10.1016/j.pscychresns.2010.08.006.

95. Farb NA, Segal ZV, Mayberg H, Bean J, McKeon D, Fatima Z, et al. Attending to the present: mindfulness

meditation reveals distinct neural modes of self-reference. Soc Cogn Affect Neurosci. 2007;2(4):313–22. doi:10.1093/scan/nsm030.

96. Farb NA, Anderson AK, Mayberg H, Bean J, McKeon D, Segal ZV. Minding one's emotions: mindfulness training alters the neural expression of sadness. Emotion. 2010;10(1):25–33. doi:10.1037/a0017151.

97. Vettese LC, Toneatto T, Stea JN, Nguyen L, Wang JJ. Do mindfulness meditation participants do their homework and does it make a difference? A review of the empirical evidence. J Cogn Psychother. 2009;23(3):198–225. doi:10.1891/0889-8391.23.3.198.

98. Del Re AC, Fluckiger C, Goldberg SB, Hoyt WT. Monitoring mindfulness practice quality: an important consideration in mindfulness practice. Psychother Res. 2013;23(1):54–66. doi:10.1080/10503307.2012.729275.

99. Snippe E, Nyklicek I, Schroevers MJ, Bos EH. The temporal order of change in daily mindfulness and affect during mindfulness-based stress reduction. J Couns Psychol. 2015;62(2):106–14. doi:10.1037/cou0000057.

100. Crane RS, Kuyken W, Hastings RP, Rothwell N, Williams JMG. Training teachers to deliver mindfulness-based interventions: learning from the UK experience. Mindfulness. 2010;1:74–86. doi:10.1007/s12671-010-0010-9.

Mindfulness-Based Cognitive Therapy in Women with Breast and Gynecologic Cancers

5

Lesley Stafford, Naomi Thomas, and Elizabeth Foley

A Clinical Case

Jane was a 50-year-old married woman with two children. She had recently been diagnosed with early-stage ovarian cancer. Her cancer treatment comprised hysterectomy, oophorectomy, and chemotherapy. Her intention for attending the mindfulness-based cognitive therapy (MBCT) program was to learn to live in the moment. Referring to the cancer, she said "I will beat this. I will live." In the first stage of the program, Jane spoke about how she tended to keep busy and noticed that she was not in the present very often. She said "I have noticed this week that I sit with my family for dinner every night and for as long as I can remember, I have quickly finished eating, without hearing the conversation or even seeing my family, always in a rush to get things done before bed." She began to realize

how her "leaning" forward in life was depriving her and her family of the present. By midway in the program, Jane was able to see that she had been feeling "out of control" since her diagnosis and that she had made herself busy as a way of coping. She realized that this busyness was making her feel lonely and more stressed. Jane had noticed that her body was tense all the time and she wanted things to be different, calmer. As Jane began to slow down, she realized that she had been fighting against the idea of having cancer. She decided to try to allow the cancer to "be there" and to put her energy into her relationships instead. At the end of the program, Jane reported feeling more grounded and more connected to herself and to those around her.

Theoretical Rationale of MBCT in Oncology Settings

It is well established that the diagnosis and treatment of cancer are associated with substantial challenges to quality of life (QOL) and high rates of psychological distress [1, 2]. As survival rates continue to improve and more cancer patients are living longer, identifying effective, cost-efficient psychosocial interventions for individuals with cancer is increasingly important. Group-based meditative practices such as mindfulness-based stress reduction (MBSR) and MBCT, which employ training in mindfulness skills are increasingly

L. Stafford, Ph.D. (✉) • N. Thomas, Ph.D.
Centre for Women's Mental Health, Royal Women's Hospital, Locked Bag 300, Corner Grattan Street and Flemington Road, Parkville, VIC 3052, Australia
e-mail: Lesley.stafford@thewomens.org.au; Naomi.thomas@thewomens.org.au

E. Foley, Ph.D.
Mind Potential, Shop 2/ 52 President Avenue, Caringbah, NSW 2229, Australia
e-mail: elizabeth@mindpotential.com.au

popular in oncology settings and their effectiveness is supported by a burgeoning empirical evidence base [3]. There are several aspects of the cancer experience that are well-suited to a mindfulness-based approach. This is described in a recent review by Carlson [4] who notes that loss of control, uncertainty, and constant change are often the most challenging aspects of coping with cancer and that attempts to negotiate these difficulties with problem-focused coping strategies are likely to be unsuccessful. Instead, emotion-focused strategies are needed to manage the existential challenges of a cancer diagnosis and this is where mindfulness approaches are particularly useful. With its focus on present moment awareness, self-compassion, acceptance, and turning toward rather than away from painful emotional experiences, mindfulness training may be an antidote to worrying about the future that is commonly experienced by individuals with cancer. The development of equanimity through mindfulness practice may directly target the reactive processes that can cause and worsen psychological distress [5]. It is noted that acceptance in this context does not mean "giving up" or declining treatment; instead, it is an acknowledgement of the reality and inevitability of loss and change that allows one to live more fully in the present [4]. This concept is illustrated in the following case vignette from the group MBCT program.

Stella had avoided looking at her chest and breasts since her lumpectomy 2 years ago for early-stage breast cancer. She was aware of negative thoughts she had about her body and labeling her breasts as "damaged" and "not whole." Through the use of body scan meditation, Stella learned how to be present with her physical experience and became more compassionate toward herself and her body. By the fourth session, Stella was no longer avoiding her chest during her daily body scan mediation and was using the breath to help her make room for difficult emotions that arose during meditation. She told the group "I now feel that I can be present with my body, my *whole* body, the way it is without struggling to avoid reminders of what I went through."

MBSR or MBCT?

Most empirical data in the oncology setting concern MBSR, a systematic 8-week mindfulness program shown to improve mood, sleep, stress, and physical wellbeing [3, 6–9]. Much less is known about the potential benefits to cancer patients of MBCT, which is a relatively recent refinement of MBSR that specifically targets the cognitive processes associated with relapse to depression [10]. Like MBSR, MBCT emphasizes daily mindfulness meditation as a key component, is facilitated through eight weekly sessions of 2 h duration, and routinely offers a full-day session of meditation practice in the later stages of the program [10, 11]. MBCT and MBSR also share an attitudinal framework of kindness, curiosity, and willingness to be present.

Although the evidence for MBSR in oncology settings is excellent and MBSR and MBCT are clearly very similar, our belief is that MBCT differs in a number of ways that make it more appropriate for individuals with cancer. For instance, whilst MBSR is routinely offered to large groups of individuals with mixed presentations (e.g., cancer, arthritis, chronic pain, diabetes), MBCT is offered to small groups of up to 12 participants and tends to have participants with a presenting issue in common (e.g., type of cancer). The smaller group allows more time for each participant and therefore a deeper holding experience for each participant and a greater opportunity to tailor the intervention for individual experiences. The small group size also offers containment of the often high level of suffering in this population. The provision of generous inquiry time for each participant may be especially valuable as individuals with cancer often report not having other places in which to express and share their experience with such honesty. By limiting the group membership to individuals with a shared presenting issue (in this instance, to women with breast and gynecologic cancer), specific formulations of the utility of mindfulness can be explored.

Another difference between MBSR and MBCT is that in the middle weeks of the MBCT program, participants are trained in using mindfulness to work with difficulties by suspending the meditation practice, encouraging thought about a current challenge and then resuming the meditation with guidance to work with any reactions. These exercises are practical training in applying mindfulness to challenging experiences. Undoubtedly, the central difference between MBSR and MBCT is the explicit focus on cognition within the latter: early in the program participants are provided with psycho-education on the association between thoughts and mood and the link between cognition and functioning is emphasized throughout. Participants learn how to recognize patterns of rumination; repetitive, passive thinking or brooding about aspects of negative experience without taking action to remedy the situation [12]. The specific focus on rumination and the significance of one's relationship to common thinking themes is especially useful in addressing the high level of psychological distress in this population, and can assist in alleviating or even preventing ongoing distress. Other differences between MBSR and MBCT are that the latter includes instruction in a short meditation practice (the 3 min breathing space), which is particularly beneficial as it makes mindfulness training "portable"; options for skilful action (e.g., nourishing activities), and relapse prevention (identifying signs of relapse and action planning) [10], both of which have an existential value for this population who can be re-evaluating their identity. Essentially, MBCT offers an integration of MBSR and cognitive therapy in a more intimate, supported group environment.

Evidence for MBCT in Oncology Settings

As noted above, the vast majority of literature relating to mindfulness in oncology settings pertains to MBSR. Existing publications of MBCT in oncology settings are limited but encouraging [13–17]. In 2010, the first randomized controlled trial (RCT) of MBCT in individuals with cancer reported significant improvements in distress, depression, and anxiety with gains maintained 3 months post-intervention in this group of mixed diagnosis patients [15]. Subsequently, two other RCTs have been published, one showing improvement in chronic fatigue and wellbeing in

a mixed diagnosis sample [17] and the other, a brief mindfulness-based cognitive behavioral intervention, reporting improved sexual response in women with gynecologic cancer [18]. At least one large RCT of MBCT to improve psychological wellbeing among individuals with cancer is currently underway [19]. Finally, two small pilot studies, one of 12 men with prostate cancer [14] and the other of 16 patients with mixed diagnoses [16] showed significant improvements in anxiety [14, 16], mindfulness [14, 16], avoidance [14], and depression [16], with gains maintained 3 months after the completion of treatment.

MBCT for Women with Breast and Gynecologic Cancer: A Pilot Study of Effectiveness and Feasibility

Together, breast and gynecologic cancers account for the majority of cancer diagnoses in Australian women [20]. Evidence shows that the experience of these conditions, which may include disfiguring and painful treatments, is associated with significant negative changes in bodily functional ability and QOL [21]. For many women, psychological distress may be chronic and protracted [22–24]. A program like MBCT that teaches independent coping and emotion regulation skills such as those outlined above may be an effective and cost-efficient intervention for this population.

Our centre, a tertiary women's hospital in metropolitan Australia, provides services to women with breast and gynecologic cancer. It was in this setting that we investigated the effectiveness and acceptability of MBCT with a view to possible inclusion of the program in routine clinical care [25]. It was of particular interest to us to facilitate MBCT groups that included women with both types of cancer diagnosis, at all stages of disease and recovery ranging from newly diagnosed to palliative, and with varying levels of psychological distress (excluding serious mental illness such as psychosis and mania). Our clinical experience has shown that attempts to coordinate group-based psychosocial interventions stratified by tumor stream, disease severity, and distress levels are both unwieldy and inefficient, and impractical for routine care. As such, we purposefully set out with generous inclusion criteria.

MBCT was designed to target unhelpful relationships to thoughts (such as rumination). Given that the development and maintenance of psychological distress can be significantly attributed to ruminative processes [5] and MBCT has been shown to decrease rumination [26, 27], the primary hypotheses were that the MBCT intervention would be associated with improvements in distress and QOL. As secondary outcomes, it was hypothesized that MBCT would be associated with positive changes in mindfulness and posttraumatic growth (also known as benefit finding).

Recruitment and Sample Characteristics

English speaking women, aged 18 years or older with a diagnosis (new or recurrent) of breast or gynecologic cancer for which treatment or active follow-up was currently being received, were recruited. Recruitment outcomes and study participation are depicted in Fig. 5.1 and are described elsewhere [25]. In total, 42 women (84% of attendees) completed the MBCT program (i.e., attended at least six of the eight sessions, or 75%)

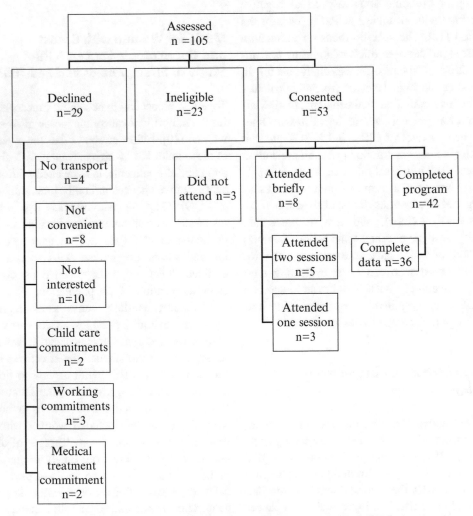

Fig. 5.1 Recruitment and study participation flow diagram for the MBCT pilot intervention. Figure reproduced with permission from Springer. Original source: Mindfulness-based cognitive group therapy for women with breast and gynecologic cancer: a pilot study to determine effectiveness and feasibility. Authors: Lesley Stafford, Elizabeth Foley, Fiona Judd, Penny Gibson, Litza Kiropoulos, Jeremy Couper. Supportive Care in Cancer, November 2013, Volume 21, Issue 11, pp3009–3019

among whom 30 (71%) had a diagnosis of breast cancer and 12 (29%) had gynecologic cancer ($n=1$ cervical, $n=6$ ovarian, $n=1$ vaginal, $n=3$ endometrial). Ten women (24%) had recurrent cancer. Median and mean (SD) time since cancer diagnosis were 33.1 weeks and 48.2 (47.0) weeks, respectively with a range from 5.9 to 236.0 weeks. At the time of commencing the program, 11 (26%) women were undergoing chemotherapy, 9 (21%) were having radiotherapy, 12 (29%) were having endocrine treatment, and 9 (21%) were receiving targeted therapy. Mean (SD) age of participants was 50.15 (10.0) years with a range from 31 to 66 years. A total of 38 (90%) women lived in the metropolitan area, 24 (57%) were employed in some capacity, 26 (62%) were married or cohabiting, 25 (60%) had educational qualifications beyond secondary schooling, 9 (21%) lived alone, 26 (57%) reported a past history of anxiety or depression, and 23 (55%) were receiving treatment for anxiety or depression at the time of commencing the intervention. Of the 42 women who completed the program, complete data were available for 36 ($n=1$ deceased, $n=5$ did not return all questionnaires).

Measures

Participants completed validated self-report assessments at three times over the course of the study: prior to the start of the MBCT program (T1), immediately after completion of the program (T2) and then 3 months subsequently (T3). Distress was measured with the 21-item Depression, Anxiety, Stress Scale short form (DASS-21) [28]. QOL was measured with the Functional Assessment of Cancer Therapy-General (FACT-G) [29], a 28-item self-report measure comprising subscales relating to physical, social, emotional, and functional well-being. Mindfulness was measured with the 14-item Freiburg Mindfulness Inventory (FMI) [30]. Posttraumatic growth was measured with the Post-Traumatic Growth Inventory (PTGI) [31], a 21-item scale measuring positive changes and benefit finding following traumatic events (i.e., cancer). On all measures except the DASS-21, higher scores denote better outcome. Self-report measures at T2 included questions about the relative acceptability and benefit

of specific components of the program and the program overall. At T3, participants were asked about the extent to which mindfulness practice had been maintained and to comment on factors that influence the frequency of mindfulness practice. Women were also asked to comment on the experience of participating in a group with women of varying degrees of illness.

Data Analysis

Data were analyzed using repeated-measures ANOVA and pairwise comparisons with Bonferroni adjustment were used to examine differences between each time point. Since we purposively recruited women from two diagnostic groups and were inclusive with regard to physical and psychological status at study entry, we investigated variations in outcome of these variables. To examine variations in outcomes based on cancer diagnosis and psychological status, tumor stream (breast vs gynecologic) and receipt of current formal mental health treatment (receiving treatment vs not) were used as a between-subjects factors, respectively. To determine the effect of physical health on outcomes, a median split of the Physical Wellbeing subscale (which includes items relating to nausea, energy, pain, treatment side effects, needing to spend time in bed and being able to meet family needs) of the FACT-G at T1 was performed and entered as a between-subjects factor. This analysis was not performed for the repeated-measures ANOVA of QOL as measured by the FACT-G total score because this total score is an aggregate score of, *inter alia*, the Physical Wellbeing Score. Cross-sectional associations between mindfulness and other outcomes were analyzed with simple bivariate correlations.

Modifications of MBCT for Women with Breast and Gynecologic Cancers

Treatment was based on the original MBCT manual that had been previously modified for use in oncology settings by the third author [15].

These modifications included the replacement of depression-specific parts of the manual (in sessions 2, 4, and 6) with those relevant for cancer, by including instructions for working with treatment-related discomfort during meditation and allowing discussion of current existential issues raised by the participants (e.g., grief and loss, identity changes, suffering, and death issues). As in the original MBCT program, the intervention involved intensive training in mindfulness meditation, the provision of theoretical material and extensive group discussion; and the program was delivered across 8 weeks in 2-h sessions. Sessions were delivered by two facilitators with experience in oncology, personal, long-term meditation practice, and professional training in MBCT. Facilitators received weekly clinical supervision. Participants were provided with a workbook summarizing each weekly session, a copy of Jon Kabat-Zinn's book, *Full Catastrophe Living* [11], which discusses the main themes of the MBSR/MBCT program and two meditation CDs with 40 min recordings of classic mindfulness meditations (i.e., the body scan, a moving meditation, and a mixed mindfulness practice). Daily homework of up to 1 h of mindfulness meditation was recommended. Home practice also included optional reading and periodic cognitive and behavioral exercises. An optional (health permitting) extended mindfulness practice session of 6 h of meditation was offered between weeks 6 and 7 of the program. Table 5.1 shows an overview of MBCT for individuals with cancer, outlining the main themes of each session as well the home practice component.

A Participant's Experience of the MBCT Program

Theresa was a middle-aged married mother of three adult children. She had been diagnosed with invasive ductal carcinoma of the left breast and had undergone a mastectomy followed by chemotherapy. During the group program, Theresa described a pattern of rushing in and trying to fix relationship problems between her children. She felt unable to sit with unpleasant emotions or the experience of discomfort in her body that was created by disharmony within her family. Through regularly practicing body scan mediation, Theresa became more aware of when she was present and connected with her body and when she was reacting to discomfort through distraction and "keeping busy." In session we practiced Moving Meditation as a group and this was a powerful experience for Theresa. She reported "feeling as if my mind is in my feet" and for the first time felt present with the motion of walking and the sensations in her feet as she took each step. Over time, Theresa was able to become more connected with her body in the present moment. She noticed that she could make space for unpleasant bodily sensations when her children had disagreements without feeling the urgency to orchestrate a quick resolution. To her surprise, her children started to work through problems on their own and her time with them became much more enjoyable.

Evidence of MBCT for Women with Breast and Gynecologic Cancers

Distress, QOL, Mindfulness, and Posttraumatic Growth

The results from the pilot intervention confirmed our hypotheses and provided further support for the use of MBCT in oncology settings. Results of the repeated-measures ANOVAs including means, F, and effect sizes for the primary and secondary outcomes are shown in Table 5.2. There were significant improvements in distress over time. Pairwise comparisons showed significant differences between T1 and T2 ($P = .007$) scores as well as T1 and T3 scores ($P = .001$). QOL scores also significantly improved over time with pairwise comparisons showing improvements between T1 and T3 ($P = .003$) and T2 and T3 ($P = .038$). There were significant changes in mindfulness and posttraumatic growth over time (Table 5.2). Pairwise comparison showed that mindfulness scores improved significantly from T1 to T2 ($P < .001$) and also

Table 5.1 Overview of MBCT for individuals with cancer

Session number	Session theme	Content overview	Meditation component	Recommended home practice component
1	Stepping out of automatic pilot	Rationale for course Defining mindfulness and "automatic pilot" Introducing the body as a focus	Eating meditation Breath and body scan	Mindfulness of everyday activities Formal practice (body scan)
2	Dealing with barriers	Identifying common barriers Thoughts and feelings exercise	Body scan Mindfulness of breath	Mindfulness of everyday activities Mindfulness of breath Formal practice (body scan) Pleasant events calendar
3	Attending to the present	Identifying the "doing" mode and the "being" mode	Mindfulness of seeing, hearing and breath Mindful stretching and walking	Formal practice (alternate body scan and moving meditation) Mindfulness of breath Unpleasant events calendar
4	Taking a wider perspective	Aversion and attachment Focus on reactions to distress including reactions to cancer experience	Mindfulness of seeing, hearing, breath and body, sounds and thoughts 3 min breathing space	Formal practice (alternate mixed meditation and moving meditation) 3 min breathing space Notice automatic reactions to stress
5	Allowing/letting be	Group discussion about allowing/letting be "Introducing a difficulty" and noticing physical and psychological reactions	Mindfulness of seeing, hearing, breath and body, sounds and thoughts 3 min breathing space with coping instruction	Formal practice (mixed meditation) 3 min breathing space
6	Thoughts are not facts	Group discussion including identifying common thinking themes Breathing space as the first step toward a wider view	Mindfulness of seeing, hearing, breath and body, sounds and thoughts with difficulty introduced 3 min breathing space	Formal practice (mixed meditation) 3 min breathing space Cultivate awareness of thinking themes
7	Taking care of myself	Exploring link between activity and mood Integrating mindfulness into daily schedule Recognizing signs of personal distress and how to respond Breathing space as the first step toward mindful decisions	Mindfulness of seeing, hearing, breath and body 3 min breathing space	Relapse prevention exercises – increasing mindfulness in daily schedule and responding to stress Formal practice (participant choice) 3 min breathing space
8	Acknowledging efforts and planning for future struggles	Review of program Plans for future practice and strategies for maintaining momentum Personal reflections	Body scan Closing meditation	

Table 5.2 Results of repeated-measures ANOVAs showing means, F, and effect sizes for primary and secondary outcome variables in the MBCT pilot intervention

Outcome variable	T1 Pre-MBCT[a] M (SD)	T2 Post-MBCT M (SD)	T3 3 Months Post-MBCT M (SD)	F	P	Effect size (partial eta squared)
DASS-21[b]	38.22 (19.47)	28.33 (17.96)	24.22 (22.60)	10.95	<.001	.238
FACT-G[c]	65.81 (17.15)	70.30 (16.32)	74.80 (17.46)	9.0	.001	.204
FMI[d]	40.0 (7.33)	46.76 (6.39)	46.15 (7.03)	18.23	<.001	.363
PTGI[e]	53.50 (22.31)	68.22 (16.16)	62.08 (22.75)	11.24	<.001	.243

[a]Mindfulness-based cognitive therapy
[b]Depression anxiety stress scale short form
[c]Functional assessment of cancer therapy-general
[d]Freiburg mindfulness inventory
[e]Post-traumatic growth inventory

Table 5.3 FMI scores correlated with DASS-21, PTGI, and FACT-G scores in the MBCT pilot intervention

		DASS-21[a] scores		FACT-G[b] scores		PTGI[c] scores	
		r	P	r	P	r	P
FMI[e] scores	Pre-MBCT[d]	−.388	.013	.363	.021	.331	.037
	Post-MBCT[d]	−.415	.008	.375	.017	.525	<.001
	3 months post-MBCT[b]	−.665	<.001	.630	<.001	.474	.004

[a]Depression anxiety stress scale short form
[b]Functional assessment of cancer therapy-general
[c]Post-traumatic growth inventory
[d]Mindfulness-based cognitive therapy
[e]Freiburg mindfulness inventory

from T1 to T3 ($P<.001$). Scores on the PTGI improved significantly from T1 to T2 ($P<.001$). There were no significant interactions between time and diagnostic group or current receipt of mental health treatment in analyses for QOL, distress, post-traumatic growth, and mindfulness. There was also no interaction effect between low versus high T1 physical wellbeing at baseline and improvement over time for all outcomes other than QOL.

Table 5.3 shows that there were significant correlations between mindfulness and levels of posttraumatic growth, distress, and QOL at each respective time point indicating that increased levels of mindfulness were associated with decreased levels of distress and higher levels of posttraumatic growth and QOL.

Acceptability and Benefit of the Intervention

Participants' perceptions of the helpfulness of different components of the program are shown in Table 5.4. Most women (93 %) found the overall program to be *quite a bit helpful* or *very helpful* and all individual components of the program were similarly endorsed by the majority of women. All women (100 %) said that they would recommend the program to other individuals with cancer and also to other women with breast or gynecologic cancer. In answer to the open-ended question of how participants experienced participation in a program with women of varying degrees of wellness, most ($n=32$) responses were positive without qualification. For instance:

Table 5.4 Participants' views of the MBCT pilot intervention

	n (%)				
	Not at all helpful	*A little bit helpful*	*Somewhat helpful*	*Quite a bit helpful*	*Very helpful*
Getting to know other women with breast or gynecologic cancer	1 (3)	5 (15)	5 (13)	9 (23)	18 (46)
Becoming more aware of my body, thoughts and feelings	–	–	3 (8)	9 (23)	27 (69)
Knowing that I am not alone in my experiences	–	1 (3)	4 (10)	10 (26)	24 (62)
Learning how to live more in the present moment	–	1 (3)	4 (10)	10 (26)	24 (62)
Learning how to meditate	–	1 (3)	3 (8)	13 (33)	22 (56)
Finding ways to cope with difficult thoughts, feelings or bodily sensations	–	2 (5)	3 (8)	10 (26)	24 (62)
Overall, how helpful did you find it to attend the therapy?	–	–	3 (6)	12 (30)	25 (63)
	I disliked this aspect a lot	*I disliked this aspect a little bit*	*I neither liked nor disliked this aspect*	*I liked this aspect a little*	*I liked this aspect a lot*
Listening to other people talk about their experiences	–	1 (3)	1 (3)	9 (23)	28 (72)
Doing the course as part of a group (rather than one-to-one)	–	–	1 (3)	2 (5)	36 (92)
Meditating	–	–	–	7 (17)	32 (82)
Emphasis on home-based practice	–	–	4 (10)	12 (31)	23 (59)
Experiences that arose as a result of practicing mindfulness	–	1 (3)	2 (5)	10 (26)	26 (67)
Time commitment required	–	4 (10)	9 (23)	11 (28)	15 (39)

"It was rewarding in a way…made me appreciate my own situation and also be aware of what others are going through and appreciate the positive support of others."

"Comfortable…I felt useful to those at the beginning of their journey and I could lean on those who were further down the track."

Two women noted that it was *"challenging"* or *"confronting"* at first but both felt this became less of an issue as the group progressed. Two women took a pragmatic view, stating that this is *"part of life"*, *"a realistic part of any group,"* and *"a reflection of how we live in the world."*

Maintenance and Frequency of Meditative Practice

Prior to the intervention, 9 (21%) women reported having some form of meditative practice. At T2, 15 (36%) women reported their likelihood of maintaining a mindfulness practice as *quite likely* and 27 (46%) said it was *very likely*. At T3, three women (8%) reported daily meditative practice, 14 (39%) meditated every few days, 10 (28%) meditated once a week, 7 (19%) meditated once a month, and 2 (6%) reported that they never meditated. The most commonly reported reason for not meditating was lack of time (*n* = 15). Other reasons included lack of discipline (*n* = 4), circumstances such as pain, fatigue, and illness (*n* = 6), and only feeling the need to meditate when extremely stressed or worried (*n* = 4).

Summary of MBCT for Women with Breast and Gynecologic Cancer

As hypothesized, the MBCT intervention was associated with significant improvements with large effect sizes in distress, QOL, mindfulness and posttraumatic growth, and these gains were maintained 3 months after program completion. Participants found the program beneficial and attrition was low. Improvements in QOL, distress, mindfulness, and posttraumatic growth did not differ based on tumor stream or whether women were receiving other, concurrent psychological treatment. Similarly, physical well-being at baseline did not interact with improvement over time for all outcomes other than QOL as measured by the FACT-G (for which the equivalent analysis was not performed because of use of the Physical Wellbeing subscale of the FACT-G as the between-subjects factor). In sum, our findings provide preliminary evidence that MBCT is as an effective and acceptable psychosocial intervention for women with breast and gynecologic cancer.

Practical Considerations of MBCT for Women with Breast and Gynecologic Cancers

The Development of an Alternative, Abbreviated Group-Based Mindfulness Meditation Program (MMP)

There has recently been a call for research on simplified mindfulness interventions that are briefer and more flexible [3]. When evaluating the feasibility of the MBCT program we also saw a need for a simpler and more cost-effective approach as the resources required to implement and evaluate the MBCT program in terms of clinician time and service costs rendered it too expensive to incorporate into routine cancer care at our centre. We followed best practice guidelines when implementing the MBCT program, such that the facilitators had ongoing personal mindfulness practice, received supervision from an experienced mindfulness teacher, and attended annual mindfulness retreats [10, 11]. This expertise was not available on site and staff had to be hired to ensure trial fidelity. Furthermore, to ensure the smooth running of the program, a group coordinator who organized venues, followed up on patients who do not attend, and arranged for completion of paperwork was required. This is an additional cost consideration.

Consequently, in late 2011, 6 months after the completion of the MBCT trial, an alternative, abbreviated group-based mindfulness meditation program (MMP) was developed by the second author to be trialed at our hospital [32]. The MMP was designed to be less resource-intensive and could be delivered across 6 weeks in 90 min sessions. Rather than 22 contact hours of therapy as in the MBCT program, the MMP comprises 9 contact hours of therapy. The MMP program had smaller numbers of participants per program compared to the MBCT program. The intervention content focused specifically on the meditative practices found in MBCT but did not include the cognitive components. Like our original MBCT program, MMP recruited women seen in routine care without reference to their tumor stream, stage of disease, or psychological status with the continuing rationale that in our busy clinical setting, it is inefficient to coordinate psychosocial interventions when stratified by these variables. Additionally, evidence from our MBCT trial as cited above showed that there were no barriers to combining women who differed on these characteristics.

Differences Between the MMP and MBCT Interventions

While both programs were based on the original MBCT manual [10] and involved training in mindfulness meditation, provision of theoretical material and group discussion, they differed in several respects. These differences were: (1) The MBCT program followed the original manual more strictly in terms of structure and content, e.g., program delivery across eight 2-h sessions, the inclusion of the extended meditation practice toward the end of the program, and the focus on cognition including periodic cognitive and behavioral exercises prescribed as part of homework (e.g., Pleasant and Unpleasant Events Calendars); (2) The greater time allocation in the MBCT program meant that more meditations were taught and more time was devoted to enquiry and group discussion; (3) Participants in the MBCT program viewed a documentary film showing the MBSR program in action; (4) Facilitators of the MBCT intervention received weekly clinical supervision from a mindfulness expert and attended annual mindfulness retreats, whereas the MMP facilitator did not.

Features shared by the two interventions were: (1) Facilitators for both interventions had clinical experience in oncology (the MMP facilitator had more experience) and their own mindfulness practice (the experience of the MBCT facilitators was more extensive); (2) Both groups received written information summarizing the weekly sessions and describing homework, meditation CDs with recordings of classical meditations (although the range of meditations was smaller in the MMP group), and copies of *Full Catastrophe Living*

[11], which prescribed as optional reading homework; (3) Both interventions were delivered in small groups with 8–10 participants in the MBCT groups and a maximum of 8 in the MMP groups; (4) The content of both interventions was modified for oncology patients to include awareness of treatment-related discomfort and distress in areas of the body affected by cancer and its treatment, and acknowledgement of this discomfort during meditation practice; and (5) Time allowed for discussion of existential issues such as role changes, relationship difficulties, concern for their children, changes in identity, and fears regarding mortality, pain and suffering, was included in both groups. Table 5.5 provides an overview of the themes, main content, meditative practice, and homework component of the MMP.

A Participant's Experience of the MMP Program

Kate was a 40-year-old mother of two young children who had separated from her husband 3 years prior to her cancer diagnosis. After the separation, Kate felt overwhelmed by juggling all the demands and responsibilities of work, running a household, and parenting with little social support. Eighteen months prior, she was diagnosed with Stage 3 ovarian cancer and underwent a hysterectomy and oophorectomy, followed by six cycles of chemotherapy. Her active treatment was completed 9 months before the commencement of the group program. In the first group session Kate described feelings of intense loneliness and frustration at how distracted and impatient she had become. She no longer felt connected to anything or anyone and had noticed that she was largely focused on "just getting through the day." The concept of being in autopilot mode resonated with Kate and she identified an absence of present moment awareness of herself in her experience. She said she felt like her mind was always split between what she was doing and what she was planning to do next. Participants were asked for homework to do one activity mindfully a day, to purposefully pay attention to what they were doing in the present moment in an accepting and

Table 5.5 Overview of MMP for women with breast and gynecologic cancer

Session number	Session theme	Content overview	Meditation component	Recommended home practice component
1	Stepping out of automatic pilot	Introduction to mindfulness with a specific focus on breast/gynecologic cancer Defining mindfulness and "automatic pilot" Present moment awareness Cost of being reactive to inner experiences	Eating meditation	Eating meditation Awareness of moving into and out of autopilot Present moment awareness of thoughts, feelings and body sensations
2	Breath and body as the focus	Identifying common barriers Three elements of experience: Awareness of thoughts, feelings, body sensations Introducing the breath and body as a focus	3 min breathing space Body scan meditation	Body scan meditation 3 min breathing space
3	Present moment awareness Foundations of mindfulness	Present moment awareness Attitude and intention of mindfulness practice Identifying the "doing" mode and the "being with" mode	"The Pause" Body scan meditation Mindfulness of everyday activities Mindful movement meditation	Body scan meditation 3 min breathing space Moving meditation
4	Patterns of rumination Breath as the focus	Traps of rumination Reactions to stress and rumination: Being responsive versus reactive Observer stance and observer self Breath as a focus and anchor	3 min breathing space Body scan meditation Mindfulness of the breath meditation	Alternate body scan meditation with mindfulness of the breath meditation 3 min breathing space Notice automatic reactions to stress
5	Allowing/letting be	Allowing/letting go reviewed Working with the wandering mind Letting go of thoughts and worry	Mindfulness of the breath meditation Leaves on a stream meditation	Alternate body scan meditation with mindfulness of the breath meditation Leaves on a stream meditation 3 min breathing space

Session number	Session theme	Content overview	Meditation component	Recommended home practice component
6	Summary and relapse prevention planning	Review of program Building mindfulness into daily schedule Plans for future practice and strategies to combat potential barriers Breathing space (and The Pause) as the first step toward mindful decisions Group exercise: What drains us and nurtures us (relapse prevention planning) Personal reflections	3 min breathing space Body scan meditation (if time permits)	Considering how to build mindfulness into one's daily schedule and respond to stress Relapse prevention planning

Tables reproduced with permission from Springer

Original sources

Tables 5.1, 5.2, 5.3 and 5.4

Mindfulness-based cognitive group therapy for women with breast and gynecologic cancer: a pilot study to determine effectiveness and feasibility

Authors: Lesley Stafford, Elizabeth Foley, Fiona Judd, Penny Gibson, Litza Kiropoulos, Jeremy Couper

Supportive Care in Cancer, November 2013, Volume 21, Issue 11, pp. 3009–3019

Table 5.5

Comparison of the acceptability and benefits of two mindfulness-based interventions in women with breast or gynecologic cancer: a pilot study

Authors: Lesley Stafford, Naomi Thomas, Elizabeth Foley, Fiona Judd, Penny Gibson, Angela Komiti, Jeremy Couper, Litza Kiropoulos

Supportive Care in Cancer, April 2015, Volume 23, Issue 4, pp. 1063–1071 non-judgmental way. Kate shared with the group her experience of mindfully washing her daughter's hair. Her account highlighted that there is *power* in simply being present. Kate said "We had just gotten home from soccer. The kids were wet and cold and needed a bath. I felt rushed and irritated because we were due at a birthday party in an hour and I thought we were going to be late again. But instead of rushing the bath, I chose to mindfully wash my daughter's hair. As I did this I became aware of the feel of her hair and the softness of her neck and forehead. I remembered how much my daughter loves to have her back rubbed, so I took a little bit longer washing her back. When we looked at each other I felt for the first time since my diagnosis that I was present with my little girl and I realized how much I had missed her. I noticed how much she was enjoying me being with her in this way. She looked at me with a sense of relief in her eyes, relief that she had her mum back." As a group, we discussed how Kate's account was an example of stepping out of "*doing* mode" into "*being with* mode" and how it created an opportunity to reconnect with her daughter.

Sample, Procedure, Measures. and Evaluation of the MMP

Inclusion criteria for the MMP trial were identical to those employed in the earlier MBCT trial. Recruitment strategies for these two consecutive trials were also the same. As in the MBCT trial, participants completed self-report assessments measuring distress, QOL, and mindfulness (the same questionnaires as in the MBCT trial) prior to the start (T1) of the MMP and again immediately after completion of the MMP (T2). Post-traumatic growth was not investigated in the MMP trial and there was also no long-term follow-up (i.e., 3 months post-completion of the intervention). Otherwise, participants in both trials were asked the same questions about their perceptions of the benefits and acceptability of the intervention, the maintenance and frequency of meditative practice, and thoughts on including women with varying stages of illness. Similar

clinical and sociodemographic information was collected in both intervention groups. We hypothesized that there would be no statistically significant differences between the improvements brought about in levels of distress, QOL and mindfulness by the respective interventions and that participants would not perceive a difference in their respective acceptability.

Comparison of the Outcomes of the MMP and MBCT Interventions

The complete results of the comparison of these two interventions are described elsewhere [32]. In sum, a total of 24 women (75 % of all attendees) with breast and gynecologic cancer completed the MMP (i.e., attended at least five of six sessions, or 80 %). There were no significant differences between the characteristics of women from the MMP and MBCT trials in terms of age, whether living alone, tumor stream, marital status, educational status, self-reported physical wellbeing, receipt of endocrine treatment, radiotherapy and chemotherapy, frequency of past or current meditative practice and receiving formal treatment for anxiety or depression at study enrolment. The only significant difference was that women who had attended the MBCT program were more likely than women in the MMP program to report a past history of receiving formal treatment for anxiety or depression, resolved at study enrolment (52 % vs 26 %, $P = .01$). ANCOVA showed that the improvements in scores from T1 to T2 on distress, QOL, and mindfulness were significant for both intervention groups and there was no main effect for type of intervention. Similarly, there were no significant differences in patient perceptions of the acceptability and benefits of the respective interventions. For instance, some 88 % of women in the MMP found the overall program to be *quite a bit helpful* or *very helpful* (compared to 93 % in the MBCT group). There were also no significant differences in responses to the maintenance of meditative practice with 96 % of women in the MMP group reporting the likelihood of maintaining a mindfulness practice as *quite likely* or *very likely* (compared to 95 % in the MBCT group). Finally, respondents in the MMP group reported similarly positive views of participating in a therapeutic group with women at different stages of illness.

Summary of Comparison Between the MMP and MBCT for Women with Breast and Gynecologic Cancer

We compared a formal 22-h MBCT program to an abbreviated, less intensive meditation program (MMP) comprising 9 h of therapy contact, among heterogeneous groups of women with breast and gynecologic cancer. As hypothesized, both the formal MBCT program and the abbreviated MMP were associated with significant improvements in QOL, distress and mindfulness and neither intervention was shown to be (statistically) significantly superior in the amount of improvement observed. Changes from pre- to post-intervention for mindfulness and distress were dependent on their respective pre-intervention scores indicating that there was more improvement when there was more capacity for improvement. There were no differences in participant perceptions of acceptability based on intervention type.

Summary and Conclusions

This chapter describes a successful trial of formal MBCT in women with breast and gynecologic cancer as well as evidence for the utility of a brief mindfulness intervention, the MMP, for improving distress and QOL in this population. While these data are very encouraging, there are several limitations to consider. These include small sample size with attendant lack of power, non-randomized study design, and unknown representativeness of the sample: The samples were highly self-selected, likely comprising very motivated women who were open to learning new skills. Many participants were tertiary educated, a finding consistent with reviews of mindfulness interventions in cancer care [3, 33].

As noted by others [3, 34], the exact component(s) of the group-based mindfulness interventions associated with the observed improvements is not clear. MBCT comprises components of mindfulness, cognitive therapy and supportive peer interaction, any of which, alone or in combination, may be integral to the success of the intervention. The MMP includes two of these components. Certainly, the perceived benefit of peer support was demonstrated in both trials with the vast majority of both samples expressing a preference for completing the respective programs as a group rather than individually. This finding is consistent with other reports [14] and warrants more scrutiny. Potentially, the more interesting issue is the apparent parity of the MMP and MBCT in benefit observed, at least in the short term, despite the substantially lower quantity and intensity of meditation and the absence of cognitive therapy in the MMP.

Abbreviated interventions are certainly attractive for under-resourced environments and may present a less daunting commitment to potential participants with terminal illness or undergoing intensive treatment. There is indeed evidence for abbreviated class time with a recent review reporting non-significant correlations between in-class MBSR hours and mean effect size for psychological distress among clinical and non-clinical samples [35]. It may be, though, that the benefit of the formal, extended program would become evident in the maintenance of gains, an outcome that was not measured in the MMP trial or in the review [35]. Similarly, the advantage of including the cognitive therapy component may only become apparent in the maintenance of improvement over time, particularly since MBCT participants received an intervention specifically targeting rumination, which is directly implicated in preventing relapse to depression. Furthermore, increased contact time itself may be important to the development of the proposed mechanistic factors of mindfulness interventions, such as greater self-compassion, a construct not measured here or elsewhere [35].

At least two other issues deserve more attention: The skill of the mindfulness facilitator and the role of adherence to home practice of meditation are both thought to be important in determining the outcome of mindfulness interventions. Although the MMP facilitator did not meet all the requirements asked of the MBCT facilitators, she was highly experienced and the short-term parity of the two interventions may potentially be attributable to her clinical skill set and her familiarity with many of the group participants from her involvement in the hospital outpatient and inpatient oncology service. This variable has not been directly studied but it is plausible that such highly skilled instructors are necessary to achieve optimal benefits in abbreviated interventions. In terms of adherence, participants were not required to record their home practice in our trials and so it is not possible to investigate a dose–response relationship. The necessity for daily home practice of meditation is certainly an important feature of MBCT but its association with positive outcomes is a complex issue [8, 34, 36, 37]. Another point of consideration is that the MMP program had smaller group numbers which could have created a greater holding environment and allowed for the content to be tailored more to the individual needs of the participants.

Future studies incorporating a randomized design with one or more alternate conditions as comparison is required to clarify the essential or active ingredient of a successful group psychosocial program. The specific effects of peer interaction, cognitive therapy, proposed putative mechanisms such as increased mindfulness and decreased rumination, facilitator skill, and participant adherence require further study. In the interim, these preliminary findings add to the limited existing data on MBCT in oncology settings and show the potential benefits of this intervention in a heterogeneous group of women with cancer.

Acknowledgments This work was supported by generous financial contribution from the Collier Charitable Trust and the Preston and Loui Geduld Trust. The Centre for Women's Mental Health is supported by the Pratt Foundation.

Conflict of interest

The authors do not have a financial relationship with the Pratt Foundation, the Collier Charitable Trust or the Preston and Loui Geduld Trust.

References

1. Carlson LE, Bultz BD. Cancer distress screening: needs, models and methods. J Psychosom Res. 2003;55:403–9.
2. Zabora J, BrintzenhofeSzoc K, Jacobsen P, et al. A new psychosocial screening instrument for use with cancer patients. Psychosomatics. 2001;42:241–6.
3. Shennan C, Payne S, Fenlon D. What is the evidence for the use of mindfulness-based interventions in cancer care? A review. Psychooncology. 2011;20(7):681–97.
4. Carlson L. Mindfulness-based cancer recovery: the development of an evidence-based psychosocial oncology intervention. Oncol Exchange. 2013;12:21–5.
5. Thomsen DK. The association between rumination and negative affect: a review. Cognit Emot. 2006;20:1216–35.
6. Carlson LE, Speca M, Patel KD, Goodey E. Mindfulness-based stress reduction in relation to quality of life, mood, symptoms of stress, and immune parameters in breast and prostate cancer outpatients. Psychosom Med. 2003;65:571–81.
7. Carlson LE, Speca M, Patel KD, Goodey E. Mindfulness-based stress reduction in relation to quality of life, mood, symptoms of stress and levels of cortisol, dehydroepiandrosterone sulfate (DHEAS) and melatonin in breast and prostate cancer outpatients. Psychoneuroendocrinology. 2004;29:448–74.
8. Shapiro SL, Bootzin RR, Figueredo AJ, Lopez AM, Schwartz GE. The efficacy of mindfulness-based stress reduction in the treatment of sleep disturbance in women with breast cancer: an exploratory study. J Psychosom Res. 2003;54:85–91.
9. Hoffman CJ, Ersser SJ, Hopkinson JB, Nicholls PG, Harrington JE, Thomas PW. Effectiveness of mindfulness-based stress reduction in mood, breast- and endocrine-related quality of life, and well-being in stage 0 to III breast cancer: a randomized, controlled trial. J Clin Oncol. 2012;30:1335–42.
10. Segal ZV, Williams JMG, Teasdale JD. Mindfulness-based cognitive therapy for depression: a new approach to preventing relapse. New York: Guilford Press; 2002.
11. Kabat-Zinn J. Full catastrophe living: using the wisdom of your body and mind to face stress, pain and illness. New York: Delacorte; 1990.
12. Nolen-Hoeksema S. Responses to depression and their effects on the duration of depressive episodes. J Abnorm Psychol. 1991;100:569–82.
13. Brotto LA, Erskine Y, Carey M, et al. A brief mindfulness-based cognitive behavioral intervention improves sexual functioning versus wait-list control in women treated for gynecologic cancer. Gynecol Oncol. 2012;125:320–5.
14. Chambers SK, Foley E, Galt E, Ferguson M, Clutton S. Mindfulness groups for men with advanced prostate cancer: a pilot study to assess feasibility and effectiveness and the role of peer support. Support Care Cancer. 2012;20:1183–92.
15. Foley E, Huxter M, Baillie A, Price M, Sinclair E. Mindfulness-based cognitive therapy for individuals

whose lives have been affected by cancer: a randomized controlled trial. J Consult Clin Psychol. 2010;78:72–9.

16. Sharplin GR, Jones SB, Hancock B, Knott VE, Bowden JA, Whitford HS. Mindfulness-based cognitive therapy: an efficacious community-based group intervention for depression and anxiety in a sample of cancer patients. Med J Aust. 2010;193:S79–82.

17. van der Lee ML, Garssen B. Mindfulness-based cognitive therapy reduces chronic cancer-related fatigue: a treatment study. Psycho-Oncology. 2012;21:264–72.

18. Brotto LA, Erskine Y, Carey M, et al. A brief mindfulness-based cognitive behavioral intervention improves sexual functioning versus wait-list control in women treated with gynecologic cancer. Gynecol Oncol. 2012;125:320–5.

19. Chambers S, Smith D, Berry M, et al. A randomised controlled trial of a mindfulness intervention for men with advanced prostate cancer. BMC Cancer. 2013;13:89.

20. Australian Institute of Health and Welfare. Cancer in Australia 2010: an overview. Canberra, Australia: Australian Institute of Health and Welfare; 2010.

21. Pearman T. Quality of life and psychosocial adjustment in gynecologic cancer survivors. Health Qual Life Outcomes. 2003;1:33.

22. Arndt V, Merx H, Stegmaier C, Ziegler H, Brenner H. Persistence of restrictions in quality of life from the first to the third year after diagnosis in women with breast cancer. J Clin Oncol. 2005;23:4945–53.

23. Hoffman KE, McCarthy EP, Recklitis CJ, Ng AK. Psychological distress in long-term survivors of adult-onset cancer: results from a national survey. Arch Intern Med. 2009;169:1274–81.

24. Mols F, Vingerhoets AJ, Coebergh JW, van de Poll-Franse LV. Quality of life among long-term breast cancer survivors: a systematic review. Eur J Cancer. 2005;41:2613–9.

25. Stafford L, Foley E, Judd F, Gibson P, Kiropoulos L, Couper J. Mindfulness-based cognitive group therapy for women with breast and gynecologic cancer: a pilot study to determine effectiveness and feasibility. Support Care Cancer. 2013;21:3009–19.

26. Wolkin JR. Cultivating multiple aspects of attention through mindfulness meditation accounts for psychological well-being through decreased rumination. Psychol Res Behav Manag. 2015;8:171–80.

27. Eisendrath SJ, Delucchi K, Bitner R, Fenimore P, Smit M, McLane M. Mindfulness-based cognitive therapy for treatment-resistant depression: a pilot study. Psychother Psychosom. 2008;77:319–20.

28. Henry JD, Crawford JR. The short-form version of the Depression Anxiety Stress Scale (DASS-21): construct validity and normative data in a large non-clinical sample. Br J Clin Psychol. 2005;44:227–39.

29. Cella DF, Tulsky DS, Gray G, et al. The Functional Assessment of Cancer Therapy (FACT) Scale: development and validation of the general measure. J Clin Oncol. 1993;11:570–9.

30. Walach H, Buchheld N, Buttenmuller V, Kleinknecht N, Schmidt S. Measuring mindfulness: the Freiburg Mindfulness Inventory (FMI). Personal Individ Differ. 2006;40:1543–55.

31. Tedeschi RG, Calhoun LG. The Posttraumatic Growth Inventory: measuring the positive legacy of trauma. J Trauma Stress. 1996;9:455–71.

32. Stafford L, Thomas N, Foley E, et al. Comparison of the acceptability and benefits of two mindfulness-based interventions in women with breast or gynecologic cancer: a pilot study. Support Care Cancer. 2015;23:1063–71.

33. Ledesma D, Kumano H. Mindfulness-based stress reduction and cancer: a meta-analysis. Psycho-Oncology. 2009;18:571–9.

34. Speca M, Carlson LE, Goody E, Angen M. A randomized, wait-list controlled clinical trial: the effect of a mindfulness meditation-based stress reduction program on mood and symptoms of stress in cancer outpatients. Psychosom Med. 2000;62:613–22.

35. Carmody J, Baer R. How long does a mindfulness-based stress reduction program need to be? A review of class contact sizes and psychological distress. J Clin Psychol. 2009;65:627–38.

36. Carlson LE, Speca M, Faris P, Katel KD. On year pre-post intervention follow-up of psychological, immune, endocrine and blood pressure outcomes of mindfulness-based stress reduction (MBSR) in breast and prostate cancer outpatients. Brain Behav Immun. 2007;21:1038–49.

37. Vettese LC, Toneatto T, Stea JN, Nguyen L, Wang JJ. Do mindfulness meditation participants do their homework? And does it make a difference? A review of the empirical evidence. J Cogn Psychother Int Q. 2009;23:198–225.

The Application of Mindfulness-Based Cognitive Therapy for Chronic Pain

6

Melissa A. Day

Clinical Case Study

Maria is a 48-year-old female who is married and has 1 young son approaching high school. Maria has experienced chronic migraine pain since her early teenage years and she considers the pain to have "robbed" her of a large part of her life. Due to the pain, and her feeling of lack of control of when a pain flare up will occur, Maria often cannot go with her husband to social events and frequently misses her son's soccer games. Although Maria continues to work in administration at the local university, she finds her job incredibly stressful as she has difficulty concentrating due to the pain, and is constantly "playing catch up" due to her need to stay home at least once a week due to migraine. Moreover, her boss recently approached her to discuss the possibility of her needing time off, and potentially considering applying for disability because of her large number of missed work days. Maria feels that her life is "unraveling" and she feels "useless" and shows symptoms of anxiety and depression. Maria has tried a multitude of different analgesic pain medications and regimens such as botox to "fight the pain," however she has experienced minimal long-term symptom relief. As a last resort, she has decided to attend an 8-week mindfulness-based cognitive therapy course for headache pain management.

The description of Maria's experience above is similar to that reported by clients living with heterogeneous chronic pain conditions, the territory of which often entails a range of social, financial, emotional, cognitive, and physiological ramifications. Pain, as well as the encompassing territory of its nature, has been shown to be highly amenable to psychological treatments designed to improve coping and self-management. In this chapter we will return to this case scenario to show how MBCT may be successfully applied to target these core symptoms, thought processes, and behavioral and emotional responses so that pain does not get in the way of living a valued, meaningful life.

The Problem of Persistent Pain

Chronic pain is defined by the International Association for the Study of Pain (IASP) as "An unpleasant sensory and emotional experience associated with actual or potential tissue damage, or described in terms of such damage" [1] that continues beyond the expected normal tissue healing time (typically 3 to 6 months depending on the definition, although quantifying the "end" of healing is often difficult) [2]. Chronic pain

M.A. Day, M.A.(Clin.), Ph.D. (✉)
School of Psychology, The University of Queensland, 330 McElwain Building, Brisbane, QLD 4072, Australia
e-mail: m.day@uq.edu.au

affects millions of individuals worldwide and is a debilitating, costly public healthcare concern. In the United States alone, recent point estimates suggest approximately one-third of all adults report a chronic pain condition [3], with the associated total annual financial costs of this in lost work days, medical expense and other benefit costs estimated to range from $560 to $635 billion in 2010 constant dollars [4]. By its very nature, chronic pain is refractory to traditional biomedical treatments; however, despite this, chronic pain is among the most common complaints presenting in medical settings with 18 million physician visits per year accounted for by headache pain alone in the United States [5]. Moreover, efforts to cope with persistent pain and its impact on function can contribute to emotional, psychological, and social upheaval.

Traditionally, pain has been understood from a purely biomedical perspective in that the amount of pain experienced was conceptualized to be a 1:1 relationship with the amount of underlying tissue damage. However, the current widely accepted understanding is biopsychosocial in nature, recognizing, as in the) IASPs definition above, the role of cognitive, emotional, and social factors in influencing pain perception. In their revolutionary Gate Control Theory of pain, Melzack and Wall [6, 7] theorized the mechanisms by which these factors influence pain. Specifically, their original theoretical model proposed that descending inhibitory signals from the brain modulate pain via a gating mechanism in the spinal column that controlled the amount of pain signals that are transmitted to the brain. The Gate Control Theory (and the subsequent neuromatrix model of pain) [8, 9] reconceptualized the experience of pain away from the historically predominant mechanistic and reductionist biomedical perspectives to suggest that psychological processes in the brain actually shape how painful stimuli are interpreted by the brain.

As technological advances in brain imaging emerged, functional magnetic resonance imaging (fMRI) studies corroborated Melzack and Wall's theory and showed that pain, and chronic pain especially, is closely connected to supraspinal cortical activity and processes rather than peripheral

activity [10–12]. Specifically, pathways associated with pain perception have been found to travel through brain regions that process cognitive and emotional activity and these areas have the capacity to enhance or inhibit the pain signal processing. Most closely associated with the experience of pain is the prefrontal cortex, anterior cingulate cortex, primary and secondary sensory cortices, and insula [12]. These advances in theory and empirical evidence functioned to expand the potential points of intervention for pain beyond purely the biomedical domain (such as surgery, narcotics, etc.) to include psychological interventions that target most, if not all of these cognitive and emotional areas of the brain. Over the past several decades, biopsychosocial treatments have been successfully developed and applied to a variety of chronic pain conditions. While the beneficial effects of these treatments are modest on average, they have been reliably shown to be effective and have been found to be at least as efficacious as medically based treatments, and are cost-effective relative to surgery and medication management [13].

The Theoretical Rationale for Mindfulness-Based Cognitive Therapy for Pain

Mindfulness-based cognitive therapy (MBCT), originally developed by Segal, Williams, and Teasdale to target depression relapse [14, 15], is based on a rich theoretical tradition that incorporates empirically supported psychological principles. MBCT for chronic pain integrates core components of cognitive-behavioral therapy (CBT) and mindfulness-based stress reduction (MBSR) theoretical models to place an explicit emphasis upon cognitions, and to concurrently explicitly target emotions and bodily sensations, such that each of the multifaceted elements that interconnect in the experience we call "pain" are addressed. To understand the theoretical rationale of MBCT as applied to pain, it is helpful to first break the theoretical components down into their constituent parts, as understood within the field of pain, and then to explain how the MBCT model seamlessly integrates them to form a streamlined protocol.

Cognitive-Behavioral Therapy (CBT)

Of the psychological approaches that have been applied to pain, CBT has arguably emerged as the current gold standard approach. Based on the widely held cognitive perspective, CBT theoretically holds that emotions and behavior are largely determined by cognitive perceptions of the world [16]. CBT aims to promote more positive and realistic reappraisals of pain and situations initially judged as stressful, such that negative automatic thoughts (such as pain catastrophizing) are addressed *before* they cascade and potentially instigate poor pain-related outcomes. Thus, a key theoretical mechanism of CBT for pain is reduction (via cognitive restructuring as a core technique) in maladaptive cognitive content (i.e., *what* clients believe about pain/stress). In the case of Maria, a CBT therapist would apply cognitive restructuring to change her unhelpful thoughts such as "Pain has robbed me of my life" and "My life is unraveling" and her core belief "I am useless" and to replace these with more helpful, adaptive, realistic thoughts and beliefs. A large body of research has documented the efficacy of CBT-based interventions for a wide range of chronic pain conditions [13]. Moreover, in headache populations, many professional organizations endorse CBT alongside pharmacotherapy as a first-line treatment approach [17]. However, a recent systematic review reported that effect sizes for CBT are modest, and not all individuals respond to CBT with clinically meaningful symptom reduction [13].

Mindfulness-Based Approaches

Although it has yet to be conclusively shown if CBT does truly work via the reasons specified by theory, it has been questioned as to whether changing cognitive content (as in CBT) per se should indeed be the critical treatment target.

Segal, Williams, and Teasdale [14, 15] hypothesized that this may be less important than changing cognitive processes (i.e., *how* individuals think about pain/stress) for symptom relief. Mindfulness, defined as "…the awareness that emerges through paying attention on purpose, in the present moment, and non-judgmentally to the unfolding of experience, moment by moment" (p. 145) [18] is one form of cognitive process that is the target and central theorized mechanism of MBSR. Meditation is taught in MBSR as the core technique to cultivate mindful awareness and acceptance of the full range of inner experiences, including thoughts, emotions, and bodily sensations, including pain. For Maria, this would entail her learning, through meditation, to relate to all thoughts as simply mental events, regardless of their content, and not THE TRUTH. Moreover, the practice of returning to present moment experience in meditation addresses Maria's fear and future-oriented mindset (i.e., the thought of losing her job and applying for disability), which is adding to her stress. The acceptance cultivated in this process would ultimately allow Maria to let go of futile attempts to "fight the pain" (which only make pain worse) and to give the pain space to allow it to be present, as it already is. A steady body of preliminary evidence is building supporting the efficacy of MBSR for a variety of painful conditions. To date, most trials have compared group MBSR to standard care and found MBSR to be beneficial with respect to pain intensity, pain coping, and measures of affect immediately post-treatment and also at follow-up [19, 20].

Mindfulness-Based Cognitive Therapy

MBCT for pain builds upon both the CBT and MBSR frameworks to directly incorporate key techniques from these approaches [18, 21] to explicitly target both cognitive content *and* cognitive process. MBCT for pain, as in the original protocol [14, 15], maintains one of the strengths of CBT-based protocols in that it includes cognitive exercises that facilitate awareness of—and the links between—cognitions, emotions, behaviors, and physical sensations (including pain). The intention of these cognitive exercises in MBCT is purely to heighten *awareness* of these experiences, without attempts to change them in any way. Practical exploration of the mind and body through a variety of mindfulness meditation practices and yoga is taught as a means to further increase awareness of mind patterns. Moreover, meditation trains the mind to disengage from unhelpful automatic thinking patterns, to simply observe them, and to purposefully place attention on anchoring bodily sensations (e.g., the breath) and other perceptive experiences (e.g., sounds). Theoretically, meditation is proposed to accelerate the shift toward relating *to* thoughts (as objects of awareness) rather than *from* thoughts (as necessarily reflecting reality) [22]. Hence, via the integration of cognitive exercises and meditation, MBCT teaches people to have increased awareness (as opposed to functioning mostly on autopilot) and to observe their experiences (including pain) with a non-judgmental, attentive approach such that they are accepted as transient experiences with natural variation. In Maria's situation, a MBCT for pain therapist would optimize the use of the cognitive therapy-oriented techniques to enhance awareness of her automatic thought processes (i.e., "Pain has robbed me of my life"; "My life is unraveling"; "I am useless"). Simultaneously, Maria would be trained in the meditation technique such that she learns to deidentify from such thoughts and associated emotions (such as fear, sadness, and anxiety) and respond with mindfulness and acceptance, letting go of the need to fight her pain. Given the MBCT for pain explicitly targets the mechanisms theorized to be central to *both* CBT and MBSR (i.e., cognitive content and cognitive process), the exciting possibility exists that MBCT may be a streamlined, efficient, and highly efficacious treatment for many individuals living with persistent, daily pain.

Adapting MBCT for Pain

Although both MBSR and MBCT have roots in Buddhism, these treatments are secular in nature [14, 18, 23]. This is a fundamental point as in delivering MBCT for pain, it is important that the meditation component not be taught as a spiritual practice—rather in this clinical context, MBCT is first and foremost delivered as a treatment for pain management. Given the growing popularity of meditation in the general public and popular media, it is helpful to come back to this basic premise, as otherwise it may be easy to "get caught up in the hype" and stray away from the grounding principal that in this context, this is a pain management intervention.

In the manualized protocol developed for one of the first MBCT for pain pilot studies in the field that I conducted with Professor Beverly Thorn and colleagues [23], I attempted to stay as close as possible to the originally described MBCT approach, while tailoring it and adapting it specifically to meet the individual needs of individuals living with pain [21]. As in the original MBCT approach, prior to the first session, clients are given a packet of reading materials to peruse that provides information on chronic pain (adapted for the specific form of chronic pain the clinician is working with, e.g., headache, back pain, etc.), treatment of chronic pain (again, adapted to the specific pain population), the MBCT for pain rationale, the importance of homework/practicing meditation, and on potential difficulties that may be encountered with the practice. All eight of the 2-h (typically group delivered) weekly MBCT for pain sessions follow the same session format: (1) Pre-session process check (except for session 1) and pain measure; (2) Orientation and theme for session; (3) In-session practice of both cognitively oriented and meditation-based exercises, and discussion; (4) Assign homework and summary; and (5) Post-session process check. A guided inquiry of experience with practices taught is included in all sessions; a homework review is incorporated in to all sessions, except session 1.

Specific pain-related content covered in the sessions includes psychoeducation on the Gate Control Theory in sessions 1 to convey clearly the rationale for this treatment for pain. The Stress-Pain-Appraisal model is also included as a means to illustrate the importance of stepping out of "automatic pilot"; this is covered in session 2. Session 4 introduces Mindful Movement (yoga) and walking meditation. The mindful movement practice should be led by a certified yoga instructor if including yoga poses or if working with a vulnerable/highly disabled group. Personally, if I am leading the group (and I am not a certified yoga instructor), this meditation is modified from the original MBCT protocol to consist of a series of basic movements that would not comprise more than an individual with chronic pain might engage in during day-to-day living (e.g., noticing the tension in raising and lowering an arm, and the contrast once the arm is relaxed by one's side). All other activities from the original MBCT for depression relapse protocol that are designed specifically for working with that population should also be revised to be suitable for pain; for example, in session 7, red flags for relapse is adapted to be an exploration of red flags for pain and stress flare-up.

Homework assignments include meditation practice with guided mindfulness meditation CDs, a guided yoga CD, brief cognitive-behavioral exercises, exercises to integrate mindfulness into everyday life, and weekly reading materials/handouts. Clients are encouraged to practice meditation in between group sessions for 45 min, 6 days per week; however, it is recommended that in the MBCT for pain program, clients also be given a 20-min version so they can gradually build to this recommended dose. Additionally, a brief 3-min breathing space meditation is also taught and becomes homework (3 times, scheduled, per day and in response to stressful situations).

Following each in-session meditation practice (and during the homework review), an important element of the protocol is for the therapist to engage clients in a guided inquiry of their experience. During this inquiry, it is most helpful to start discussion by staying as close as possible to feedback on the practice that has just ended. The clinician should elicit feedback about the practice using open questions (e.g., "What was that experience like for you?" and "What did you notice during that practice?"). By asking these open-ended questions the discussion is grounded in moment-to-moment experience. Conducting this inquiry also provides an opportunity for the therapist to embody and model the exact qualities

that the treatment is designed to cultivate in clients: curiosity, present moment attentiveness, openness, kindness, and a non-judgmental attitude. For example, Maria might likely report early on in treatment that "I really struggled with the practice, I was just thinking, thinking, thinking…"; the clinician might respond "Well, just that you were aware that you were thinking Maria is really mindfulness in and of itself! And even if you were only able to notice you were thinking and return to the object of meditation just one time in a whole meditation practice, that IS mindfulness. This is the practice, just training our mind, non-judgmentally and with kindness, to return, over and over again. Like training a puppy to 'stay' it takes training, kindness and practice…" Any obstacles or challenges in the practice should also be discussed (e.g., "What, if any, difficulties or challenges did you experience?"). Finally, it is important during the inquiry to relate the practice back to coping with pain, perhaps by asking "What connection do you think this practice has to living with chronic pain?", this primes clients to consider the application of their techniques in managing and coping with their pain.

Efficacy of MBCT for Chronic Pain

The body of empirical research devoted to examining mindfulness and interventions based on mindfulness principles has grown exponentially over recent decades. In a recent paper I wrote with my colleagues [24], we reported that between 1990 and 2006 the number of published scientific articles on mindfulness went from fewer than 80 to over 600, and at the time we completed that article (October 22, 2013) there existed over 1200 research articles in PubMed devoted to the topic. In terms of the broad psychotherapy literature, studies examining the efficacy of MBCT specifically have emerged for a variety of populations (e.g., depression, anxiety, insomnia), and findings uniformly indicate that MBCT is beneficial [19]. Although some studies have implemented elements of MBCT into a mindfulness protocol for pain [25, 26], to the best of my knowledge, at the time of writing this text (July, 2015) there are only three published randomized controlled trials (RCTs) examining the efficacy of a formal MBCT protocol for chronic pain.

In a pilot RCT of MBCT for pain that my collaborators and I conducted, we examined the feasibility and efficacy of this approach compared to a treatment as usual, delayed treatment control (DT) within a headache pain population [23]. Results indicated that MBCT was feasible, tolerable and acceptable to participants. Intent-to-treat analyses ($N=36$) showed that compared to DT, MBCT resulted in significantly greater improvement in pain interference, headache pain management self-efficacy, and pain acceptance, and a tendency toward greater reductions in pain catastrophizing (p's < .05). Results of the completer analyses ($N=24$) produced a similar pattern of findings; additionally, compared to DT, MBCT completers reported significantly improved catastrophizing and a trend toward a steeper decline in daily peak headache pain intensity ratings. In terms of the sizes of effects among individuals who completed treatment, results demonstrated large benefits for pain intensity (ds = .80 for both average and peak intensity) as well as for pain interference, pain acceptance, pain catastrophizing, and headache pain management self-efficacy (ds = 1.29, 1.22, .94, and 1.65, respectively), which is comparable to the range of effect sizes seen with other psychosocial interventions, such as CBT [13].

Around the same time that we were conducting our study with a headache pain sample, Parra-Delgado and Latorre-Postigo were in Spain conducting a similar pilot RCT to examine the efficacy of MBCT in reducing the impact of fibromyalgia, as well as improving depressive symptoms and pain [27]. MBCT was compared to a DT control condition with a sample of female individuals with fibromyalgia ($N=33$). Intent-to-treat analyses found that MBCT resulted in significant improvement in the impact of fibromyalgia, and depressive symptoms compared to DT, and these effects were maintained at 3-month follow-up. A slight decrease in pain intensity was found for the MBCT group at post-treatment but differences were not significant. Of note, theoretically, mindfulness-based interventions for pain target an individual's relationship to pain, so they can observe the pain mindfully and accept it; the aim is not reduction of pain intensity per se [18, 24]. Thus, pain interference is emerging in the literature as the recommended primary outcome variable in mindfulness trials [28]. In Parra-Delgado and Latorre-Postigo's study, interference was not examined. In future trials, it will be important to examine this theoretically relevant construct as a primary outcome for determining the efficacy of MBCT for chronic pain.

It has long been recognized that chronic pain is underdiagnosed and undertreated, and access to effective multidisciplinary treatment is often limited for a variety of reasons (e.g., lack of services, cost, rurality, lack of transportation, or physical disability that hinders mobility, just to name a few) [29, 30]. To address these barriers, Dowd and colleagues [31] recently developed a computerized, Internet-delivered MBCT program and conducted a pilot RCT to examine its efficacy compared to a psychoeducation control condition within a heterogeneous, non-cancer pain population. Intent-to-treat analyses ($N=124$) found both groups reported significant improvements in pain interference, pain acceptance, catastrophizing, and pain intensity from pre- to post-treatment. Participants in the MBCT group showed greater improvements in subjective well-being, present pain intensity, and emotion regulation indicators. Most of these effects were maintained at 6-month follow-up. Given the increasing public demand for access to online healthcare resources [32], there is a need for more research devoted to examining innovative treatment delivery interfaces such as the one implemented by Dowd and colleagues, and to determine if specific pain population subgroups might be more or less suitable.

Mechanisms of MBCT for Chronic Pain: How and for Whom?

There has been a call from experts in the field of psychological approaches for pain management to move beyond the first-order question of simply seeking to establish the *efficacy* of treatment, and to gain insight into the second-order question of the *mechanisms* of treatment [33, 34]. A scarcity of research has examined the mechanisms of MBCT for pain. However, recently my colleagues and I developed a theoretical model of the hypothesized mediators of mindfulness-based interventions for pain, including MBCT, based on the available evidence [24, 33] and in our recent research we have begun examining the theorized pathways. So far, we are the only research group reporting data on the mechanisms of MBCT for pain; it will be important for research in this area to expand and grow in the coming decade.

In our initial MBCT for headache trial described above [23], we found that, as theorized, MBCT resulted in significantly improved cognitive process (pain acceptance) and cognitive content (pain catastrophizing and headache management self-efficacy), as compared to the DT control. In a recently completed secondary analysis examining the potential mechanism role of these factors, we found that of these potential mediators, pain acceptance emerged as the sole significant mediator of the MBCT intervention to improved pain interference relation [35]. We found a similar pattern of results in a mixed methods analysis of MBCT treatment responders compared to non-responders, with responders reporting greater improvement than non-responders in pain acceptance ($d = .64$) [36]. These findings suggest that pain acceptance may be a critical cognitive process variable for the efficacy of MBCT in improving pain intensity and interference in a headache population.

We have also begun to investigate the potential mechanism role of common factors. Consistent with our review of the potential mechanisms of mindfulness [24], in the mixed methods analysis study we conducted (described above), we also found a medium effect size difference for therapeutic alliance between MBCT treatment responders and non-responders, with responders reporting higher alliance than non-responders [36]. Further, in a closer examination of the potential environmental/common factors that may mediate MBCT effects, we found that working

alliance, therapist adherence to protocol, and therapist quality were all positively associated with client satisfaction at post-treatment [37]. In this same study, we also found that more positive pre-treatment expectations and motivation were associated with greater pre- to post-treatment improvement in pain interference. While limited research has examined dose–response relations in the broad MBCT literature, we found in our original MBCT for headache pilot that the average daily meditation dose was 25 min; for those participants who completed MBCT, the average daily dose was 40 min [23]. Interestingly, we also found that therapist-rated client engagement *during session* predicted the amount of meditation practice participants engaged in during their at-home practice [37]. However, none of the dose indicators used in our research so far have been significantly associated with pain outcomes [37]. Determination of the optimal dose of number of treatment sessions and recommended at home practice is a critical next step in the field.

Practical Considerations

Evidence on the utility and efficacy of MBCT for pain is building, and given the rapidly increasing popularity of mindfulness approaches in the media, among researchers, therapists, and also patients, it is likely that in the coming decade growth in this area will be substantial. However, there are a number of practical considerations when deciding whether to implement MBCT within your own clinical practice. Careful consideration of these factors is essential for optimal client care.

Who Might Be Most Suitable for MBCT for pain?

When collaboratively deciding with a client if MBCT might be an appropriate treatment plan, it is important to discuss what the treatment entails and the associated time commitment (which is quite substantial given the recommended daily meditation practice for homework). In our MBCT for headache trial, a number of participants dropped out prior to treatment completion [23], and the time commitment of participating in treatment was reported as a common barrier [36]. This finding is consistent with unpublished research by Carmody (as cited in Carmody and Baer [38]) that found 45 % of eligible individuals who declined to participate in a mindfulness intervention cited time as the primary limiting factor. An additional consideration stems from our research (described above in the *Mechanisms of MBCT for Chronic Pain* section) that has found that those individuals who enter MBCT for pain with more positive expectations and motivation report better outcomes at post-treatment [37]. Related to this, clients may hold concerns about a meditation-based approach due to cultural, personal, or religious reasons [39]; to allay these concerns and prevent them from impacting alliance, explicitly discussing the secular nature of MBCT prior to treatment starting can be helpful. Further, if you are working with a client that is not at a stage where they are motivated to commence MBCT, it may be wise to first implement a preparatory pre-MBCT intervention (such as motivational interviewing) to enhance readiness to change [40].

What Is the Best Treatment Format and Mode of Delivery for MBCT?

As described above (in the *Adapting MBCT for pain* section), the standard treatment format is a group-delivered, 8-week protocol (one session per week), with each session lasting 2 h, and at-home practice and other homework exercises encouraged for between each session. This format mirrors the original MBCT for depression relapse protocol [14], which in turn mirrors the format of the MBSR protocol developed by Kabat-Zinn [18]. However, it has not been empirically established as to whether this is the *best* or most efficacious treatment format. Within the context of the building body of research identifying that the time commitment to participate in MBCT is a barrier for treatment engagement, there has been a call for examination of brief mindfulness interventions [38]. Some research has found a positive association between daily dose of meditation and certain salutatory effects

[41]. However, potentially a shorter practice might be just as clinically effective, and likely might be more feasible and acceptable for many people [24]. In terms of the most appropriate mode of delivery, MBCT for pain is typically delivered in a group setting and based on clinical experience, an ideal group size is between approximately 6 and 10 individuals. Although it is certainly an option to deliver MBCT in an individual therapy setting (and in my own clinical practice I have done so with great effect), research suggests that group factors, such as group cohesion and social learning, can become agents of change in and of themselves [42, 43]. A promising alternative to traditional in-person treatment delivery modalities is the use of technology to enhance treatment access, such as Internet-based, telephone or Therapeutic Interactive Voice Response approaches [31, 44]. Based on the findings by Dowd and colleagues described above (in the *Efficacy of MBCT for Chronic Pain* section) [31], Internet-delivered MBCT for pain may be a feasible and efficacious alternative.

What Form of Therapist Training Is Needed?

In considering implementing MBCT for pain, as with any other intervention, evidence-based practice and relevant codes of ethics direct clinicians to first obtain the needed skills and expertise to competently deliver the approach in order to maximize benefit and minimize potential harm. Although no formal certification process is *required* for delivering MBCT for pain, ethical standards mandate clinicians practice within the bounds of competence [45]. Thus, to ensure professional competence and ethical practice, practitioners considering regularly implementing MBCT for pain management should consider obtaining formal MBCT training in conjunction with familiarizing oneself with the available literature. The UCSD Center for Mindfulness, *Mindfulness-Based Professional Training Institute* website is a good starting resource that provides professional trainings, the option of a certification process for advancing expertise, as well as a comprehensive list of recommended resources containing various published texts relating to a wide range of specific populations [46]. In addition to the matter of competence and ethical standards, a core constituent of mindfulness-based interventions is the recommendation that therapists have a personal, established meditation practice prior to implementing these approaches clinically [18]. An established, personal practice in meditation places the therapist in a better position to genuinely model for clients the qualities of mindfulness, acceptance, kindness, and a non-judgmental attitude that clients are cultivating in engaging in the MBCT treatment and this is hypothesized to strengthen therapeutic alliance.

Summary and Conclusions

The case scenario of Maria at the start of this chapter is indicative of the life lived by millions of individuals worldwide who live with pain on a daily basis. Although CBT is still considered the gold standard psychological approach to pain, "one size does not fit all" and we need other alternative, theoretically sound, efficacious treatments available. A rapidly increasing body of research is documenting the efficacy of MBCT for a variety of conditions, and in the realm of pain specifically, it seems a tipping point may have been reached in that this approach is becoming a topic of investigation across a number of prominent research groups worldwide. MBCT is an innovative treatment approach and shows considerable promise for pain management; however, current research investigating its use across various pain conditions is preliminary and more research is needed. Moreover, it is not enough to simply determine that MBCT *works*. To demonstrate the true public health value of this approach, we also need to understand the mediators (i.e., how does the treatments work?) and the moderators (i.e., for whom does the treatment work?) of MBCT for pain. Identification of the specific mediators of MBCT for pain will determine if this treatment does work via the reasons specified by theory; this information will inform the capacity to further streamline the protocol to maximize efficacy and efficiency. Concurrent identification of those client characteristics that might deem an individual most suitable to MBCT (i.e., sometimes referred to as Aptitude X Treatment Interactions [47]) will allow for optimization of resources via the devel-

opment of patient-treatment matching algorithms. Further, determining "how much is enough" will optimize the dissemination and widespread use of the pain self-management techniques taught in MBCT by making this approach feasible and acceptable to a diversity of individual client needs and lifestyles. Clearly, great strides have been made in the area of chronic pain management in the last several decades. MBCT represents an additional promising treatment that has the capacity to lessen the suffering associated with chronic pain so individuals can learn to live a meaningful life, with pain and all.

Acknowledgments I would like to acknowledge and express my sincere appreciation for Professor Beverly Thorn, for her valued collaborations and insightful contributions in working with me to develop a line of research examining MBCT for pain.

References

1. IASP Task Force on Taxonomy. Classification of Chronic Pain, Second Edition. Merskey, H., Bogduk, N., editors. Seattle, Washington: IASP Press; 1994.
2. IASP Subcommittee on Taxonomy, Classification of chronic pain. Descriptions of chronic pain syndromes and definitions of pain terms. Pain. 1986;3:S1–226.
3. Johannes CB, Le TK, Zhou X, Johnston JA, Dworkin RH. The prevalence of chronic pain in United States adults: results of an internet-based survey. J Pain. 2010;11(11):1230–9.
4. Gaskin DJ, Richard P. The economic costs of pain in the United States. J Pain. 2012;13(8):715–24.
5. Schwartz BS, Stewart WF, Simon D, Lipton RB. Epidemiology of tension-type headache. JAMA. 1998;279(5):381–3.
6. Melzack R, Wall PD. Pain mechanisms: a new theory. Science. 1965;150(699):971–9.
7. Melzack R, Wall PD. The challenge of pain. New York: Basic Books; 1982.
8. Melzack R. Pain and the neuromatrix in the brain. J Dent Educ. 2001;65:1378–82.
9. Melzack R. Evolution of the neuromatrix theory of pain. The Prithvi Raj Lecture: presented at the third World Congress of World Institute of Pain, Barcelona 2004. Pain Pract. 2005;5:85–94.
10. Apkarian AV, Baliki MN, Geha PY. Towards a theory of chronic pain. Prog Neurobiol. 2009;87(2):81–97.
11. Apkarian AV, Hashmi JA, Baliki MN. Pain and the brain: specificity and plasticity of the brain in clinical chronic pain. Pain. 2011;152(3 Suppl):S49–64.
12. Jensen MP. A Neuropsychological model of pain: research and clinical implications. J Pain. 2010;11:2–12.
13. Williams AC, Eccleston C, Morley S. Psychological therapies for the management of chronic pain (exclud-

ing headache) in adults. Cochrane Database Syst Rev. 2012;11, CD007407.

14. Segal Z, Williams JM, Teasdale J. Mindfulness-based cognitive therapy for depression: a new approach to preventing relapse. New York: Guilford Press; 2002.

15. Segal ZV, Williams JMG, Teasdale JD. Mindfulness-based cognitive therapy for depression. New York: Guilford; 2013.

16. Turk DC, Meichenbaum D, Genest M. Pain and behavioral medicine: a cognitive-behavioral perspective. New York: Guilford Press; 1983. p. 452. xii.

17. Penzien DB. Stress management for migraine: recent research and commentary. Headache. 2009;49(9):1395–8.

18. Kabat-Zinn J. Full catastrophe living: using the wisdom of your body and mind to face stress, pain and illness. New York: Delacourt; 1990.

19. Fjorback LO, Arendt M, Ornbol E, Fink P, Walach H. Mindfulness-based stress reduction and mindfulness-based cognitive therapy: a systematic review of randomized controlled trials. Acta Psychiatr Scand. 2011;124(2):102–19.

20. Grossman P, Niemann L, Schmidt S, Walach H. Mindfulness-based stress reduction and health benefits. A meta-analysis. J Psychosom Res. 2004;57:35–43.

21. Thorn BE. Cognitive therapy for chronic pain: a step-by-step guide. New York: Guilford Press; 2004.

22. Safran JD, Segal ZV. Interpersonal process in cognitive therapy. New York: Basic Books; 1990.

23. Day MA, Thorn BE, Ward LC, Rubin N, Hickman SD, Scogin F, et al. Mindfulness-based cognitive therapy for the treatment of headache pain: a pilot study. Clin J Pain. 2014;22(2):278–85.

24. Day MA, Jensen MP, Ehde DM, Thorn BE. Towards a theoretical model for mindfulness-based pain management. J Pain. 2014;15(7):691–703.

25. Cathcart S, Galatis N, Immink M, Proeve M, Petkov J. Brief mindfulness-based therapy for chronic tension-type headache: a randomized controlled pilot study. Behav Cogn Psychother. 2014;42:1–15.

26. Garland EL, Thomas E, Howard MO. Mindfulness-oriented recovery enhancement ameliorates the impact of pain on self-reported psychological and physical function among opioid using chronic pain patients. J Pain Symptom Manag. 2014;48(6):1091–9.

27. Parra-Delgado PM, Latorre-Postigo JM. Effectiveness of mindfulness-based cognitive therapy in the treatment of fibromyalgia: a randomised trial. Cogn Ther Res. 2013;37:1015–26.

28. Veehof MM, Oskam MJ, Schreurs KM, Bohlmeijer ET. Acceptance-based interventions for the treatment of chronic pain: a systematic review and meta-analysis. Pain. 2011;152(3):533–42.

29. Day MA, Thorn BE. The relationship of demographic and psychosocial variables to pain-related outcomes in a rural chronic pain population. Pain. 2010;151(2):467–74.

30. Tait RC, Chibnall JT. Racial and ethnic disparities in the evaluation and treatment of pain: psychological perspectives. Prof Psychol Res Pract. 2005;36(6):595–601.

31. Dowd H, Hogan MJ, McGuire BE, Davis MC, Sarma KM, Fish RA, et al. Comparison of an online mindfulness-based cognitive therapy intervention with

online pain management psychoeducation: a randomized controlled study. Clin J Pain. 2015;31(6):517–27.

32. Griffiths F, Lindenmeyer A, Powell J, et al. Why are health care interventions delivered over the internet? A systematic review of the published literature. J Med Internet Res. 2006;8.

33. Jensen MP. Psychosocial approaches to pain management: an organizational framework. Pain. 2011;152(4):717–25.

34. Thorn BE, Burns JW. Common and specific treatment mechanisms in psychosocial pain interventions: the need for a new research agenda. Pain. 2011;152(4):705–6.

35. Day MA, Thorn BE. The mediating role of pain acceptance during mindfulness-based cognitive therapy for headache. Under Review.

36. Day MA, Thorn BE, Rubin N. Mindfulness-based cognitive therapy for the treatment of headache pain: a mixed-methods analysis comparing treatment responders and treatment non-responders. Complement Ther Med. 2014;15(3):278–85.

37. Day MA, Halpin J, Thorn BE. An empirical examination of the role of common factors of therapy during a mindfulness-based cognitive therapy intervention for headache pain. Clin J Pain. In Press.

38. Carmody J, Baer RA. How long does a mindfulness-based stress reduction program need to be? A review of class contact hours and effect sizes for psychological distress. J Clin Psychol. 2009;65(6):627–38.

39. Day MA, Eyer J, Thorn BE. Therapeutic relaxation. In: Hofmann SG, editor. The Wiley handbook of cognitive behavioral therapy: a complete reference guide volume 1: CBT General Strategies. 1: Wiley-Blackwell; 2013. p. 157–80.

40. Day MA, Ehde DM, Jensen MP. Psychosocial pain management moderation: the limit, activate and enhance model. J Pain. New York 2015;16(10):947–60.

41. Carmody J, Baer RA. Relationships between mindfulness practice and levels of mindfulness, medical and psychological symptoms and well-being in a mindfulness-based stress reduction program. J Behav Med. 2008;31(1):23–33.

42. MacKenzie KR. The alliance in time limited group psychotherapy. In: Safran JD, Muran JC, editors. The therapeutic alliance in brief psychotherapy. Washington, D.C.: American Psychological Association; 1998. p. 193–215.

43. Yalom ID, Leszcz M. The theory and practice of group psychotherapy. 5th ed. New York: Basic Books; 2005.

44. Naylor MR, Keefe FJ, Brigidi B, Naud S, Helzer JE. Therapeutic interactive voice response for chronic pain reduction and relapse prevention. Pain. 2008;134(3):335–45.

45. Association AP. Ethical principles of psychologists and code of conduct: 2010 amendments 2010. Accessed 29 May 2015. From: http://www.apa.org/ethics/code/.

46. Mindfulness TUCf. Mindfulness-Based Professional Training Institute. Accessed 29 May 2015. From: http://mbpti.org/.

47. Dance KA, Neufeld RW. Aptitude-treatment interaction research in clinical settings: a review of attempts to dispel the "patient uniformity" myth. Psychol Bull. 1988;104:192–213.

Mindfulness-Based Cognitive Therapy: Medically Unexplained Symptoms

7

Hiske van Ravesteijn and Lone Fjorback

Two Clinical Case Studies

A 40-year-old woman from Eastern Africa entered the room; she was very neatly dressed and she had tightly combed hair. For a couple of years she had chronic headaches and she frequently experienced palpitations of the heart for which no physical cause was found. And more recently she was diagnosed with high blood pressure. For these symptoms she used painkillers and antihypertensive medication; they provided some relief, but the symptoms did not resolve over time. Although she often did not feel well, she always went to work. She was a hard-working secretary in a big company.

She had heard about our study examining the effects of mindfulness for medically unexplained symptoms and she wondered whether mindfulness training could be helpful to her. Together we decided that it was worthwhile to examine what mindfulness training could mean for her. She took part in an 8-week MBCT class together with other patients with chronic medically unexplained symptoms.

During the first two sessions she did not share much with the group. But in the third session, after an exercise of attentive listening, she started to speak. While she was listening attentively to the sounds in the room and the birds outside, the church bells rang. At once she became clearly aware of the fact that she was not "at home." She was in a country that was not her home country, a very different place from where she grew up, far away from her family. She realized that she felt lonely and she cried. The group was silent. After a while she spoke again. She wondered whether she had been hiding from this feeling of loneliness by working very hard.

In the following weeks she started to take breaks at work and she even put up a sign not to be disturbed on her office door. She did some of her mindfulness practices during this time. To her surprise, her colleagues accepted that she was not continuously available. In addition, she started to listen to her favorite music while driving the car. She noticed that she felt less stressed, and her headaches and the heart palpitations diminished over time.

She felt more at ease, had more attention for her surrounding, and experienced more moments of joy; she started to treat herself in a more caring way. Remarkably, her looks changed during the MBCT course: her hair was not tightly combed anymore; she now had big frizzy hair.

H. van Ravesteijn, M.D., Ph.D. (✉)
Department of Psychiatry, Radboud University
Nijmegen Medical Centre, PO Box 9101, 6500 HB
Nijmegen, The Netherlands
e-mail: Hiske.vanRavesteijn@radboudumc.nl

L. Fjorback, M.D., Ph.D.
Danish Center for Mindfulness, Aarhus University
Hospital, Barthsgade 5, 8200 Aarhus N, Denmark

Another 40-year-old woman used to work as a schoolteacher in Denmark. For 5 years she suffered from headache, nausea, concentration difficulties, impairment of memory, fatigue, muscular, and abdominal pain. She had unexplained physical symptoms since early childhood and recurrent infections and migraine since early youth. She was diagnosed with irritable bowel syndrome, fibromyalgia, chronic fatigue syndrome, and migraine. In her previous job, 5 years ago, she had had three longer periods of sick leave because of stress. She had tried many different therapies for her symptoms, e.g., physiotherapy, craniosacral therapy, acupuncture, chiropractor, diets (avoidance of sugar and gluten), psychotherapy, and medication (painkillers and an antidepressant). In the present state she was in bed 5 days a week and had a very limited social life. She decided to attend mindfulness therapy, a course specifically designed for patients with severe bodily distress.

Five months after the mindfulness therapy she wrote a note to thank us for the process which she had gone through: "I can't understand that I feel SO much better in a just a few months. I was a diligent student, fully committed to becoming well—and it seems I've succeeded. Feeling how I am has become second nature—stop, one thing at a time, not be perfect, go slowly and feel the ground beneath my feet, etc. I've become excellent at 'discovering' if my mind is too busy with 'other' things while I am doing routine tasks. I challenge my limits by seeing how much I can, and gradually I've become very secure with the situation—I feel more and more that I have gotten my life back! I can go on and on … a lot less pain, six weeks between migraines; which are milder, a lot of faith in the future, I have a social life again …"

The Problem of Medically Unexplained Symptoms

Medically unexplained symptoms are highly prevalent. In primary care 20–50% of the physical symptoms remain medically unexplained. Often, these symptoms resolve over time. However, in a minority of the patients these symptoms persist. Patients with persistent MUS suffer from psychological distress, functional impairment, and social isolation. The impairments of MUS are comparable with those of depressive disorders or a general medical disease.

Societal costs associated with persistent medically unexplained symptoms are substantial [1]; they mainly consist of health care costs and costs of lost productivity. Health care costs of patients with persistent medically unexplained symptoms are high due to high consultation rates in both primary and secondary care [2] and due to often unnecessary medical procedures to rule out medical conditions with the potential for iatrogenic harm. Disabilities caused by medically unexplained symptoms lead to diminished employment participation: patients with persistent medically unexplained symptoms are more on sick leave and have higher rates of unemployment [3]. The traditional tools offered by medicine, including psychiatry, are often intended to fix or attack patients' symptoms, not to release suffering or promote vitality.

At present, cognitive behavioral therapy is the intervention of choice for persistent medically unexplained symptoms. Several studies have shown modest improvements in somatic symptoms, psychological distress, and functional impairment [4]. However, many patients with medically unexplained symptoms do not easily accept psychological treatment. Probably, an intervention that has a body-oriented focus is more acceptable to patients with chronic medically unexplained symptoms. They experience physical symptoms and are often afraid for an underlying disease. In a recent trial on the effectiveness of a group cognitive behavioral intervention for medically unexplained symptoms, physical health improved significantly whereas mental health did not show a strong improvement [5].

Patients with medically unexplained symptoms are often stigmatized, and effective treatment is rarely delivered, leaving these patients isolated, left by themselves, vulnerable to costly and potentially harming medical and alternative treatments. Consequently, there is still a need for more acceptable and effective treatment options. There is a need for non-harming practical tools in order to help patients to take responsibility for their own health and well-being.

Theoretical Rationale of MBCT for Medically Unexplained Symptoms

Patients with medically unexplained symptoms are suffering, and mindfulness attempts to work with the stress and pain that causes suffering [6]. From a traditional Buddhist point of view, suffering is a basic premise of life. The principal underlying cause of suffering is assumed to be attachment or clinging. By definition, there is no known cause of medically unexplained symptoms. However, the co-occurrence of negative affect and pain is well recognized. An impaired ability to evaluate and categorize painful sensations could indicate a problem in the regulation of pain perception in patients suffering from medically unexplained symptoms. This is probably related to changes in the parietal and prefrontal cortex, which are the areas that sustained training of mindfulness can improve. Impairments of sensory processing may lead to repetitive overloading, which may in turn lead to fear of movement and unhealthy coping strategies.

Certain behavioral, cognitive, and emotional patterns are overrepresented in patients with chronic medically unexplained symptoms. Patients often describe that they shift between ignoring and being totally overwhelmed by somatic symptoms. The following patterns are often seen in patients with chronic medically unexplained symptoms: patterns of not paying careful attention to body signals, or on the contrary patterns of continuously focusing on each body signal. Other patterns that are frequently present are emotional patterns of anger, anxiety, and depression due to trauma or affective neglect. Patients with medically unexplained symptoms often have difficulty with setting boundaries towards others, or put simply: they have difficulty with saying "no."

Through mindfulness training patients are invited to step out of their ordinary life and their automatic patterns. They are asked to stop, to observe what is going on. They are invited to listen to their body. By experiencing their own physical sensations, thoughts, emotions, and behavioral tendencies, they can learn to step out of their automatic patterns. This is done in a group setting that provides safety and careful attention. Often, standing still in the current moment is less frightening than the patient had thought. Patients can experience that they are able to tolerate what is present. They can observe their own tendencies without directly reacting to their tendency. There is time to observe how symptoms, thoughts, and emotions come and go. These new experiences can lead to new insights, which are not taught by the trainer, but which the patient has discovered himself or herself.

Mindfulness has a body-focused and experiential approach, which is different from more cognitive approaches used in cognitive behavioral therapy. Mindfulness training can help participants in developing the ability to tolerate symptoms while at the same time not letting the symptoms dictate behavior [4].

Modifications of MBCT for Medically Unexplained Symptoms

Two versions have been developed of mindfulness training for patients with medically unexplained symptoms. One version stays close to the original MBCT format. It has been developed in the Netherlands and it has been tested on patients with moderate-to-severe medically unexplained symptoms.

This version of MBCT for patients with MUS consists of eight weekly sessions of 2.5 h plus a 6-h silent day [7]. Preferably, the group has 10–14 patients. In this way there is sufficient time to share experiences in the group and to learn from others. In addition to the group sessions, participants are instructed to practice 6 days a week for approximately 45 min a day. The training protocol is based on the MBCT format for patients with recurrent depression [8]. Adaptations were made to the MBCT training protocol to make it suitable for patients with physical symptoms. In all sections where "depression" or mental health problems are mentioned, we changed this into "physical symptoms." The program consists of formal meditation exercises such as body scan, sitting meditation, walking meditation, and mindful movement. Participants are also encouraged to cultivate awareness of everyday activities, such as eating or taking a shower. In addition, the program includes cognitive techniques such as psycho-education, monitoring and scheduling of activities, and identification of negative automatic thoughts. In the section on psycho-education, we included information about respecting physical and mental boundaries and dealing with impairments. In line with the original mindfulness-based stress reduction format, a silent day is incorporated to give participants the opportunity to deepen their mindfulness practice. To support home practice, patients receive a folder with information about the individual sessions, homework assignments, and forms to keep a record of their practice, together with CDs with guided meditations and movement exercises. The homework exercises are identical to those of the MBCT course.

In Denmark another version has been developed: Mindfulness Therapy [9]. This version includes more psycho-education about medically unexplained symptoms than the abovementioned version. This version has been tested on patients with severe medically unexplained symptoms.

The sessions take eight weekly 3.5-h sessions and one follow-up session. The MBSR manual developed by Jon Kabat-Zinn is closely followed, except the all-day retreat, which lasted only 3.5 h. It includes psycho-education, symptom registration, and a model for graded exercise. The psycho-education covers the following themes: registration and differentiation of fluctuating symptoms; diagnostic labels for medically unexplained symptoms (fibromyalgia, chronic fatigue syndrome, and somatization disorder); biological, psychological, and social factors contributing to the development and maintenance of medically unexplained symptoms; connecting bodily symptoms, emotions, thoughts, and behaviors; restoring sleep; diffusion of inflexible symptom attributions, and impact of negative illness perceptions; identifying cognitive distortions; and recapitulation of the above in the last session. The workbook of mindfulness therapy is available at www.mindfulness.au.dk.

In randomized controlled trials both treatment protocols have been proven to be effective [10, 11]. For mild-to-moderate symptoms the first protocol might be sufficient. For patients who have become severely disabled due to their medically unexplained symptoms, the 3.5-h version, named mindfulness therapy, is probably most suitable. For some patients, the mindfulness training is not sufficient; for some it is just the beginning of a longer lasting process of change. An individual treatment could follow, for example with a psychomotor therapist or a psychotherapist, depending on the process and preferences of the patient.

We recommend offering homework practice for 15–45 min per day. It is important not to force people to do homework; it is an invitation. It is desirable to spend 45 min per day on formal practice; however, if this is too intense for patients, the amount of practice should be lowered to fit the patient's abilities.

The trainer should be experienced both in providing mindfulness training and in working with patients with medically unexplained symptoms. The trainer should be able to distinguish between symptoms that need acute medical care and symptoms that can be tolerated without acute medical care. The trainer might be a psychologist, a psychotherapist, a medical doctor, psychiatrist, a psychomotor therapist, or another healthcare worker with experience in both mindfulness training and medically unexplained symptoms.

Evidence of MBCT for Medically Unexplained Symptoms Including Mechanisms of Change

During the last two decades at least 15 scientific studies have been performed examining the effectiveness of mindfulness-based therapies for medically unexplained symptoms. An extensive review and meta-analysis of these studies has been written by Lakhan and Schofield [12]. They included 13 randomized controlled trials with a total of 1092 patients. All studies used mindfulness-based therapy as the intervention; this could be mindfulness-based stress reduction (MBSR), mindfulness-based cognitive therapy (MBCT), or an eclectic or unspecified mindfulness-based therapy. The control conditions consisted of a waitlist condition or support groups. Some of the studies focused on a specific syndrome, such as fibromyalgia, chronic fatigue syndrome, and irritable bowel syndrome. The main outcomes were pain, severity of symptoms, quality of life, depression, and anxiety.

Patients who received mindfulness-based therapy experienced less pain, a decrease in the severity of symptoms, less depression, a decrease in anxiety, and an increase in the quality of life, compared to patients in the control conditions. When the researchers examined the effects for each syndrome separately, they found that the mindfulness-based therapies were most effective in the irritable bowel syndrome. Another finding was that the studies in which mindfulness-based stress reduction (MBSR) or mindfulness-based cognitive therapy (MBCT) was used had better results than studies in which eclectic or unspecified mindfulness-based therapies were used.

One of the 15 studies that were included in the abovementioned review was the randomized controlled trial by Fjorback et al.[11]. They combined MBSR with cognitive behavioral therapy, and specifically treated patients with severe medically unexplained symptoms. The treatment was named mindfulness therapy, it consisted of eight weekly sessions of 3.5 h and one follow-up session of 3.5 h. One hundred and nineteen patients were included. Mindfulness was compared to an active control group entitled "specialized treatment" in which an individual treatment was planned in collaboration between the patient and a medical doctor specialized in medically unexplained symptoms and psychiatry. Mindfulness therapy was comparable to specialized treatment in improving the quality of life and the symptoms of the patients with medically unexplained symptoms at 15-month follow-up. However, in the mindfulness therapy group, the physical functioning significantly changed at the end of the treatment and this change remained at 15-month follow-up, whereas no significant change was seen in the specialized treatment group until the 15-month follow-up. Mindfulness therapy produced greater and more rapid improvement than specialized treatment.

The economic effects of the mindfulness therapy [13] were evaluated by the use of original register data from the 119 enrolled patients and a matched control group of 5950 individuals. Mindfulness therapy had substantial socioeconomic benefits over specialized treatment. The disability pensions were significantly lower in the mindfulness therapy group than in the specialized treatment group over a 15-month follow-up period; 25% from the mindfulness therapy group received disability pension compared with 45% from the specialized treatment group. In conclusion, mindfulness therapy may have significantly improved physical functioning, seemed to prevent further social decline, and led to reduced societal costs.

A randomized controlled trial that was conducted more recently examined the effectiveness of MBCT for patients with medically unexplained symptoms who frequently attended their family physician for these symptoms [10]. One hundred and twenty-five patients were included in the trial; they were randomized to receive either MBCT or enhanced usual health care. Although the physical functioning did not differ between the two conditions, mental functioning improved significantly in patients who had received MBCT. Patients indicated to experience more vitality and better social functioning. During the year in which the study took place, a cost-effectiveness study was done by using diaries for health care use and presence at work [14]. In this study there was no significant influence of MBCT on the presence at work. But total hospital costs were lower for patients who had received MBCT, whereas the use of mental health care had increased in the MBCT condition.

Alongside this study a longitudinal interview study was done with 12 patients who were interviewed before, directly after, and a year after the MBCT [15]. During the year the patients went through a process of change. This started with awareness of the present moment. They became more aware of sensory experiences, thoughts, and emotions. Patients described that they became better able to accept their experiences, rather than resisting them. Awareness and acceptance of painful symptoms and emotions were key factors in this process. Also, patients started to recognize their own behavioral patterns. And some were able to change them, thus improving self-care. Some patients indicated that they visited their family physician less frequently, as they had become less anxious and better able to tolerate symptoms for a while. An increase in self-compassion resulted from the newly gained insights, and at the same time it seemed to facilitate the process of change. Main barriers were concurrent social problems, such as the loss of a partner, and the inability or unwillingness to accept symptoms. For two patients the MBCT seemed effective on the short term, but on the long term the changes did not last. They probably needed individual treatment to reach a longer lasting change.

Another longitudinal interview study, with 22 patients, examined how mindfulness-based therapy for patients with chronic medically unexplained symptoms influenced patients' stress experiences and coping strategies [16]. Before the mindfulness-based therapy, most patients were struggling with existential themes. In this study this was indicated as "an existential crisis." They felt insecure about their social identity, and insecure about the causes, consequences, and management of their illness. In addition, they had difficulties in identifying and expressing cognitions, emotions, and feelings. They experienced a low awareness of the body and the experience of self. The interviewed patients often used avoidant coping, which made them more vulnerable to stress. After the mindfulness therapy, which consisted of eight weekly sessions of 3.5 h, patients indicated that they felt more self-confident. In relation to their symptoms, they felt recognized as "really" ill. The patients had a clearer view upon the nature, management, and future prospects of their illness. Generally, they used more flexible coping strategies to reduce their daily stress experiences. The patients experienced an increased awareness of body and mind, were better able to relax by using mindfulness techniques, and described an improved ability to identify and express needs and feelings of distress. Half of the patients experienced an increased sexual drive; they described how their relations had improved both sexually and communicatively.

Conclusions

The term mindfulness, which derives from the pāli word *sati*, means to "remember"; remember the body, the mind, and the heart. This is obvious and trivial, but it may, nevertheless, be exactly what is called for in modern medicine. Teaching how to feel whole, physically present, mentally clear, and emotionally balanced may, indeed, be an integrated part of modern medical practice. Mindfulness-based therapies are an effective approach to deal with stress via enhanced body awareness and insight into automatic patterns.

Mindfulness training is valuable for patients with medically unexplained symptoms. It can open up a path of awareness of the body and it can help patients to stay out of avoidance strategies. At the same time it can prevent patients from identifying too much with their symptoms. By experiencing the body, and being conscious of thoughts and emotions, patients gain new ways of experiencing themselves. Often, this leads to a more friendly way of taking care of oneself. It improves the ability to express needs and feelings of distress and can lead to more active communication with others.

Mindfulness training offers non-harming practical tools which can help patients to take responsibility for their own health and well-being. Although mindfulness does not simply "clear away" the physical symptoms, it does offer a way of treating oneself in a more friendly manner. Mindfulness training can help in developing the ability to tolerate symptoms while at the same time not letting the symptoms dictate behavior. This leads towards more psychological flexibility and a better mental health.

References

1. Konnopka A, Schaefert R, Heinrich S, Kaufmann C, Luppa M, Herzog W, et al. Economics of medically unexplained symptoms: a systematic review of the literature. Psychother Psychosom. 2012;81(5):265–75.
2. Barsky AJ, Orav EJ, Bates DW. Somatization increases medical utilization and costs independent of psychiatric and medical comorbidity. Arch Gen Psychiatry. 2005;62(8):903–10.

3. Edwards TM, Stern A, Clarke DD, Ivbijaro G, Kasney LM. The treatment of patients with medically unexplained symptoms in primary care: a review of the literature. Ment Health Fam Med. 2010;7(4):209–21.
4. Deary V, Chalder T, Sharpe M. The cognitive behavioural model of medically unexplained symptoms: a theoretical and empirical review. Clin Psychol Rev. 2007;27(7):781–97.
5. Zonneveld LN, van Rood YR, Timman R, Kooiman CG, Van't Spijker A, Busschbach JJ. Effective group training for patients with unexplained physical symptoms: a randomized controlled trial with a non-randomized one-year follow-up. PLoS One. 2012;7(8):e42629.
6. Kabat-Zinn J. Full catastrophe living, how to cope with stress, pain and illness using mindfulness meditation. New York, NY: Bantam Doubleday Dell; 1990.
7. Ravesteijn HJ. Mindfulness-based cognitive therapy for patients with medically unexplained symptoms. Nijmegen: Radboud University Medical Center; 2013.
8. Teasdale JD, Segal ZV, Williams JM, Ridgeway VA, Soulsby JM, Lau MA. Prevention of relapse/recurrence in major depression by mindfulness-based cognitive therapy. J Consult Clin Psychol. 2000;68(4):615–23.
9. Fjorback LO. Mindfulness and bodily distress. Aarhus: Aarhus University; 2012.
10. van Ravesteijn H, Lucassen P, Bor H, van Weel C, Speckens A. Mindfulness-based cognitive therapy for patients with medically unexplained symptoms: a randomized controlled trial. Psychother Psychosom. 2013;82(5):299–310.
11. Fjorback LO, Arendt M, Ornbol E, Walach H, Rehfeld E, Schroder A, et al. Mindfulness therapy for somatization disorder and functional somatic syndromes – randomized trial with one-year follow-up. J Psychosom Res. 2013;74(1):31–40.
12. Lakhan SE, Schofield KL. Mindfulness-based therapies in the treatment of somatization disorders: a systematic review and meta-analysis. PLoS One. 2013;8(8):e71834.
13. Fjorback LO, Carstensen T, Arendt M, Ornbol E, Walach H, Rehfeld E, et al. Mindfulness therapy for somatization disorder and functional somatic syndromes: analysis of economic consequences alongside a randomized trial. J Psychosom Res. 2013;74(1):41–8.
14. van Ravesteijn H, Grutters J, olde Hartman T, Lucassen P, Bor H, van Weel C, et al. Mindfulness-based cognitive therapy for patients with medically unexplained symptoms: a cost-effectiveness study. J Psychosom Res. 2013;74(3):197–205.
15. van Ravesteijn HJ, Suijkerbuijk YB, Langbroek JA, Muskens E, Lucassen PL, van Weel C, et al. Mindfulness-based cognitive therapy (MBCT) for patients with medically unexplained symptoms: process of change. J Psychosom Res. 2014;77(1):27–33.
16. Lind AB, Delmar C, Nielsen K. Searching for existential security: a prospective qualitative study on the influence of mindfulness therapy on experienced stress and coping strategies among patients with somatoform disorders. J Psychosom Res. 2014;77(6):516–21.

Mindfulness-Based Cognitive Therapy application for People Living with Chronic Disease: the case of HIV

8

Marian González-García, Xavier Borràs, Javier González López, and Kim Griffin McNeil

Abbreviations

AIDS	Acquired immune deficiency syndrome
ART	Antiretroviral therapy
HIV	Human immunodeficiency virus
MBCT	Mindfulness-based cognitive therapy
MBIs	Mindfulness-based interventions
MSM	Men who have sex with men
PLWH	People who live with HIV
RCT	Randomized controlled trial

The real voyage of discovery consists not in seeking new landscapes, but in having new eyes

Marcel Proust

M. González-García, Ph.D. (✉)
Department of Psychology, European University of the Atlantic, Santander, Spain

BalanCe Center for Psychology & Mindfulness, Santander, Spain
e-mail: marian.gonzalez@uneatlantico.es

X. Borràs, Ph.D.
Stress and Health Research Group (GIES), Faculty of Psychology, Universitat Autònoma de Barcelona, Barcelona, Spain

J.G. López, M.S.
BalanCe Center for Psychology & Mindfulness, Santander, Spain

K.G. McNeil, Ph.D.
Department Chair of Translation and Interpretation, European University of the Atlantic, Santander, Spain

A Brief Overview of HIV/AIDS

Around 1950, penicillin, antibiotics, and vaccinations freed humanity from the fear of death caused by infectious diseases [1]. Three decades later, an article that appeared in *The New England Journal of Medicine* refuted the supposed triumph indicating that it had all been a mere illusion in the eternal competition to survive among the different life forms on Earth [2]. This article described the first cases of a new syndrome that would become the great epidemic of the twentieth century [3].

After more than three decades of history, the Human Immunodeficiency Virus/Acquired Immune Deficiency Syndrome (HIV/AIDS) epidemic continues to be a global health issue. It is estimated that 35 million people live with the disease, and the number is increasing as more people live longer due to antiretroviral therapy (ART). In spite of the worldwide tendency toward decreasing numbers, in Western Europe and North America people continue to become infected through unprotected sexual activity. In fact, contagion increased by 6% since 2001 [4]. This represents a paradox of having access to information and protection measures, yet the way the infection is perceived is not enough to prevent new instances of the disease.

HIV is a lentivirus belonging to the *Retroviridae* family [5] that multiplies by using the genetic material from lymphocytes T CD4, a type of immune defense system cells. From the moment that the virus penetrates the human body, HIV spreads out in search of these cells, invades them and multiplies, liberating virions that continue to infect and destroy CD4 cells. In this way, HIV progressively decreases immune competence through a long process without provoking any specific symptomatology. This is why it was named the "silent killer" and as many as 19 million of the estimated current 35 million PLWH are not even aware that they are HIV-positive [4]. HIV continues to destroy immune competence to the level of compromising health at 200 cells/mm³. (A healthy person possesses approximately 1000 cells/mm³.) Once achieved this point, the immune system can no longer defend itself and ends up producing an illness caused by so-called "opportunistic infections" (a term that refers to infections that take advantage of a weakened organism in order to invade it). This is the case of illnesses such as *Pneumocystis carinii* or *Kaposi* sarcoma. The final stage of the process is called AIDS, and without proper treatment the patient will die within approximately 1 year. While in the USA a diagnosis of AIDS is made when the CD4 cell count reaches 200 cells/mm³, in Europe it is diagnosed as soon as an opportunistic infection is detected. The conversion of an HIV infection to AIDS takes an average of 10 years, in some patients the process passes more quickly from one stage to the other. Nevertheless with proper ART, PLWH have a considerably greater life expectancy.

Actually the introduction of the combined ART in 1996 represented a major historical change in the treatment of the infection, as much as it ceased to be considered a terminal illness and became a chronic but manageable disease. Through treatment the viral replication decreases considerably and it facilitates partial recovery of the CD4 cell count [6]. However, treatment is only effective if patients adhere strictly to medical orders. Those who do not adhere to adequate ART levels may experience treatment failure, immunological deterioration, and may even develop drug resistances that limit therapy options [7, 8]. Furthermore, once the treatment begins, it must be followed consistently, which

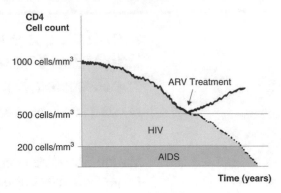

Fig. 8.1 Difference between HIV infection and AIDS, and ART effects on CD4 cell count

represents an added degree of toxicity to the organism. For this reason, clinical guides recommend delaying ART until the point where HIV has reduced the number of CD4 to below 500 cells/mm³. As shown in Fig. 8.1, the initiation of ART produces the maintaining of CD4 cell levels in a safety margin, avoiding the onset of AIDS.

Current Challenges for PLWH

The success of ART in making HIV a chronic disease, created the illusion that we were witnessing health recovery for PLWH. Nevertheless, recent results show that this is still far from being a reality. PLWH age much more quickly than normal rates. As a consequence they experience a higher level of age-related neurocognitive, cardiovascular, osteopathic, and metabolic diseases, as well as non-AIDS related cancers, in comparison to their non-AIDS infected peers [9–11]. In spite of successful ART, their life expectancy is between 10 and 15 years less than those who are free from infection [12–14]. Furthermore, HIV infection is a prototype of chronic vital situational stress. During the infectious process, patients must cope with numerous stressors that can be categorized as either biological or psycho-emotional.

At the *biological level*, they must cope with stressors such as HIV infection and the toxicity derived from years of being exposed to ART. Moreover, as aging takes place, they need more medication to treat comorbidities, resulting in polypharmacy that increases potential drug-to-drug interactions [15]. The overload of stressors can reduce the body's capacity of resistance. In fact, some studies show that PLWH experience frailty, a decreased capacity to confront biological stress due to aging [16] similar to HIV-negative subjects who are 10 years older [17]. All these biological stressors are thought to potentiate physiological aging as they share common detrimental pathways that lead to early immunosenescence, mainly immune activation and persistent inflammation [18]. Indeed, inflammation—indexed by proinflammatory cytokines such as IL-6 levels—has been identified as an etiological factor for premature or early aging in PLWH [11]. This persistent inflammation may lead to a reduced ability to adapt to metabolic stress [19] and biological stressors, leading to an increase of the vulnerability to develop comorbidities [20].

At the *psycho-emotional level* an HIV diagnosis brings with it a host of potentially stressful experiences including physical health concerns, the need to interact with a complex health care system, stigma, and the challenge to come to terms with a new identity as someone living with HIV [21]. Moreover, facing a chronic life-threatening condition, financial burden, social isolation, pressure to strictly adhere to a medication regime [22], and the uncertainty about symptoms associated with aging [23] add to the stress of PLWH. It is precisely the uncertainty associated with a lack of therapeutic response to premature aging that constitutes the main challenge for PLWH who live in developed countries. The accumulation of all of these stressors impact mental and physical health-related quality of life [24] and may contribute to depression [25, 26]. Research indicates a high level of diagnosed depression in PLWH reaching 22% [27], 35% [28] and up to 50% [29]. A meta-analysis concluded that the risk of being diagnosed with depression was 50% higher in PLWH than the non-infected cohort [30]. Furthermore, older adults living with HIV/AIDS are "doubly stigmatized" because of their advanced age and HIV-positive status, increasing their risk for depression [31, 32]. In addition, a number of people lack proper diagnosis because the symptoms of depression simulate the same effects that HIV causes. As an example, apathy is considered one of the symptoms of the neuropathology of HIV [33].

In turn, psychological stress can affect biological processes that may contribute to HIV disease progression [34]. Numerous, classical studies carried out in the field of psychoneuroimmunology (PNI) have established that stress and depression are potential causal factors of inflammation [35, 36]. In the HIV population, psychological stress has been associated with high levels of inflammation—indexed by IL-6 levels—[37]. Also, cortisol, a hormone related to stress and depression, has been associated with greater T cell activation, a known risk factor for accelerated progression of HIV [38]. Closing the circle, inflammation may amplify psychological distress, as proinflammatory cytokines induce depressive symptoms and increase anxiety [39]. In addition, psychological stress may also implicate indirect mechanisms that can impact HIV disease progression through behavioral factors [40] such as poor nutrition and sleep, that, in turns, may lead to further inflammation [41, 42].

As seen in the previous text, physiological effect of stressors displayed by PLWH, both biological and psycho-emotional, shares a common denominator: the condition of chronic *inflammation* of the immune system. In sum, these stressors can potentiate each other causing increased risk for age-related morbidity and mortality. Along these same lines, in a recent proposal, our subjective perception of social threats, such as those observed in PLWH, can elicit the same physiological mechanisms as real physical threats, creating an increase in risk for inflammation-related disorders, depression, infection, accelerated biological aging, and early mortality [26]. For the above cited reasons we consider it a priority to provide PLWH with resources to be able to successfully face these stressors, thereby preventing the occurrence of "allostatic load," the cumulative wear and tear on the body and brain due to an overactive or inefficiently managed stress response [43, 44].

Theoretical Rationale of MBCT for HIV

As previously explained, in PLWH biological and psycho-emotional stress may exacerbate each other, thereby increasing inflammation resulting in accelerated aging and an impaired health status. High levels of stressors, along with the prevalence of depression observed in this population, supports Mindfulness-Based Cognitive Therapy (MBCT) as a promising therapy; one that address the main challenges present. MBCT correlates highly with the stress management program called Mindfulness-Based Stress Reduction (MBSR), developed by Jon Kabat-Zinn [45], and has particular specificity to prevent and treat depressive symptoms. Other reasons for its potential usefulness include its non-pharmacological properties (given the treatments-derived toxicity in PLWH), as well as its cost-effectiveness (given the high cost of ART itself, added to that of the medication needed to treat comorbidities). Another characteristic of this program and that makes it especially appropriate for this population, is that it is associated with group support. PLWH often experience emotional loneliness and lack of social support. It is well known that social support is positively related to better adjustment [46] and health outcomes [24] among adults living with HIV.

Many reasons exist to justify the application of mindfulness to PLWH, such as the elevated number of stressors faced by PLWH, the devastating effect of stress on health, and the efficiency demonstrated by mindfulness as a stress management technique [47]. Research indicates that mindfulness training is proposed to promote self-regulation such as homeostasis by protecting the internal milieu from the harmful effects of stressors [48]. In addition, the value of investigating mindfulness training as a method to promote successful aging has been proposed [49]. Certain evidence supports mindfulness training as a form of cognitive training that could create cognitive reserve and protect against neurodegeneration [50]. A number of studies demonstrate the effectiveness of the MBSR program in improving psychological well-being [51–54], emotional well-being [55], self-reported medical symptoms [54], immune function [56], buffer CD4 cell loss [51], improve CD4 cell count [53, 54], and reducing adverse effects of ART [57]. (See [58] for a complete review.) Regarding MBCT, according to our knowledge only two published studies have examined its effects on HIV. The first one, carried out by Nicholas Wood

in form of a pilot single group dissertation, showed promising benefits in terms of depression, quality of life (QoL), and mindfulness skills, despite some methodological limitations [59]. The second one, a randomized controlled trial (RCT) carried out by our team in 40 long-term diagnosed and treated HIV-infected persons, showed a large effect size of MBCT on QoL, psychological stress, depression and anxiety levels. Moreover, during follow-up, MBCT group members showed an increase in CD4 cell count [60]. These results suggest that MBCT may promote successful aging in those living with HIV.

Modifications of MBCT for HIV

In general, psycho-educational interventions with the HIV population have a high dropout rate. Regarding mindfulness-based interventions (MBIs) dropout rate tends to register at approximately 25 % [61], and in PLWH specifically has been measured at between 40 % [51] and 50 % [55]. In the case of MBCT in HIV population, the previously mentioned first published study shows an 80 % dropout rate [59]. In our RCT [60] the dropout rate was surprisingly low (2.5 %). Later MBIs that we have carried out have maintained a low dropout rate. As we see it, the success of keeping participants in the program depends on the ability to make them feel accepted, understood, and accompanied, facilitating better self-acceptance and the ensuing self-regulation toward positive change.

The MBCT original program [62] is flexible, in that it allows for adapting some of the elements needed to address specific needs of the target population, maximizing its effectiveness. In this sense, we attempt to reach the greatest number of patients; not only those who have a history of depression, but all of those who might be experiencing psychological or emotional difficulties that affect their quality of life and the self-management of their health. Therefore, compared to the original program, the discourse that we use, does not concentrate exclusively on depression, rather refers also to stress, anxiety, and other psychological or emotional difficulties in order to help all participants to feel recognized.

Oftentimes, this constitutes true prevention of the development of episodes of depression derived from the burden of stressors.

One of the ways that we strengthen the effectiveness of MBCT is to adapt the language that we use as well as discussions about aspects relative to the challenges faced by PLWH. In general, to present the contents of each session we use slides to help participants focus their attention on critical issues. It is our experience that the elements that make them feel the most understood are *metaphors* and narration of adapted *examples*. In our program, the main modification that we include is precisely this adaptation, presenting the contents in such a way as to adapt to the reality that PLWH experience. Special changes with regard to the original program are made in sessions 3, 4, and 5.

Session 3 is dedicated almost exclusively to yoga exercises. Yoga exercises grounded in classic Hatha Yoga are a helpful tool to promote well-being. Quite often PLWH feel a significant disconnection from their bodies. In some cases, the discomfort, symptoms, and outward signs such as lipodystrophy lead them to hide their bodies. In other cases, they show it as if it were a showcase, a sign of beauty, almost as if it were a product carrying it to extremes and suffering high levels of anxiety at the first sign of a wrinkle or an ounce of fat on their waistline. Leading them to feel their body helps them to reconcile with themselves, and on the other hand disarms thought patterns and automatic reactions. In this sense, practicing yoga helps to introduce the key concepts of mindfulness, such as acceptance, non-force, and kindness, in a gentle and metaphorical manner that prevents psychological resistance.

In sessions 4 and 5, we do not show the videotape "Healing from within" as is done in the original program. Instead, we focus on emotional tolerance. We show participants specific neuroscience findings in an easy way. We present slides about the role of amygdalae as the center for impulsive reactions and prefrontal cortex as the center for effective response. We have adapted the 3-min breathing space-coping version (in which participants are taught to become aware of their situation, redirecting their attention to breathing as an anchor and expanding awareness around the breathing whenever they notice unpleasant feelings) by including a previous step before expanding further, in which we guide participants to explore with curiosity the sensation that emotion produces in themselves describing it as an impartial observer, without judging. By doing this they stop conceiving emotions as a static place, in which they lose their minds in thought, and begin to disidentify from emotions. As they remain connected with the changing physical sensations derived from emotions, they begin to adopt a new way of relating to them, accepting their feelings. Next we present slides to explain that this easy step acts as a trick, which might turn off the amygdalae and restore activation in the "freedom center," the prefrontal cortex. These and other simple explanations about the brain, help the person to go from feeling like a victim to empower themselves, taking responsibility about how they manage emotional states. We also provide participants an audio recording with this practice, which is one of the most highly valued exercises in our groups as being the most helpful. A common difficulty experienced by PLWH revolves around feeling isolated and a lack of social support. To address this issue, in session 5 we present slides about different styles of communication along with tips to encourage assertiveness and, in general, spread mindfulness abilities to the arena of social relationships.

In the rest of the sessions, we follow the same content as the original program. In the following clinical cases we describe the modifications in a greater detail.

Clinical Case Studies: Anna and John

These following clinical cases were selected as they illustrate current HIV main challenges and relevant issues in the application of MBCT in PLWH. "Anna" and "John" will be used as pseudonyms in order to protect the individuals' privacy. These cases were selected as part of a larger study [63] conducted in the Germans Trias i Pujol University Hospital (Badalona, Spain) where the first author of this chapter worked as a psychologist and mindfulness trainer for 5 years leading the MBCT groups. The second author contributed throughout the research giving advice regarding practical considerations and determining the theoretical background for mindfulness application and research. The third author assisted as co-therapist during the intervention and assisted in preparing the sessions.

Anna goes regularly to the HIV Unit of the cited Hospital for clinical care. There she has been treated by an interdisciplinary team for 21 years. When we personally first interviewed her, in 2010, Anna was a 46-year-old widow, mother of two uninfected children, ages 20 and 18, who were unaware that their mother was HIV-positive. Of her family, only David, her second husband, knew about her condition. Anna has been in ART since 1997 as well as taking other drugs for comorbidities. She also has osteoporosis and lipodystrophy. In her fight against the infection, she has experienced several bouts with depression, some diagnosed while others went undetected. The latest episode, dating back to 2009, has not been overcome. What precipitated this episode was the realization that her health was increasingly deteriorated, to the point where she could no longer continue to work as a cleaning woman. Since then she has been receiving disability benefits. She has recently begun to express feelings of uselessness and discomfort due to age-related conditions such as fatigue, general pain, and dryness of the skin.

Anna's history is that of a fighter who has survived the epidemic. She was diagnosed in 1994, when her first husband, who became infected through injection drug use, was diagnosed with *Pneumocystis carinii* and subsequently died of AIDS. She, who had never used drugs nor had engaged in sexual activity with anyone but her husband, did not fit any of the stereotypes associated with HIV. Needless to say, the diagnosis came as a tremendous shock. She believed that if people around her found out about the diagnosis, they would mistakenly think that she was a drug addict and would reject her. So she decided to cope on her own keeping her condition a secret from everyone. Anna concentrated all of her efforts on bringing up her two children, while living with the uncertainty of the illness that threatened to kill her. She began to be treated with the first ART, which caused the secondary effect of lipodystrophy (a syndrome that affects the distribution of body fat making visible the signs of the illness). As time passed, she began taking new medications, and almost without noticing, began to age. The aging process became truly devastating for her. The fact that she would not actually die from the illness, as she initially believed, but instead would age while still suffering from it, contributed to sending her more deeply into depression. In spite of several attempts to bring her out of the depressive state through antidepressants and cognitive-behavioral therapy, she is still depressed.

In 2010, we recommended her participation in an MBCT course. In the individual pre-intervention interview, the fact that people could identify her as HIV-positive came out as the main obstacle in to participate. She had been hiding her condition for 15 years, so that participating in the course would mean admitting in front of others for the first time ever that she was HIV-positive. In the interview we repeatedly presented this obstacle as an opportunity to get to know people who, just as she, had been hiding for years, and therefore would understand perfectly her feelings. We also explored the difficulties that she was encountering in this moment of her life, revolving around the fact that she was aging. We explained that participation in the course would be a way to help her to manage these difficulties better. We used, as an example, the results of some studies that had been carried out with MBCT in older people. After this session, Anna agreed to participate but she came to the first session with reticence and was very reserved. In the presentation before the group, she defined her goals as wanting to love herself more and to make her pain less disruptive. In this first session, dedicated to the concept of "automatic pilot" we explained: "The habitual working of the mind is to be on automatic pilot, a tendency to go through life without being truly conscious of what we are thinking, feeling, or doing, like an automaton. For example, have you ever gone to the doctor only to realize that you forgot what you were supposed to ask him or her? Or, do you sometimes forget whether you have taken your medication?" Anna and other participants responded by saying that these things did happen to them constantly and that they believed that this was the consequence of becoming older and losing their faculties. The facilitators continue: "Sometimes this is not because of getting older, but rather because our heads are so filled with worry that we cannot take any more. When we live on automatic pilot our attention works in a fragmented way and we are not aware of the harmful effect of our thoughts. Automatic pilot is made up of unconscious brain activation patterns that have been strengthened by the effect of repetition. It is like the course of a river. Over time the current cuts a deeper path making it easier for the water to flow. That is why we constantly repeat the same worrisome thoughts and impulsive reactions. In this training we will learn to carve alternative paths that nurture our well-being. Automatic pilot is made up of our patterns that are similar to molecules made up of 3 different types of atoms: thoughts, sensations, and emotions. These three are interrelated and feed off of each other. Let's take a look at an example: I get up in the morning and realize that my back hurts (sensation). Then I start to think things like the following: 'if my back keeps hurting I won't be able to go to work, I will have to call my boss, and he will surely suspect that I am HIV-positive and will fire me. If I get fired I will no longer be able to pay rent…' These thoughts generate a characteristic type of emotions, similar to frustration or anger that in turn feed the sensation of pain. Therefore, the pain, that was initially manageable, has now worsened because of the thoughts and has become unbearable. Our thoughts are constantly travelling back and forth between the past and the future and not only prevent us from enjoying the present but also act as amplifiers that increase the intensity of sensations and emotions. If we stop feeding our thoughts, we can reduce our pain (physical or emotional) and keep it at manageable levels. This is precisely the aim of the course; to learn how to manage our thoughts to be able to cope with emotions and sensations in a healthier way. The next step, as in the original program, the participants carry out the "body scan" exercise

(in which they are taken on a guided tour through their body by focusing their attention on each part as an impartial observer).

In the debate at the beginning of the second session, upon reviewing her homework, Anna said that sometimes the "body scan" relaxed her, but other times her negative thoughts prevented her from practicing it. The instructors respond to her as follows: "The mind works this way, pulling us out of the present moment over, and over again. Our mind when on automatic pilot doesn't want to relinquish the control over our life and finds many excuses to prevent us from taking command. So when you realize that your attention has gotten lost in harmful thought patterns and you decide to return to the present moment, you weaken those old automatic pilot patterns. Each time that you realize that you are in one of these thought patterns can be taken as an opportunity to weaken them and gain power over your own life. Sometimes after doing the exercises we feel relaxed, but that is only a side effect. When we practice we are not seeking relaxing but training our minds. There is no place to go to, nor special plane to arrive at. The only thing that is important is to keep on training our minds to come home." In the exercise during session 2, we introduce the cognitive model of depression (following the example "You are walking down the street, and on the other side of the street you see somebody you know. You smile and wave. The person just doesn't seem to notice and walks by"). Answers given by PLWH tend to show their perception of stigma, which is one of the greatest challenges that they face. This is why we include explicit references to HIV. For example: "What would happen if you thought that that person knew about the HIV and did not greet you because of it? What if you were 100 % sure that the person did not know about the HIV? What if you found out that that person was HIV-positive? What would happen if you did not have HIV? What would you think? How would you react? How would you feel?" We usually finish this exercise with the following reflection: "Everyone in this room has HIV, but each one reacts in a different way. The HIV virus can exacerbate problems that we have in our lives, but not all of our problems come from being HIV-positive. If they did, everyone would react in the same way. Through MBCT we can learn about how to keep these problems from limiting us." It is here where we introduce an interesting metaphor: "We all see the world through glasses tinted by our thoughts. The color of the lenses distorts reality causing us to react unconsciously according to how we interpret the world. For example, when we wear dark glasses, things seem worse than they really are. When we wear rose-colored glasses, we interpret reality better than it truly is. Dark and rose-colored are only examples. As we have seen in the cognitive model exercise, there are multiple possible colors to interpret reality. In our day-to-day lives, we interpret the world according to colored lenses composed of our thoughts and beliefs. That is why it is said that we do not see reality as it is, but as we are. If we try to wear the same colored glasses, these become our automatic pilot color, and this pattern gains strength in our lives governing our reactions almost without our realizing it. This is the case of a person who suffers depression and interprets reality with dark glasses. The simple act of being aware of the color of the lens of our glasses in a given moment has a liberating effect. Only by noticing the color of our glasses can we neutralize automatic patterns and create the freedom to respond instead of reacting impulsively." In the debate of the third session, Anna makes the following comment: "This week I have done the exercises every day and I have noticed that I feel calmer. I always believed that my thoughts showed me the sole truth. Now I have begun to see that sometimes I can change the lens of my glasses. When I do, reality changes. Last week, I realized that there are other people in worse situations. Yet, they handle it better because of the glasses that they wear." This comment shows the process through which Anna has begun to develop cognitive flexibility and relates in a different way to her thoughts. In the review of the week of the fourth session she comments: "When I do the 'body scan' I feel totally capable of accepting the present, even the discomfort and pain. I am beginning to feel OK under my skin." As she continued to accept her body sensations in the present, she began to accept her current life as well as her life history, thereby initiating the real

job of working through her diagnosis. Anna had great difficulty in accepting her illness. She acknowledged that she still experienced an internal battle with the feelings of guilt for being infected, anger toward her first husband, and general resentment toward life. In her own words: "By paying attention to my thoughts these past weeks, I came to realize that I was constantly blaming myself about my condition. I learned to stop fighting against myself. Knowing that keeping my past in the present mades me suffer, and living in the present without fighting to make it different, helped me to really live." The contents of session 5 regarding communication styles (that we have included as a modification) had a great impact on Anna, who began to be conscious of the automatic patterns that she followed in her relationships. In session six, Anna told us: "The other day I was with my husband in the car and we found ourselves in a traffic jam. We were in a hurry and it was hot. He started to protest because of being in the jam and I started to get nervous. Normally I would have started arguing with him to try to convince him that it wasn't my fault that we were in a traffic jam. That used to go on for hours. But this time I observed our pattern in a mindful way. He stopped, look at me and smiled. This time I knew that we could get through these things that we don't like in life, in a different way…even smiling! This week I have been thinking about this, and I have realized that many times I argue with him because I think that if he complains so much it is because he is not happy with me and he might leave me. That is only in my thoughts, but it might not be true." The instructor used this example to explain the importance of becoming aware. "As you may noticed during last weeks, sometimes becoming mindful of certain things is uncomfortable, but it is good for us. In the Anna's commentary we can see that she has come to realize how her emotions and thoughts set off old patterns of behavior. By paying attention to the uncomfortable situation of the traffic jam, she was able to begin to use mechanisms of emotion regulation, which in turn sets off mechanisms of self-regulation in the couple's relationship. This self-regulation allows them to adapt, passing through the situation without creating additional problems, as they attempt to resolve the original problem, the traffic jam."

This change in relationship with her thoughts continued to translate into a change in behavioral self-regulation. At the end of the sixth session, she suggested to the rest of the group that they go out for coffee together afterwards. This change in Anna's behavior showed a turning point in her evolution. Realizing that she could actively participate in a group without being rejected and even daring to take the first step meant a personal rebirth. In Anna's words, in session 7: "I have realized that I have spent my live in isolation out of fear of being rejected. I have been so alone that the only solution that I saw was to die. I used to spend all of my time before doctor's appointments trying to avoid being seen going into the office, as if I were a criminal avoiding the police. Now I am calm, happy with myself, and even looking forward to having someone to chat with."

At the end of the program in week 8, she explained: "For me this course has defined a before and an after. I believe that I have always been judging myself, and what is even worse, I didn't even realize it. I have spent years fantasizing about going back to who I was before the illness. Now I can say that even with this illness I feel better than I did before I became infected. Now I am happy with who I am... for the first time in my life I love myself, something that I had never known before. I really begin to enjoy my life." When we asked her which part of the program helped her the most, she responded: "hearing how things are fine just like they are, and learning to connect with my present, with its pros and cons. From the first weeks it has helped me to feel a peace like I have never felt before. Before the pain always stopped me in my tracks, but now I have a tool to manage the pain and that makes me really feel prepared to live my life and face the future with hope." Anna's case can serve as an example of the situation that some PWLH experience; however, there are other profiles that are quite different, as we will see in the next case.

"John" is a 35-year-old man who works in the area of advertising and is an MSM. He lives in Barcelona, a city well known for its gay activism. He is single and has a promiscuous sexual life-

style. In June of 2009 John takes a rapid HIV test that came out positive. He was referred to us for psychological consultation as protocol dictates. During the consult he did not appear to be affected by the diagnosis. He had been told that nowadays being HIV-positive was similar to having diabetes. Nowadays, this kind of comparison continues impeding many people to take care of their HIV-infection, that it is much more devastating, both at biological and psychoemotional levels, than diabetes. His discourse is superficial and he continually plays down the implications that a chronic infection and its treatment has on an organism. This image of the HIV infection coincides with the general idea that most of the MSM community in Barcelona has. John demonstrated a high level of worship of the body and physical appearance. This was reflected both in his conversation as well as in his way of dressing that accentuated his sculptured body as the result of time spent in the gym. He said that his life was like an advertisement and that the only thing that he was concerned with was how to maintain his lifestyle. After 6 months, his CD4 cell count showed that he should begin to take medication. He continued with his dizzying party lifestyle, promiscuity, and recreational drug use, all of which not only put his health at risk, but also the health of those with whom he has unsafe sex. He did not take his medication regularly and did not come to the medical appointments because he did not want anyone to suspect anything at work. After months in this situation, his CD4 levels became seriously low and he began to feel physically ill, so that he no longer could attend parties like before and even had stopped going to the gym. His party friends numbered only two, who were taking care of him. This situation made him hit bottom, showing primarily symptoms of anxiety. We suggest that he participate in an MBCT course and he accepted.

In the presentation of the first session, he expressed his goal as wanting to reduce the limitations caused by his fear of losing everything that he had gained. Although he did not explain it to the group, he was referring to his physique and his social status. In the practical part of session one, it was very difficult for him to follow the "body scan." He opened his eyes, and changed his posture constantly. In the round of post-exercise questions, he said that this was just not for him. We told him that he didn't have to like it, that the goal of the exercise is to train his muscles, but the mental ones this time. We also said that he has his whole life in front of him with this body, and that it would be a big help to him to learn how to listen to his body in order to treat it better. Besides, just as working out physically causes sore muscles, working the mind does too; except that this soreness appears as a subtle resistance, in the form of thoughts such as "This is not for me, or this is not going to work." In the second session, he commented that he gots out of breath when he focused on his breathing. The instructor responded to him: "At times when we pay attention to breathing we breathe with more difficulty. But we may trust that our body knows how to breathe. The proof is that we have been breathing all of our life without paying any attention to it… Sometimes the attempt to control breathing may be a reflection of the need to control other aspects of our lives. In this sense breathing in a mindful way may represent a good opportunity to letting go of the need to push and control, letting things be as they are. Beginning to be confident that it is ok to opening ourselves to life as it unfolds moment by moment, without forcing ourselves to breathe in a certain way." In the third session, practicing yoga, John showed the first signs of insight. By the fourth session, he showed actual surprise. In the group debate he commented that he was feeling more animated. With the yoga exercise he had become aware of his body: "As long as I can remember I have made a huge effort to be good-looking and in shape. This week I have realized through yoga, that I have never really been in my body. My whole life I have used it as an instrument for enjoyment, but I have never been conscious of it." Yoga provided the opportunity for John to be in touch and accept himself. That gave him a framework to focus on the effect that his habits have on him, and to activate mechanisms of self-regulation: "I have realized that killing myself at the gym is not always good for me. For example, I have observed that lifting weights hurts my lower back, and this week I have changed weight-lifting for yoga because that way I can take care of my outer self without neglecting my inner self."

In session 4, as previously explained, we focused more specifically on emotions. We explained the following: "When you realize that there are emotions within you, the key is to describe the characteristics as if you were a witness inside your own body. The first step is naming it the best way you can. For example, aha, I'm feeling… sad. The next step is to describe the sensation without judging it. For example, this is a sensation in my heart, in the left side. It is like a jab, like something is moving inward… By doing this simple trick you are taking up the reins of your life, turning on the freedom center (prefrontal cortex) and turning down your impulsive reaction center (amygdalae). During this exercise, your mind may flood you with thoughts. And, as you know through personal experience, trying to control feelings with thoughts like "I don't want to feel like this," is not an effective way to do so. Now, each time that you realize that you are thinking, you can go back to focusing on describing the real sensations that emotion provokes in your body. After this you can expand your attention and make a space for it inside of you, helping your feelings to mature in their passing through you." This exercise was especially helpful to John, who became aware of automatic patterns that limited his life, as he shared in the fifth session: "There is something inside of me, a sensation that I would call insecurity, that forces me to have to go out and pick up partners in order to demonstrate to myself that people like me. Sometimes I have taken drugs like Ecstasy or Viagra just to be able to be more successful in satisfying other people's expectations of me. I don't know how to fix this." The instructors respond to this comment as follows: "Sometimes we feel an emotion and in the attempt to get rid of it, we create more problems for ourselves. It is the same with physical pain. Something hurts and we start to complain, to drink more or whatever to fight against it all. The harder we fight, the more we hurt, because we create more tension around the pain. It is as if we were trying to remove an arrow by sticking another arrow in. That way we have to fight against two arrows (the feeling and the impulsive reaction consequences). For now, just handling with one arrow (the feeling) is enough." In the sixth session, he tells us that he has managed to maintain this sensation without reacting for most of the week. On Saturday though, he realized that he was doing the same things such as drinking too much or staying up late in order to cover up his emotions. This made him feel like a failure. We answered him with the following words: "The path to free ourselves from the automatic patterns begins by becoming aware. The important thing is that now you know what is happening. It is this feeling that triggers your reactions. And this is the true difference from the other times that you have done this. To be able to change it is necessary that you first take care of your feeling of insecurity." By the way during the last sessions John managed to do the breathing exercise. By doing this, he realized that sometimes things went better for him when he was not trying to control them. This has produced a cascade effect that allowed him to reduce his obsession with his physique and began to take better care of him mentally and emotionally. In his own words: "I was frightened of losing my 'showcase' body, and I was having very dark thoughts. But now I feel better inside, and that is what is really important to me, that I can always return to my body and find peace." In the follow-up a month later at the end of the course he said: "In the past I had always tried to control uncertainty by demanding too much of myself, forcing myself to have a perfect body, a perfect life. I thought that if I had that, the time would come when I would be happy because others would value me. But that moment never came. In trying to control everything I lost confidence in myself. In this course I learned to trust myself and to manage the thoughts of being perfect that were keeping me from enjoying life." When we asked him what he thought had helped him the most, he responded: "Listening that there is nothing to force, nowhere to arrive, that everything is just fine the way it is. Those words come into my head at times when I find myself fighting against the inevitable. I don't even try it just comes to me. Now I know that I am doing things better and losing a part of my physique, but I don't care so much because I feel better about my body now than five years ago. It was also revealing to learn how my mind works and to know that I have a tool to deactivate my amygdalae makes me feel confident about myself." As this book was being

published we contacted him to see how he was doing and he told us that he continued to practice mindfulness, and especially yoga. He was still making changes toward a healthier lifestyle. He was taking his medication regularly and had stopped smoking. He told us that he remembered the course: "I have maintained more or less what I learned, and I practice it often, although not quite so formally. The best has been to discover the power to transform the huge ball of problems, daily frustrations, and problems that had accumulated and against which I had no defenses, into a small ball, that I can manage. Knowing that I have tools to manage my problems makes me feel confident about myself. Thank you for showing me how to do it."

The two cases that we have presented here illustrate two of the main HIV-patient profiles that can be found in the clinical practice according to how individuals cope with stress. The first, portrayed by Anna, amplifies the gravity of the illness very seriously and although she uses problem-focused coping strategies taking her medicine regularly, at the same time she may have coping strategies (such as self-blame) that cause impediments. At the other extreme, we find those who minimize the implications of the virus, like John, and adopt coping devices that lead them to unsafe lifestyles and habits putting themselves, and others, directly at risk. As coping research shows, the strategies used by Anna and John such as blaming oneself for stressful events, escape-avoidance, and distancing, may seem useful in the short term as a way of reducing distress, but in the longer term, they are clearly detrimental and can be associated with negative outcomes, such as deeper depression [64]. These two profiles represent two sides to the same coin, because both have finally had to face up to the same reality and similar challenges. The job of the psychologist or health care provider is to help them find the point of equilibrium at which their level of awareness is adequate enough to take measures that are necessary to adapt to the challenges presented by being HIV-positive. In this sense MBCT training can be helpful. Indeed, a recent study found that dispositional mindfulness is inversely related to escape/avoidance and self-blame forms of coping [65]. Previous studies suggest that turning attention to the present moment's experiences provides an important momentary pleasure that helps to restore the individual's resources and enables them to continue coping with what from the outside appears to be unendurable stress [64].

Practical Considerations of MBCT for HIV

We will describe some practical considerations to take into account when adapting MBCT or MBIs to specific populations.

Group Size and Format

In Spanish hospitals, this population is served through the public health system. Sometimes the courses must adapt to the availability of resources, and therefore might not be under ideal conditions. This is why we have experimented with different group sizes that range from single individuals to groups of up to 20 people. In all cases the program has been successful, although we have observed that the ideal group size is between eight and ten participants. With this size, the sessions are more dynamic and the facilitator can be sure that all of the participants join the debate about the topics dealt with in each session. We generally recommend the group format, although on occasion if a person cannot or does not want to attend group sessions, we offer the option of individual training. This format can combine MBCT with psychotherapy, adapting the proposed concepts to the individual's problems. It is our experience that this format is also effective.

Patient Selection

We generally admit into the PLWH groups anyone with or without symptoms and history of depression. To avoid possible confounding variables, we exclude people from the treatment if they are already involved in some other psychotherapeutic intervention, or if they have a concomitant psychiatric disorder (bipolar disorder, psychotic and/or epileptic episodes).

Facilitator Training

In our opinion, there are two requirements to be a facilitator. The first is to "preach by example," to be "mindful." We tend to use the concept "practice embodiment," because it truly refers to incarnate examples of that which we wish to transmit. To accomplish this one must practice each week what one teaches in order to keep in mind the challenges that one finds in guiding others along the right path. Also, keeping up to date on the advances in research into mindfulness, helps to understand and explain better the process of change that comes from the training. Frequently in the groups, certain delicate topics may come up regarding a person's intimate thoughts, emotions, uncertainties…that require impeccable management by the facilitator. By "impeccable" we mean that the therapist must know how to redirect the session, show support of the individual in question, all from a compassionate yet realistic perspective. For this reason, we recommend that the person who teaches the course have studied psychology or psychotherapy, as well having their own mindfulness practice.

The second requirement refers to being familiar with the unique characteristics and challenges that this population faces along with the health care professionals who take care of them. This helps the instructor to be able to guide and redirect the course of the discussions and group debates, as well as responding realistically to questions that come up.

Setting

When the intervention is carried out in a hospital setting, the fact that medical personnel know about mindfulness makes a difference in that it can greatly enhance the program's success. First, because a recommendation to take the course that comes from a health care professional can increase the confidence and commitment on the part of the patient, yielding better outcomes. Second, mindfulness can serve as an alternative when there is no pharmacological way to address challenges such as premature aging. Practicing mindfulness can also be beneficial for the health care professionals themselves, promoting practitioner well-being and resilience [66]. It is for all of these reasons that we highly recommend that hospitals offer 30-min informative sessions to all health care professionals so that they may acquire information about the nature of the program and its scientifically demonstrated effectiveness.

Home Practice

Daily practice constitutes the heart of this program. Nevertheless, frequently in the sessions we see participants who start to slack off on the amount of practice and need to be reminded of the importance of keeping to the regime. In the pre-intervention session it is important to point out the requirements of practice as well as manage psychological resistance to practice. This effort needs to be continued throughout all of the sessions. Also adapting the length of the practice in such a way as to help participants to incorporate the practice in their daily lives in formal (i.e., doing the body scan for 10 min) and informal ways (i.e., guided breathing for 1 min). In order to facilitate the maintenance of benefits it is fundamental to practice. For this reason we recommend to organize follow-up monthly sessions, sometimes termed alumni groups.

Proposed Mechanisms of Change

As both MBSR and MBCT share common core elements, it has been proposed that they may also have similar underlying mechanisms [67]. A review of recent research about action mechanisms of MBIs from the perspective of Neuroscience as well as from a theoretical-based point of view [48, 61, 68–74] reveals a certain lack of coherence partially derived from differences in nomenclature and no established order among components [71]. Besides, as mindfulness research continues to expand, it has been generated a lack of clarity of what mechanisms lead to change. In an attempt to find coherence, we have considered previous research as well as the testimony of participants in our groups of clinical and

general population over the last decade. We have developed a meta-model that tries to identify a common structure that synthesizes the main mechanisms of MBSR and MBCT (Fig. 8.2). It is a simple, transversal model that adopts a hierarchical perspective, thereby establishing order among the different mechanisms. The model proposes that when people begin to practice mindfulness, they do so by training their attention. This training generates the development of metacognitive skills that prepare the terrain to activate the self-regulation mechanisms that allow them to make changes in order to adapt better to the challenges that they face. At the same time, this contributes to how a person develops well-being at multiple levels, which in turn reinforces the practice of mindfulness. For this reason, the model can be seen not as a closed circle, but rather as a spiral in which well-being that they experience in practicing mindfulness feeds the reset of the process at a higher level. This causes a progressive increase in the level of awareness. Therefore, at the first level, the persons change aspects that are relative to their physical well-being, and progressively this change spreads (as illustrated by the next levels of the spiral in Fig. 8.2) to dimensions that are more complex and subtle in their lives, such as emotional, cognitive, relational, and even spiritual ones. In the next section we will describe the main mechanisms by reviewing previous studies and the findings based on neuroscience (Table 8.1 shows a description of these components and the brain-related areas):

Attention

Mindfulness begins with attentional training. Indeed, mindfulness is defined as intentional, non-judgmental attention to the present moment experiences [45]. Mindfulness skills require learning to direct attention in a specific way: with an attitude of kindness (without tension) and of impartial observation and equanimity. It also requires the intention to accept whatever experience is happening at the moment (a thought, a feeling, or an emotion), without judgment and without acting in an automatic way. The study of attention has identi-

Fig. 8.2 Meta model for
mindfulness mechanisms of
change

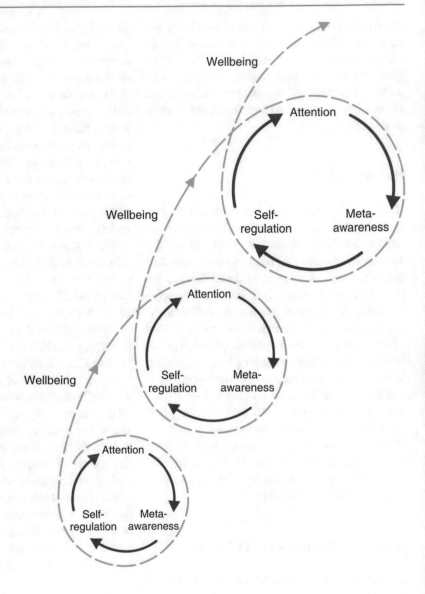

Table 8.1 Description of mechanisms of change of MBIs and associated brain areas

Mechanism	Definition	Associated brain areas
Attention	Ability to orient and maintain attention intentionally, with kindness, accepting everything as it is	Anterior cingulate cortex, striatum, dorsolateral prefrontal cortex and parietal areas
Meta-awareness	Ability to take awareness itself without identifying with self-referential processes	Insula, temporoparietal junction, medial prefrontal cortex
Self-regulation	Ability to orient one's cognitive, emotional, physiological, and behavioral responses in order to work toward a desired goal	Anterior cingulate cortex, medial prefrontal cortex

fied three different anatomical networks proposed as a framework to integrate parallel findings in psychological science [75]. These three components are alerting (achieving and maintaining a state of readiness to attend to stimuli), orienting (selecting specific stimuli from sensory input), and executive attention (monitoring and resolving conflict among thoughts, feelings, and responses) [76]. By now, there is evidence of improved attention regulation and strengthened brain activity in attentional areas following mindfulness training [74]. One systematic review that compiled these studies concludes that early phases of mindfulness training might be associated with improvements in orienting and executive attention, whereas later phases might be associated with alerting attention improvements [77].

The cerebral region that has most systematically been associated with the effects of mindfulness is the one that manages executive attention, the anterior cingulate cortex (ACC). Several studies found ACC activation during mindfulness training. Moreover, structural studies found that mindfulness meditation might be associated with greater cortical thickness [78] and enhanced white matter integrity in the ACC [79, 80].

Other attention related areas in which functional changes have been observed following this kind of training include dorsolateral prefrontal cortex (PFC, also implicated in executive attention) and parietal regions (implicated in alerting attention) (see [74] for a review of Neuroscience findings of mindfulness meditation). Following the model that we propose, this attention effect from mindfulness training facilitates acquiring the skills by the second mechanism.

Meta-awareness

It refers to the heightened self-awareness that comes with mindfulness practice in terms of increased ability to notice one's thoughts, emotions, body sensations, and behaviors. It also refers to the development of metacognitive skills through which a person changes from self-referenced processing to an open frame of mind of enhanced awareness of present moment experiences. It includes learning to see thoughts and feelings as temporary and auto-

matic events in the mind instead of as of real facts or true descriptions [45, 81]. Meta-awareness also points to the possibility of taking awareness itself as an object of attention [82]. In this kind of awareness we disidentify ourselves from our ego and reidentify with pure awareness. As a recent review proposes, this shift in awareness may be one of the major active mechanisms of change of mindfulness meditation [74]. This concept has been called decentering and is defined as the capacity to observe one's thoughts and feelings as temporary events in the mind, rather than as valid reflections of reality or central aspects of the self [62].

Mindfulness interventions have been shown to enhance activity in the main area associated with meta-awareness, the insula [72, 83, 84]. The insula has been proposed to be involved in awareness of experiences of the present moment [85–87] and of internal bodily states [88, 89], as well as in emotional processing [86]. In a recent neuroimaging study, the ability of experienced mindfulness practitioners to exert self-control was related with activity in the insula, proposing that a plausible mechanism of action for mindfulness may include the development of metacognitive skills for detached viewing of emotion [90]. In this way of thinking, some research suggests that mindfulness may represent a neural path for regulating emotions by reducing self-referential activity (associated with cortical midline and language area recruitment) and by balancing regulatory responses (with coordinated monitoring of less valenced and more sensory visceral information) [86]. There is also evidence that ties Mindfulness to a lesser activity in what is called the default mode network (DMN), a series of interconnected regions of the brain that are activated when we do not carry out specific tasks, and that induces a state of mind-wandering [91, 92]. These results fit with our proposal that meta-awareness or "becoming aware" of automatic patterns of thoughts, feelings, actions, and reactions may play a role as a previous step that makes self-regulation possible.

Self-Regulation

This is a central concept in psychology and psychopathology. According to Karoly [93] it is defined as a process that enables individuals to guide their goal-directed activities by modulation of thought, affect, behavior, or attention via deliberate or automated use of specific mechanisms. It includes the ability to focus attention on a given task, to regulate internal (thoughts, feelings) and external distractions, and to work toward a desired outcome or goal. Self-regulation is a broad concept that includes cognitive, emotional, and behavioral regulation [94]. Self-regulation at the cognitive and emotional levels represents a key component in mindfulness. This kind of self-regulation is closely related with the mindfulness facet named nonreactivity, referring to the ability to allow one's thoughts and feelings (pleasant and unpleasant) to come and go, without reacting to them [95]. Recent studies report that improvement on general psychopathological symptoms following mindfulness training was mediated by this ability [96]. In addition, a recent meta-analysis identified strong, consistent evidence for regulating cognitive and emotional reactivity as mechanisms underlying MBIs [74]. Furthermore, self-regulation at the behavioral level, the ability to respond in an adaptive manner instead of reacting impulsively, is closely related with inhibitory control, the ability to inhibit prepotent course actions and resistance to interference from irrelevant stimuli [97, 98]. Previous research has shown that mindfulness training is particularly relevant to improve this kind of inhibitory control [79, 99].

Self-regulation abilities have been associated with the anterior cingulate cortex (ACC), an area that controls the influx of information from the environment in order to avoid conflicting responses in behavior [94]. As we have mentioned earlier in this chapter, recent studies have shown that mindfulness training produces changes in this area of the brain. In this way, mindfulness has been related to increased integrity and efficiency of the white matter linking the ACC and other regions of the brain. This suggests increments in the capacity of the individual for self-regulation at the cognitive and emotional levels [100] (see also [74] for a detailed review). Most of the ACC activity, as well as activity in the PFC, encouraged by the MBIs can be associ-

ated with more control of the regions of the lower brain where initial phases of sensorial and emotional processing take place: the thalamus and the amygdalae [101].

Up to this point we have identified the three main mechanisms of change that underlies MBIs. All of these components interact closely, maintaining bidirectional relationships, thereby contributing to enhanced well-being. As numerous studies show, MBIs result in an enhanced state of well-being in emotional, psychological and physical dimensions [102–104]. Well-being has been associated with an increased ability in individuals to respond positively to difficult circumstances and experiences encountered in life. This leads to dynamic balance point between an individual's resource pool and the challenges faced, enhancing the idea of equilibrium/homeostasis [105]. This definition of well-being can provide a framework to group together the multiple effects from MBIs in the following dimensions:

- Psychological: e.g., lower levels of rumination [106] or higher levels of life satisfaction [107].
- Emotional: e.g., less depression and anxiety [103, 108, 109].
- Physiological: in terms of self-reported health [102, 104], and in terms of more objective indicators such as improving immune response to vaccination [110], reducing chronic inflammation [111], improving disease-related parameters [104], or altering expression of inflammatory genomic markers [112].

To illustrate the process, let us take a look at a brief example. Imagine the case of a man who begins to learn about MBIs. In the first sessions, he starts to train his attention intentionally and without judgment directing their bodily sensations (Attention). In doing so he realizes that he puts too much tension in a certain part of their body (Meta-awareness). Then he begins to loosen the tension (Self-regulation). He perceives this alleviation as well-being, which in turn encourages him to continue practicing. At the next level, as he continues to train his attention, he realizes how a painful feeling sets off old automatic patterns of thoughts and impulsive reactions (Meta-awareness). The fact that he realizes all of these aspects sets the stage for beginning to change his conscious response to situations instead of reacting impulsively (Self-regulation). When he realizes how those thoughts affect him, he begins to develop a self-compassion that helps him to feel more at peace with himself. This well-being feeds the process of spreading the mindfulness skills to higher dimensions and adds to a progression in their perceived ability to empower himself, gaining well-being at multiple levels of his live. In Anna and John's cases, we can see this process clearly. They began to accept the physical sensations and as they continue to practice, they began to accept their present situations, themselves and their own history (including the HIV diagnosis). In sum, this meta-model may help clinicians as well as researchers to understand and integrate the process by which MBIs produce changes at multiple levels.

Future Directions and Conclusions

Living with HIV represents a paradigmatic condition of chronic stress. Stress has been shown to deplete the self-regulation resources needed to facilitate adaptive mechanisms to cope with life challenges both at the psycho-emotional and physical levels. Moreover, as the population of PLWH over age 50 continues to grow, methods to facilitate successful aging for this population are compellingly needed. Successful aging is referred to as a process of accepting and coping with the challenges of aging [113]. Accumulated research of mindfulness, in general, and MBCT in particular, suggests that MBIs may help to replenish these vital adaptive resources, leading to improved self-regulation and well-being.

Emerging studies about MBCT application to HIV offer preliminary support to encourage advanced research in this area. We recommend that researchers conduct RCTs trials that include active control groups in order to identify specific active ingredients of MBCT. In addition, the field should move towards examining mechanisms of change and mediators of outcomes. In this way

we can pursue an increased measure of integration of multiple theories incorporating the advances in Neuroscience and adding them to research on PNI can reveal new perspectives. As previously called for, a closer collaboration between clinicians and neuroscientists is also needed in order to make advances in the clinical potential of MBIs [106]. Even though we agree that it is worthwhile to continue research in neurological mechanisms, we also believe that an exclusively neurocentric approach is not enough. In order to reach a deeper understanding of intricate mind-body mechanisms underlying MBCT and MBIs benefits, we suggest looking at them from a wider perspective, including measures of peripheral physiology such as heart rate variability (HRV), an indicator of emotional regulation and a marker for flexible dynamic regulation of autonomic nervous system flexibility [114].

Although the work that we have done so far is promising, it is also fortunate that there is still much more that we can do in bringing light to the study of human awareness. This enhanced awareness constitutes the base to be able to start to change from rigidity to a flexible state in our lives. Flexibility means finely honing the adaptive abilities at every dimension of our lives, cognitive, emotional, physiological, social, and also spiritual levels. In this sense, flexibility means balance and health and rigidity means suffering.

In our experience, accumulated through the teaching of MBIs, the process through which all, as human beings, increase our level of awareness and begin to self-regulate is basically the same. Both therapists and patients face similar challenges in order to be able to enjoy a full life. The difference lies merely in the ways that the challenges manifest themselves. It is our mission, as mindfulness guides, to impeccably manage participants' experiences in enhancing their self-awareness. It is for this reason that we are required to be disciplined enough to utilize each one of the difficulties that we encounter along the way to enhance our own self-awareness. Only through our own self-awareness, only when we are capable of managing our own difficulties honestly, are we then able to accompany others in this fascinating journey. Therefore, by learning to live our lives in a more flexible and meaningful way, each of us contributes to improving the well-being of society as a whole.

References

1. Harden VA. Aids at 30: a history. Washington, DC: Potomac; 2012.
2. Tomes N. The gospel of germs: men, women and the microbe in American life. Cambridge: Harvard University; 1999.
3. Gottlieb MS, Schroff R, Schanker HM, Weisman JD, Fan PT, Wolf RA, et al. Pneumocystis carinii pneumonia and mucosal candidiasis in previously healthy homosexual men: evidence of a new acquired cellular immunodeficiency. N Engl J Med. 1981;305:1425–31.
4. UNAIDS. The GAP report. Joint United Nations Programme on HIV/AIDS. Geneva: United Nations; 2014.
5. Coffin JM, Hugues SH, Varmus HE. Retroviruses. New York, NY: Cold Spring Harbor Laboratory; 1997.
6. Palella Jr FJ, Delaney KM, Moorman AC, Loveless MO, Fuhrer J, Satten GA, et al. Declining morbidity and mortality among patients with advanced human immunodeficiency virus infection. N Engl J Med. 1998;338:853–60.
7. Van Sighem AI, van de Wiel MA, Ghani AC, Jambroes M, Reiss P, Gyssens IC. Mortality and progression to AIDS after starting highly active antiretroviral therapy. AIDS. 2003;17:2227–36.
8. Bangsberg DR, Porco TC, Kagay C, Charlebois ED, Deeks SG, Guzman D, et al. Modeling the HIV protease inhibitor adherence-resistance curve by use of empirically derived estimates. J Infect Dis. 2004;190:162–5.
9. Bhatia R, Ryscavage P, Babafeni T. Accelerated aging and human immunodeficiency virus infection: emerging challenges of growing older in the era of successful antiretroviral therapy. J Neurovirol. 2012;18:247–55.
10. Effros RB, Fletcher CV, Gebo K, Halter JB, Hazzard WR, Horne FM, et al. Aging and infectious diseases: workshop on HIV infection and aging: what is known and future research directions. Clin Infect Dis. 2008;47:542–53.
11. Deeks SG. HIV infection, inflammation, immunosenescence, and aging. Annu Rev Med. 2011;62:141–55.
12. Lohse N, Hansen AB, Pedersen G, Kronborg G, Gerstoft J, Sørensen HT, et al. Survival of persons with and without HIV infection in Denmark, 1995–2005. Ann Intern Med. 2007;146:87–95.
13. Antiretroviral Therapy Cohort Collaboration. Life expectancy of individuals on combination antiretroviral therapy in high-income countries: a collaborative analysis of 14 cohort studies. Lancet. 2008;372:293–9.
14. May M, Gompels M, Delpech V, Porter K, Post F, Johnson M, et al. Impact of late diagnosis and treatment on life-expectancy in people with HIV-1: UK Collaborative HIV Cohort (UK CHIC) Study. BMJ. 2011;343:d6016.
15. Marzolini C, Back D, Weber R, Furrer H, Cavassini M, Calmy A, et al. Ageing with HIV: medication use and risk for potential drug–drug interactions. J Antimicrob Chemother. 2011;66:2107–11.
16. Rockwood K. Frailty and its definition: a worthy challenge. J Am Geriatr Soc. 2005;53:1069.
17. Desquilbet L, Jacobson LP, Fried LP, Phair JP, Jamieson BD, Holloway M, et al. Multicenter AIDS Cohort Study. HIV-1 infection is associated with an earlier occurrence of a phenotype related to frailty. J Gerontol A Biol Sci Med Sci. 2007;62:1279–86.
18. Nasi M, Pinti M, De Biasi S, Gibellini L, Ferraro D, Mussini C, et al. Aging with HIV infection: a journey to the center of inflammAIDS, immunosenescence and neuroHIV. Immunol Lett. 2014;162:329–33.
19. Tsoukas C. Immunosenescence and aging in HIV. Curr Opin HIV AIDS. 2014;9:398–404.
20. Freund A, Orjalo AV, Desprez PY, Campisi J. Inflammatory networks during cellular senescence: causes and consequences. Trends Mol Med. 2010;16:238–46.
21. Moskowitz JT, Wrubel J, Hult JR, Maurer S, Acree M. Illness appraisals and depression in the first year after HIV diagnosis. PLoS One. 2013;8, e78904.
22. Howland LC, Gortmaker SL, Mofenson LM, Spino C, Gardner JD, Gorski H, et al. Effects of negative life events on immune suppression in children and youth infected with human immunodeficiency virus type 1. Pediatrics. 2000;106:540–6.
23. Fumaz C, Muñoz-Moreno J, Ferrer M, Gonzalez-Garcia M, Perez-Alvarez N, Miranda C, et al. Aging-associated symptoms in the physician-patient dialogue in a group of long-term diagnosed HIV-infected individuals. J Int AIDS Soc. 2012;15:18164.
24. Ballester-Arnal R, Gomez-Martinez S, Fumaz CR, Gonzalez-Garcia M, Eduardo Remor E, Fuster MJ. A Spanish study on psychosocial predictors of quality of life in people with HIV. AIDS Behav. 2015. doi:10.1007/s10461-015-1208-6.
25. Mundt C, Reck C, Backenstrass M, Kronmüller K, Fiedler P. Reconfirming the role of life events for the timing of depressive episodes. A two-year prospective follow-up study. J Affect Disord. 2000;59:23–30.
26. Slavich GM, Irwin MR. From stress to inflammation and major depressive disorder: a social signal transduction theory of depression. Psychol Bull. 2014;140:774–815.
27. Komiti A, Judd F, Grech P, Mijch A, Hoy J, Williams B, et al. Depression in people living with HIV/AIDS attending primary care and outpatient clinics. Aust N Z J Psychiatry. 2003;37:70–7.
28. Judd F, Komiti A, Chua P, Mijch A, Hoy J, Grech P, et al. Nature of depression in patients with HIV/AIDS. Aust N Z J Psychiatry. 2005;39:826–32.
29. Bing EG, Burnam MA, Longshore D, Fleishman JA, Sherbourne CD, London AS, et al. Psychiatric disorders and drug use among human immunodeficiency virus-infected adults in the United States. Arch Gen Psychiatry. 2001;58:721–8.
30. Ciesla JA, Roberts JE. Meta-analysis of the relationship between HIV infection and risk for depressive disorders. Am J Psychiatry. 2001;158:725–30.
31. Emlet CA. "You're awfully old to have this disease": experiences of stigma and ageism in adults 50 years

and older living with HIV/AIDS. Gerontologist. 2006;46:781–90.

32. Fumaz CR, Muñoz-Moreno JA, Ferrer MJ, Gonzalez-Garcia M, Negredo E, Perez-Alvarez N, et al. Emotional impact of premature aging symptoms in long-term treated HIV-infected subjects. J AIDS. 2012;59:5–8.

33. McIntosh RC, Rosselli M, Uddin LQ, Antoni M. Neuropathological sequelae of human immunodeficiency virus and apathy: a review of neuropsychological and neuroimaging studies. Neurosci Biobehav Rev. 2015;55:147–64.

34. Cohen SE, Janicki-Deverts D, Miller GE. Psychological stress and disease. JAMA. 2007;298:1685–7.

35. Kiecolt-Glaser JK, Preacher KJ, MacCallum RC, Atkinson C, Malarkey WB, Glaser R. Chronic stress and age-related increases in the proinflammatory cytokine IL-6. Proc Natl Acad Sci. 2003;100:9090–5.

36. Glaser R, Robles TF, Sheridan J, Malarkey WB, Kiecolt-Glaser JK. Mild depressive symptoms are associated with amplified and prolonged inflammatory responses after influenza virus vaccination in older adults. Arch Gen Psychiatry. 2003;60:1009–14.

37. Fumaz CR, Gonzalez-Garcia M, Borras X, Muñoz-Moreno JA, Perez-Alvarez N, Mothe B, et al. Psychological stress is associated with high levels of IL-6 in HIV-1 infected individuals on effective combined antiretroviral treatment. Brain Behav Immun. 2012;26:568–72.

38. Patterson S, Moran P, Epel E, Sinclair E, Kemeny ME, Deeks SG, et al. Cortisol patterns are associated with T cell activation in HIV. PLoS One. 2013;8, e63429.

39. Maes M, Berk M, Goehler L, Song C, Anderson G, Gałecki P, et al. Depression and sickness behavior are Janus-faced responses to shared inflammatory pathways. BMC Med. 2012;10:66.

40. Antoni MH. Stress, coping, and health in HIV/AIDS. In: Folkman S, editor. The Oxford handbook of stress, health, and coping. Oxford: Oxford University; 2010. p. 428–42.

41. Kiecolt-Glaser JK, Belury MA, Porter K, Beversdorf DQ, Lemeshow S, Glaser R. Depressive symptoms, omega-6:omega-3 fatty acids, and inflammation in older adults. Psychosom Med. 2007;69:217–24.

42. Von Känel R, Dimsdale JE, Ancoli-Israel S, Mills PJ, Patterson TL, McKibbin CL, et al. Poor sleep is associated with higher plasma proinflammatory cytokine interleukin-6 and procoagulant marker fibrin D-dimer in older caregivers of people with Alzheimer's disease. J Am Geriatr Soc. 2006;54:431–7.

43. McEwen BS. Stress, adaptation, and disease. Allostasis and allostatic load. Ann N Y Acad Sci. 1998;840:33–44.

44. Sterling P, Eyer J. Allostasis: a new paradigm to explain arousal pathology. In: Fisher S, Reason J, editors. Handbook of life stress, cognition, and health. New York, NY: Wiley; 1988. p. 629–49.

45. Kabat-Zinn J. Full catastrophe living: using the wisdom of your body and mind to face stress, pain, and illness. New York, NY: Delta; 1990.

46. Turner-Cobb JM, Gore-Felton C, Marouf F, Koopman C, Kim P, Israelski D, et al. Coping, social support, and attachment style as psychosocial correlates of adjustment in men and women with HIV/AIDS. J Behav Med. 2002;25:337–53.

47. Logsdon-Conradsen S. Using mindfulness meditation to promote holistic health in individuals with HIV/AIDS. Cogn Behav Pract. 2002;9:67–72.

48. Vago DR, Silbersweig DA. Self-awareness, self-regulation, and self-transcendence (S-ART): a framework for understanding the neurobiological mechanisms of mindfulness. Front Hum Neurosci. 2012;6:296.

49. Turner K. The promotion of successful aging through mindfulness skills training. Doctorate in Social work (DSW) dissertations, paper 1; 2010.

50. Valiente-Barroso C. Practica de la meditación y neuroprotección frente a la demencia: profundizando en el concepto de reserva cerebral. In: Perez Serrano S, editor. Envejecimiento activo y solidaridad intergeneracional: claves para un envejecimiento activo. Madrid: UNED; 2012. p. 65.

51. Creswell JD, Myers HF, Cole SW, Irwin MR. Mindfulness meditation training effects on CD4? T lymphocytes in HIV-1 infected adults: a small randomized controlled trial. Brain Behav Immun. 2009;23:184–8.

52. Sibinga EM, Stewart M, Magyari T, Welsh CK, Hutton N, Ellen JM. Mindfulness-based stress reduction for HIV-infected youth: a pilot study. Explore (NY). 2008;4:36–7.

53. Jam S, Imani AH, Foroughi M, SeyedAlinaghi S, Koochak HE, Mohraz M. The effects of mindfulness-based stress reduction (MBSR) program in Iranian HIV/AIDS patients: a pilot study. Acta Med Iran. 2010;48:101–6.

54. SeyedAlinaghi S, Jam S, Foroughi M, Imani A, Mohraz M, Djavid GE, et al. Randomized controlled trial of mindfulness-based stress reduction delivered to human immunodeficiency virus-positive patients in Iran: effects on CD4? T lymphocyte count and medical and psychological symptoms. Psychosom Med. 2012;74:620–7.

55. Gayner B, Esplen MJ, Deroche P, Wong J, Bishop S, Kavanagh L, et al. A randomized controlled trial of mindfulness-based stress reduction to manage affective symptoms and improve quality of life in gay men living with HIV. J Behav Med. 2012;35:272–85.

56. Robinson FP, Mathews HL, Witek-Janusez L. Psycho-endocrine-immune response to mindfulness-based stress reduction in individuals infected with the human immunodeficiency virus: a quasiexperimental study. J Altern Complement Med. 2003;9:683–94.

57. Duncan LG, Moskowitz JT, Neilands TB, Dilworth SE, Hecht FM, Johnson MO. Mindfulness-based stress reduction for HIV treatment side effects: a randomized, wait-list controlled trial. J Pain Symptom Manage. 2012;43:161–71.

58. Riley KE, Kalichman S. Mindfulness-based stress reduction for people living with HIV/AIDS: preliminary review of intervention trial methodologies and findings. Health Psychol Rev. 2015;9:224–43.

59. Wood NA. Mindfulness-based cognitive therapy for the symptoms of depression in a community-based HIV/AIDS clinic: outcomes and feasibility. Chester: Widener University; 2008.

60. Gonzalez-Garcia M, Ferrer MJ, Borras X, Muñoz-Moreno JA, Miranda C, Puig J, et al. Effectiveness of mindfulness-based cognitive therapy on the quality of life, emotional status, and CD4 cell count of patients aging with HIV Infection. AIDS Behav. 2014;18(4):676–85.

61. Baer RA. Mindfulness training as a clinical intervention: a conceptual and empirical review. Clin Psychol Sci Pract. 2003;10(2):125–43.

62. Segal ZV, Williams JMG, Teasdale JD. Mindfulness-based cognitive therapy for depression: a new approach to preventing relapse. New York, NY: Guilford; 2002.

63. Gonzalez Garcia M. Mindfulness y VIH. Efecto sobre calidad de vida, estrés percibido, estado emocional y situación inmunológica. Doctoral dissertation, Barcelona: Autonomous University of Barcelona, Barcelona; 2012.

64. Folkman S, Chesney MA, Christopher-Richards A. Stress and coping in caregiving partners of men with AIDS. Psychiatr Clin North Am. 1994;17:35–53.

65. Moskowitz LG, Duncan PJ, Moran M, Acree ES, Epel ME, Kemeny FM, et al. Dispositional mindfulness in people with HIV: associations with psychological and physical health. Pers Indiv Differ. 2015;86:88–93.

66. Krasner MS, Epstein RM, Beckman H, Suchman AL, Chapman B, Mooney CJ, et al. Association of an educational program in mindful communication with burnout, empathy, and attitudes among primary care physicians. JAMA. 2009;302:1284–93.

67. Gu J, Strauss C, Bond R, Cavanagh K. How do mindfulness-based cognitive therapy and mindfulness-based stress reduction improve mental health and wellbeing? A systematic review and meta-analysis of mediation studies. Clin Psychol Rev. 2015;37:1–12.

68. Shapiro SL, Carlson LE, Astin JA, Freedman B. Mechanisms of mindfulness. J Clin Psychol. 2006;62:373–86.

69. Brown KW, Ryan RM, Creswell JD. Mindfulness: theoretical foundations and evidence for its salutary effects. Psychol Inq. 2007;18:211–37.

70. Grabovac AD, Lau MA, Willett BR. Mechanisms of mindfulness: a Buddhist psychological model. Mindfulness. 2011;2:154–66.

71. Hölzel BK, Lazar SW, Gard T, Schuman-Olivier Z, Vago DR, Ott U. How does mindfulness meditation work? Proposing mechanisms of action from a conceptual and neural perspective. Perspect Psychol Sci. 2011;6:537–59.

72. Farb NA, Segal ZV, Anderson AK. Mindfulness meditation training alters cortical representations of interoceptive attention. Soc Cogn Affect Neurosci. 2013;8:15–26.

73. Creswell JD. Biological pathways linking mindfulness with health. In: Brown KW, Creswell JD, Ryan RM, editors. Handbook of mindfulness: theory, research, and practice. New York, NY: Guilford; 2014. p. 426–41.

74. Tang YY, Hölzel BK, Posner MI. The neuroscience of mindfulness meditation. Nat Rev Neurosci. 2015;16:213–25.

75. Posner MI, Rothbart MK. Research on attention networks as a model for the integration of psychological science. Annu Rev Psychol. 2007;58:1–23.

76. Petersen SE, Posner MI. The attention system of the human brain: 20 years after. Annu Rev Neurosci. 2012;35:73–89.

77. Chiesa A, Calati R, Serretti A. Does mindfulness training improve cognitive abilities? A systematic review of neuropsychological findings. Clin Psychol Rev. 2011;31:449–64.

78. Grant JA, Courtemanche J, Duerden EG, Duncan GH, Rainville P. Cortical thickness and pain sensitivity in Zen meditators. Emotion. 2010;10:43–53.

79. Tang YY, Ma Y, Wang J, Fan Y, Feng S, Lu Q, et al. Short-term meditation training improves attention and self-regulation. Proc Natl Acad Sci U S A. 2007;104:17152–6.

80. Tang YY, Lu Q, Fan M, Yang Y, Posner MI. Mechanisms of white matter changes induced by meditation. Proc Natl Acad Sci. 2012;109:10570–4.

81. Teasdale JD, Segal Z, Williams JM. How does cognitive therapy prevent depressive relapse and why should attentional control (mindfulness) training help? Behav Res Ther. 1995;33:25–39.

82. Lutz A, Dunne JD, Davidson RJ. Meditation and the neuroscience of consciousness. In: Zelazo P, Moscovitch M, Thompson E, editors. Cambridge handbook of consciousness. New York, NY: Cambridge University; 2007. p. 499–555.

83. Lutz A, Brefczynski-Lewis J, Johnstone T, Davidson RJ. Regulation of the neural circuitry of emotion by compassion meditation: effects of meditative expertise. PLoS One. 2008;3, e1897.

84. Tang YY, Ma Y, Fan Y, Feng H, Wang J, Feng S. Central and autonomic nervous system interaction is altered by short-term meditation. Proc Natl Acad Sci. 2009;106:8865–70.

85. Farb NA, Segal ZV, Mayberg H, Bean J, McKeon D, Fatima Z, et al. Attending to the present: mindfulness meditation reveals distinct neural modes of self-reference. Soc Cogn Affect Neurosci. 2007;2:313–22.

86. Farb NA, Anderson AK, Mayberg H, Bean J, McKeon D, Segal ZV. Minding one's emotions: mindfulness training alters the neural expression of sadness. Emotion. 2010;10:25–33.

87. Farb NA, Segal ZV, Anderson AK. Attentional modulation of primary interoceptive and exteroceptive cortices. Cereb Cortex. 2013;23:114–26.

88. Critchley HD, Wiens S, Rotshtein P, Ohman A, Dolan RJ. Neural systems supporting interoceptive awareness. Nat Neurosci. 2004;7:189–95.

89. Craig AD. How do you feel – now? The anterior insula and human awareness. Nat Rev Neurosci. 2009;10:59–70.

90. Kirk U, Montague PR. Mindfulness meditation modulates reward prediction errors in a passive conditioning task. Front Psychol. 2015;6:90.

91. Brewer JA, Worhunsky PD, Gray JR, Tang YY, Weber J, Kober H. Meditation experience is associated with dif-

ferences in default mode network activity and connectivity. Proc Natl Acad Sci U S A. 2011;108:20254–9.

92. Marchand WR. Neural mechanisms of mindfulness and meditation: evidence from neuroimaging studies. World J Radiol. 2014;28:471–9.

93. Karoly P. Mechanisms of self-regulation: a systems view. Ann Rev Psychol. 1993;44:23–52.

94. Posner MI, Rothbart MK, Sheese BE, Tang Y. The anterior cingulate gyrus and the mechanism of self-regulation. Cogn Affect Behav Neurosci. 2007;7:391–5.

95. Baer RA, Smith GT, Lykins E, Button D, Krietemeyer J, Sauer S, et al. Construct validity of the five facets mindfulness questionnaire in meditating and nonmeditating samples. Assessment. 2008;15:329–42.

96. Heeren A, Deplus S, Peschard V, Nef F, Kotsou I, Dierickx C, et al. Does change in self-reported mindfulness mediate the clinical benefits of mindfulness training? A controlled study using the French translation of the five facet mindfulness questionnaire. Mindfulness. 2015;6:553–9.

97. Bjorklund DF, Harnishfeger KK. The evolution of inhibition mechanisms and their role in human cognition and behavior. In: Dempster FN, Brainerd CJ, editors. Interference and inhibition in cognition. San Diego, CA: Academic; 1995. p. 142–69.

98. Nigg JT. On the inhibition/disinhibition in developmental psychopathology: views from cognitive and personality psychology and a working inhibition taxonomy. Psychol Bull. 2000;126:220–46.

99. Chiesa A, Serretti A. A systematic review of neurobiological and clinical features of mindfulness meditations. Psychol Med. 2010;40:1239–52.

100. Tang YY, Yang L, Leve LD, Harold GT. Improving executive function and its neurobiological mechanisms through a mindfulness-based intervention: advances within the field of developmental neuroscience. Child Dev Perspect. 2012;6:361–6.

101. Zeidan F. The neurobiology of mindfulness meditation. In: Brown KW, Creswell JD, Ryan RM, editors. Handbook of mindfulness: theory, research, and practice. New York, NY: Guilford; 2014. p. 171–89.

102. Grossman P, Niemann L, Schmidt S, Walach H. Mindfulness-based stress reduction and health benefits: a meta analysis. J Psychosom Res. 2004;57:35–43.

103. Keng SL, Smoski MJ, Robins CJ. Effects of mindfulness on psychological health: a review of empirical studies. Clin Psychol Rev. 2011;31:1041–56.

104. Carlson LE. Mindfulness-based interventions for physical conditions: a narrative review evaluating levels of evidence. ISRN Psychiatry. 2012;2012:651583.

105. Dodge R, Daly A, Huyton J, Sanders L. The challenge of defining wellbeing. Int J Wellbeing. 2012;2:222–35.

106. Van der Velden AM, Roepstorff A. Neural mechanisms of mindfulness meditation: bridging clinical and neuroscience investigations. Nat Rev Neurosci. 2015;16:439.

107. Christopher MS, Gilbert BD. Incremental validity of components of mindfulness in the prediction of satisfaction with life and depression. Curr Psychol. 2009;29:10–23.

108. Brown KW, Ryan RM. The benefits of being present: mindfulness and its role in psychological well-being. J Pers Soc Psychol. 2003;84:822–48.

109. Shapiro SL, Oman D, Thoresen CE, Plante TG, Flinders T. Cultivating mindfulness: effects on well-being. J Clin Psychol. 2008;64:840–62.

110. Davidson RJ, Kabat-Zinn J, Schumacher J, Rosenkranz M, Muller D, Santorelli SF, et al. Alterations in brain and immune function produced by mindfulness meditation. Psychosom Med. 2003;65:564–70.

111. Rosenkranz MA, Davidson RJ, MacCoon DG, Sheridan JF, Kalin NH, Lutz A. A comparison of mindfulness-based stress reduction and an active control in modulation of neurogenic inflammation. Brain Behav Immun. 2013;27:174–84.

112. Kaliman P, Alvarez-López MJ, Cosín-Tomás M, Rosenkranz MA, Lutz A, Davidson RJ. Rapid changes in histone deacetylases and inflammatory gene expression in expert meditators. Psychoneuroendocrinology. 2014;40:96–107.

113. Baltes PB, Baltes MM. Psychological perspectives on successful aging: the model of selective optimization and compensation. In: Baltes PB, Baltes MM, editors. Successful aging: percpectives from the behavioral sciences. Cambridge: New York, NY; 1990. p. 1–34.

114. Thayer JF, Ahs F, Fredrikson M, Sollers 3rd JJ, Wager TD. A meta-analysis of heart rate variability and neuroimaging studies: implications for heart rate variability as a marker of stress and health. Neurosci Biobehav Rev. 2012;36:747–56.

Mindfulness-Based Cognitive Therapy for Severe Health Anxiety or Hypochondriasis

David Adam Lovas

Clinical Case Study

Derek is a 40-year-old married man who works as a custodian at a shopping mall, and who was referred to our study by his primary care physician due to his escalating presentations to the clinic with a barrage of somatic complaints and illness fears. Most recently, his fears were triggered when he was cleaning out a dumpster, and thought that he felt something sharp on one of his fingers. Derek quickly examined himself, but found no obvious hole in his rubber gloves nor puncture wound on his finger. However, he could not shake the thought that he had been stuck by a small needle. This thought quickly cascaded to the conclusion that the needle was used by an IV drug user, and that he would contract HIV. While he had a flash of self-awareness—recognizing his long-standing and agonizing pattern of illness fears dating back to adolescence—the terror

quickly won out. Derek started researching the potential consequences online. As he typed and clicked, he regularly paused to inspect and rub the potentially pricked finger, convinced it felt "weird." He also described the situation to his wife, who shook her head and told him that he was "crazy just like his mother," and who made it clear she was sick of hearing about it.

Derek took the fears to his doctor with trepidation, as he sensed that he, too, was becoming tired of his anxieties. However, Derek was able to convince the doctor to do an HIV test. He was temporarily soothed by this intervention and by the negative result. However, he knew from internet reading that there was a chance for a false-negative, so when he developed a headache he became convinced that it was caused by viral spread to the central nervous system. He made several more visits to his doctor, who examined him and assured him that there was no evidence of HIV, or abnormal neurologic signs, and that an MRI was not necessary. His fears were always only temporarily mitigated by these visits, and they gradually began to migrate to the broader differential diagnoses for the headache that he had discovered online, including brain cancer and Creutzfeldt–Jakob disease. The fears were exhausting and isolating, and he started to feel increasingly fatigued, adding more fuel to the illness-attribution fire. The fatigue, compulsive internet research, and fears about possible exposures at work, led to sick days. His doctor, who knew Derek's pattern over the years, was

D.A. Lovas, M.D. (✉)
Department of Psychiatry, IWK Children's Hospital, Dalhousie University, 5850 University Avenue, P.O. Box 9700, Halifax, NS, Canada B3K 6R8

Department of Psychology and Neuroscience, Dalhousie University, Halifax, NS, Canada
e-mail: david.lovas@iwk.nshealth.ca

© Springer International Publishing Switzerland 2016
S.J. Eisendrath (ed.), *Mindfulness-Based Cognitive Therapy*, DOI 10.1007/978-3-319-29866-5_9

considering ordering him the MRI, hoping it might appease him, when he saw the ad for the study. Derek, exhausted and frustrated by his relentless mind and its negative effects on his marriage, agreed to try "anything."

The Problem of Severe Health Anxiety/Hypochondriasis

Severe health anxiety (HA), or hypochondriasis, as is has long been known, is an often debilitating condition characterized by persistent intrusive fears of having a serious medical illness, in spite of appropriate medical work-up and reassurance. Prevalence rates of hypochondriasis can be as high as 9 % in primary care settings [1], and up to 5 % in the general population [2]. These fears can often be associated with somatic symptoms that trigger checking behaviors and reassurance seeking from friends, family, and physicians. The latter has the potential for the inappropriate use of health care resources and iatrogenic harm, as these patients often receive unnecessary tests and procedures [3]. HA is also a strong, independent risk factor for disability, and one study found that its predictive effect is comparable to that of depression [4]. Recovery from HA occurs in as few as 30 % of the afflicted [5].

It should be noted that DSM-5 has recently renamed hypochondriasis as either illness anxiety disorder (if distressing somatic symptoms are absent), or somatic symptom disorder (if distressing somatic symptoms are present). However, robust epidemiological and clinical data are not yet available for these new diagnostic labels. As a result, this chapter will continue to use the widely researched concepts of severe HA and hypochondriasis.

Theoretical Rationale of MBCT for Severe Health Anxiety/ Hypochondriasis

In one of the seminal papers on hypochondriasis, Warwick and Salkovskis [6] proposed a cognitive behavioral model, which highlighted three maintaining mechanisms: (1) selective attention to bodily sensations and HA thoughts, (2) misinterpretation of physiological arousal and bodily sensations, and (3) safety-seeking behaviors. Cognitive behavioral therapies (CBT) have been developed to address these facets, and they are often successful when patients participate (e.g., [7]). However, participants are often reluctant to participate in CBT, with enrollment rates as low as 30 % [7], and dropout rates as high as 30 % [8]. As such, the results of CBT trials have been mixed [9]. The relative recalcitrance of HA, as compared to other anxiety disorders, may be due in part to the inherent difficulty in challenging feared predictions for illnesses that may develop insidiously over years [10]. This stands in contrast to other anxiety disorders with fears of more immediate consequences—e.g., that of a panic attack. This leaves substantial room for doubt in the mind of the HA patient.

A mindfulness approach, which does not aim to challenge or change the thoughts of the HA patient, may be a useful alternative to CBT. Rather than challenging the cognitions, a mindfulness approach seeks to enhance the ability to decenter from thoughts, and recognize that "thoughts are just thoughts," and not facts. This mechanism has been associated with improvement in depression [11]. The opposite of this state—cognitive fusion—has been shown to play a significant role in HA, independent of negative affect and experiential avoidance [12]. Thus, if HA patients were able to learn cognitive defusion, or decentering, perhaps they could decrease the believability of their disease fears without directly challenging the thoughts or trying to propose alternative thoughts.

Returning to the other mechanisms of the Warwick and Salkovskis model, mindfulness-based approaches are uniquely poised to target attentional bias towards bodily sensations. Attentional regulation has been described as one of the core components of mindfulness training [13]. Furthermore, the positive effects of MBCT have been in part linked to this mechanism [11]. Mindfulness training has also been shown to improve interoceptive regulatory control, as evidenced at neural and behavioral levels of observation [14, 15]. In the mindfulness for chronic pain literature, this has also been associated with the related findings of not only improved coping, but also decreased pain intensity and decreased activation of the neural pain matrix [16, 17]. Furthermore, these improvements in interoceptive awareness and regulation have been associated with decreased autonomic arousal in those with anxiety disorders [18]. With regard to attentional bias towards HA thoughts, rumination has been shown to be a key mechanism in HA [19], and there is evidence that MBCT can decrease rumination [11, 20]. This all begs the question: Could MBCT help patients with HA better regulate their attention to interoceptive and cognitive phenomena, and in so doing, decrease autonomic arousal and somatic symptoms?

Lastly, regarding safety-seeking behaviors, there is evidence that MBCT may be an effective intervention against avoidance and reassurance seeking. Experiential avoidance has been shown to be a maintaining mechanism in anxiety broadly [21], and health anxiety specifically [12, 22]. It appears to be closely related to the fear of the somatic aspects of anxiety [22, 23]. Mindfulness training directly addresses experiential avoidance by gently teaching participants, in a graded, compassionate manner, how to directly experience the physical sensations and emotions in their bodies and the thoughts in their minds in the present moment, without judgment. Over time, this allows practitioners to be able to respond to their present condition with thoughtfulness, rather than reacting habitually or compulsively [24]. With regard to reassurance-seeking, there is evidence from a large population study that MBCT broadly (not specifically for HA), decreases health care utilization in high utilizers [25].

In sum, MBCT seems well suited to address many of the original cognitive behavioral mechanisms, as well as some of the more recent contextual mechanisms, felt to be important in the maintenance of HA.

Modifications of MBCT for Severe Health Anxiety/Hypochondriasis

MBCT for severe health anxiety/hypochondriasis was largely an adaptation of the original MBCT manual for depression [26] and its progenitor, mindfulness-based stress reduction

(MBSR; [27]), but tailored to this unique patient population and the mechanisms described above. Two research groups—ours at Harvard [28], and McManus et al. [29] at Oxford—independently developed manuals and conducted studies, but the modifications appear to have been similar (for summary of their approach see [24]).

As in the original model, the program begins with individual orientation sessions with the teacher/clinician to assess suitability and readiness (see section below). The following sessions follow the typical 2-h, weekly class format, over 8 weeks.

Sessions 1–3: There are only minimal modifications from the original manual [26]. In the first session, instead of referencing depression, we acknowledge that everyone is here due to "chronic physical symptoms" and "stress related to health," as opposed to using the words "health anxiety" or "hypochondriasis." This was done to maintain an etiology-neutral stance, so as not to challenge cognitions, and to accommodate varying levels of insight. These terms are also less stigmatizing, and thus do not carry a potentially implicit societal judgment, which might work at counter-purposes to our goal of teaching a nonjudgmental attitude. Just as in the original manual, the raisin exercise is used to illustrate the automatic nature of the conditioned mind and the potential to cultivate its opposite. The group is asked to reflect on how this exercise might be related to chronic physical symptoms or stress related to health. The Socratic questioning guides the group into discovering some of the mechanisms of HA, and how their stress may be caused in part by the mind's "autopilot." The body scan is introduced next, and further elucidates the mind's habits when confronted with sensations in the body. Participants are taught mindfulness of the breath before scanning throughout the body, and are instructed to come back to the awareness of the physical sensations of the breath should the sensations in the body prove overwhelming. The normality of the difficulty of this exercise is emphasized and the importance of kindness and a curious attitude—the same curiosity evoked in the raisin exercise. Session 2 helps to further normalize the difficulties that arise, and addresses the participants' expectations for "mindfulness," as outlined in the original manual. The body scan is often particularly difficult for HA patients, as it ostensibly functions as a form of exposure and response prevention therapy—body scanning, but not ruminating, or engaging in safety behaviors. Instead of body scanning with fear and a mind propelled into a future of dreadful outcomes, they are body scanning with curiosity, and a mind settling into the simplicity of the sensations in the present moment. This mind watches the conditioned themes of disease-fear arise, and then lets them go, returning to the present moment awareness of sensations with a nonjudgmental, gentle attitude. This session uses the "walking down the street" cognitive distortion exercise of the original manual, but again asks the participants how this may relate to their physical symptoms. The exercise and discussion introduces the "thoughts are not facts" principle. In the third session, we introduce the topic of automatic judgments and how they affect thoughts and physical sensations, laying the ground work for a fuller discussion the following week. By the end of the third session participants have learned an assortment of mindfulness techniques (eating, sitting, breathing, lying, walking, stretching, 3-min breathing space), and they are encouraged to play with what works in the moment to help them notice, and step out of, rumination.

Session 4: This session in the original manual is focused in part on "getting to know the territory of the illness." Instead of mechanisms of depression, we focus on the mechanisms of HA. We introduce the concept of the symptom–fear cycle, in which a random bodily sensation or disease-thought leads to judgment, escalating fear, more catastrophic thoughts, more fear, and intensifying thoughts and symptoms, as they are fueled by worried attention (attentional bias). Participants share their common catastrophic worries, and typical behaviors in response to them. We then invite participants to discuss how they might intervene in this cycle, employing what they have learned thus far about mindfulness practice, and the specific techniques that they feel might be most helpful.

Sessions 5–8: These sessions are again similar to the original manual, with the exception of Session 6. Session 5 focuses on acceptance and its essential role in the symptom-fear cycle. Letting go of the struggle to "fix" is a key theme. Session 6 (different in the Oxford protocol, which echos the original manual's themes for this session; Surawy et al. [24]) uses elements of the original MBSR manual and traditional CBT for HA [7] to cover the theme of "working with difficult communications." This session was meant to address some of the interpersonal elements of HA that have been shown to be maintaining mechanisms [30], and have been included in CBT protocols for HA [7]. This session introduces mindful listening, with participants being instructed to listen, but to maintain at least 30 % of their attention on their own physical sensations in the moment, watching for signs of physical and/or emotional reactions as they listen. They also discuss a difficult communications calendar that they were asked to record as part of the prior week's homework. They are asked to reflect on their recordings of the past week in terms of passive, aggressive, and assertive patterns of communication. Participants are then asked if they noticed any connections between the way they communicated and their symptoms. Participants are asked to imagine that a video camera filmed their interactions, and to consider how an observer would know who was sick if she watched the tape with the sound off? From the MBSR manual, the Aikido-based "pushing exercise" is used to illustrate the various forms of passive (stuck, afraid, helpless), aggressive (as well as passive-aggressive), and assertive/responsive interpersonal styles. Mindfulness of feelings is also emphasized as an important first step to effective and assertive communication. Sessions 7 and 8, as in the original MBCT manual, serve to prepare participants for the end of the program, and for ongoing practice in life. They also involve brainstorming about how participants can best care for themselves, and make meaningful behavioral changes in their lives to prevent a return to maladaptive patterns (e.g., looking up differential diagnoses online). The classes also guide participants in recognizing warning signs that they are slipping back into old ways.

Evidence Supporting MBCT for Severe Health Anxiety/Hypochondriasis and Delineating Mechanisms of Change

The available evidence supporting MBCT for HA stems from one open-label trial [28], one qualitative study [10], and one randomized control trial [29]. In the small open-label trial ($N=10$), we found a significant improvement from pre to post intervention in our primary outcome variable, the Whitely Index (WI; the most commonly used measure of hypochondriasis symptom severity). The clinical significance was substantial, with 3/10 of participants no longer meeting clinical level of symptom severity after the intervention, and that number increasing to 7/10 after 3 months post-intervention. The Short Health Anxiety Inventory (SHAI) was also used, and improved similarly. The randomized control trial compared MBCT plus unrestricted services ($N=36$) to unrestricted services alone ($N=38$), and used the same measures of HA [29]. They found that the MBCT plus unrestricted services significantly outperformed unrestricted services alone on the primary outcome of health anxiety, and that the effect was present in the intention to treat analysis. The effect sizes in the intention to treat analysis were just shy of medium (Cohen's $d=-0.48$) for both pre to post intervention, and pre to 1 year follow-up. In the less stringent per protocol method (which excluded three participants who withdrew from the study at post-intervention and three participants who withdrew at 1 year follow-up), the effect sizes were 0.49 and 0.62, respectively. The diagnosis of hypochondriasis in the MBCT group was halved post-intervention, and only about a third met criteria at 1-year follow-up. This was a significantly different outcome than in the controls, where three-quarters of participants maintained their diagnosis throughout.

In addition to its primary effects on HA, we found an improvement in somatic, depressive, and general anxiety symptoms post-intervention and at 3-month follow-up [28]. Overall quality of life and health satisfaction were improved at 3-month follow-up. McManus et al. [29] found improvements in depression and anxiety in the MBCT group over time, but the control group had also improved to a similar degree.

The qualitative study [10] demonstrated that practicing mindfulness meditation regularly within the group was challenging but rewarding for those who did. This required an open-minded attitude along with a willingness to practice in preparation for future difficulties (as opposed to sitting in a reactive manner to deal with present difficulties). Participants appreciated the variety and flexibility of MBCT practices. Many found the group to be validating and normalizing. Many felt empowered to break their HA cycles with the techniques learned, and, more broadly, many found that MBCT helped improve their outlook on life and their self-compassion.

In terms of mechanisms of change, we found that improvement in mindfulness was highly correlated with improvement in HA severity [28], and McManus et al. [29] replicated and extended this finding with more robust statistical study by way of meditational analysis. Although, not examined as mediators, we found a significant decrease in reassurance seeking and in the frequency and believability of hypochondriacal cognitions. Similarly, McManus et al. [31] found a decrease in the frequency of intrusive mental images related to HA. The associated distress and intrusiveness of the images also decreased post intervention and at 3-month follow-up, with medium to large effect sizes (Cohen's $d=0.75-1.50$).

Practical Considerations of MBCT for Severe Health Anxiety/Hypochondriasis Including Patient Selection, Home Practice, Group Size, Format, Facilitator Training

For the most part, these practicalities should follow the original MBCT manual [26]. For the facilitator, in addition to the strong mindfulness meditation background that is typically required, it may be beneficial to have some clinical experience with HA to better understand its formulation and the patients' struggles.

Case Follow-Up

During the baseline screen, Derek showed high levels of health anxiety, generalized anxiety, somatic symptoms, and moderate depressive symptoms. Although he had never heard of "mindfulness," his quality of life was at an all-time low, and he was willing to commit to the eight sessions and the daily homework. When he first met with the group he was encouraged to meet so many others suffering from similar fears. He found it tremendously validating, and he became a jovial contributor to group discussion.

However, Derek's enthusiasm stalled when he tried the body scan in the first class and in the first week's homework. The intensity of the physical sensations was at times overwhelming, and his mind raced with disease fears. When he returned to the second class he felt defeated, but he had practiced the homework every day nonetheless. He was surprised to learn that most of the class shared his difficulties, and that he was not alone in not finding it "relaxing" as he had hoped. Derek was also reassured to learn that everyone's body felt "noisy," and that the tingling sensations he felt in his hands and feet were experienced by many in the class, and were likely not the sign of burgeoning multiple sclerosis.

As the sessions proceeded and he learned more techniques, he was pleased to be able to find techniques that suited him during different times of the day and windows of opportunity. For instance, he often walked at work, instead of ruminating about possible HIV exposures, he practiced bringing his mind back to the simple physical sensations of lower limbs rising, falling, and making contact with the floor. He often found the moving meditations were easier than sitting meditations when he felt particularly on edge.

Initially, Derek found some of the educational content to be abstract and counterintuitive. However, with repetition and experience, he eventually understood that the goal of mindfulness was not to "relax" or "get rid of his symptoms," but rather to learn to accept and let go of habitual tendencies of the mind that lead to suffering. He sometimes still wanted to "relax away" his symptoms, but he learned to notice this judgment and reactivity, and to "breath into it" with self-compassion.

Derek found the interpersonal session helpful, as he recognized how he had learned maladaptive patterns of communication from his mother, and was enacting them with his wife, to detrimental effect. Similarly, he learned to identify the behavioral patterns that were reinforcing his anxiety, such as internet-checking and reassurance-seeking, and he started including more pleasant events in his life.

At the end of the course, Derek's health anxiety was significantly improved from baseline, and he was no longer missing work, but stress was still associated with health fears. He felt the group support was a key element of his success, and wondered if he would practice as regularly without the sense of obligation to the group. However, he felt that he was "starting to get the hang of it," and saw a benefit in his practice.

After the course, he continued to practice a few times per week, particularly enjoying the 3-min breathing spaces, given their efficacy. The body scan had also become less threatening, and sometimes he would do a scan at night if he was having difficulty falling asleep. When he was seen at 3-month follow-up his Whitely Index score was no longer in the clinically significant range, and he was very thankful for the course. He found that as he practiced the mindfulness exercises, he was better able to use the techniques in high-anxiety situations, many of which had nothing to do with illness fears.

Summary/Conclusions

MBCT for HA or hypochondriasis appears to be a useful alternative to traditional CBT. It offers a unique strategy of targeting the putative underlying mechanisms of HA in a manner that may be more acceptable to some patients. Moreover, like all mindfulness trainings, its benefits may go beyond mere symptom reduction, and towards facilitating a more engaged, present, and joyful life.

References

1. Creed F, Barsky AJ. A systematic review of the epidemiology of somatization disorder and hypochondriasis. J Psychosom Res. 2004;56:391–408.
2. Gureje O, Üstün TB, Simon GE. The syndrome of hypochondriasis: a cross-national study in primary care. Psychol Med. 1997;27(05):1001–10.

3. Barsky AJ, Ettner SL, Horsky J, Bates DW. Resource utilization of patients with hypochondriacal health anxiety and somatization. Med Care. 2001;39(7):705–15.
4. Mykletun A, Heradstveit O, Eriksen K, Glozier N, Øverland S, Mæland JG, et al. Health anxiety and disability pension award: The HUSK Study. Psychosom Med. 2009;71(3):353–60.
5. Olde Hartman TC, Borghuis MS, Lucassen PL, van de Laar FA, Speckens AE, van Weel C. Medically unexplained symptoms, somatisation disorder and hypochondriasis: course and prognosis. A systematic review. J Psychosom Res. 2009;66(5):363–77.
6. Warwick HM, Salkovskis PM. Hypochondriasis. Behav Res Ther. 1990;28(2):105–17.
7. Barsky AJ, Ahern DK. Cognitive behavior therapy for hypochondriasis: a randomized controlled trial. JAMA. 2004;291(12):1464–70.
8. Visser S, Bouman TK. The treatment of hypochondriasis: exposure plus response prevention vs cognitive therapy. Behav Res Ther. 2001;39:423–42.
9. Thomson AB, Page LA. Psychotherapies for hypochondriasis. The Cochrane database of systematic reviews. 2007;17(4):CD006520.
10. Williams MJ, McManus F, Muse K, Williams JMG. Mindfulness-based cognitive therapy for severe health anxiety (hypochondriasis): an interpretative phenomenological analysis of patients' experiences. Br J Clin Psychol. 2011;50(4):379–97.
11. van der Velden AM, Kuyken W, Wattar U, Crane C, Pallesen KJ, Dahlgaard J, et al. A systematic review of mechanisms of change in mindfulness-based cognitive therapy in the treatment of recurrent major depressive disorder. Clin Psychol Rev. 2015;37:26–39.
12. Fergus TA. I really believe i suffer from a health problem: examining an association between cognitive fusion and healthy anxiety. J Clin Psychol. 2015;71(9):920–34.
13. Tang YY, Hölzel BK, Posner MI. The neuroscience of mindfulness meditation. Nat Rev Neurosci. 2015;16(4):213–25.
14. Farb NA, Anderson AK, Segal ZV. The mindful brain and emotion regulation in mood disorders. Can J Psychiatry. 2012;57(2):70.
15. Haase L, Thom NJ, Shukla A, Davenport PW, Simmons AN, Paulus MP et al. Mindfulness-based training attenuates insula response to an aversive interoceptive challenge. Soc Cognit Affect Neurosci. 2014;nsu042.
16. Goyal M, Singh S, Sibinga EM, Gould NF, Rowland-Seymour A, Sharma R, et al. Meditation programs for psychological stress and well-being: a systematic review and meta-analysis. JAMA Intern Med. 2014;174(3):357–68.
17. Jensen MP, Day MA, Miró J. Neuromodulatory treatments for chronic pain: efficacy and mechanisms. Nat Rev Neurol. 2014;10(3):167–78.
18. Delgado-Pastor LC, Ciria LF, Blanca B, Mata JL, Vera MN, Vila J. Dissociation between the cognitive and interoceptive components of mindfulness in the treatment of chronic worry. J Behav Ther Exp Psychiatry. 2015;48:192–9.
19. Marcus DK, Hughes KT, Arnau RC. Health anxiety, rumination, and negative affect: a mediational analysis. J Psychosom Res. 2008;64(5):495–501.
20. Hawley LL, Schwartz D, Bieling PJ, Irving J, Corcoran K, Farb NAS, et al. Mindfulness practice, rumination and clinical outcome in mindfulness-based treatment. Cogn Ther Res. 2014;38(1):1–9.
21. Bardeen JR, Tull MT, Stevens EN, Gratz KL. Exploring the relationship between positive and negative emotional avoidance and anxiety symptom severity: the moderating role of attentional control. J Behav Ther Exp Psychiatry. 2014;45(3):415–20.
22. Wheaton MG, Berman NC, Abramowitz JS. The contribution of experiential avoidance and anxiety sensitivity in the prediction of health anxiety. J Cogn Psychother. 2010;24(3):229–39.
23. Bardeen JR, Fergus TA, Orcutt HK. The moderating role of experiential avoidance in the prospective relationship between anxiety sensitivity and anxiety. Cogn Ther Res. 2014;38(4):465–71.
24. Surawy C, McManus F, Muse K, Williams JMG. Mindfulness-Based Cognitive Therapy (MBCT) for health anxiety (Hypochondriasis): rationale, implementation and case illustration. Mindfulness. 2014;6(2):382–92.
25. Kurdyak P, Newman A, Segal Z. Impact of mindfulness-based cognitive therapy on health care utilization: a population-based controlled comparison. J Psychosom Res. 2014;77(2):85–9.
26. Segal ZV, Williams JMG, Teasdale JD. Mindfulness-based cognitive therapy for depression: a new approach to relapse prevention. New York: Guilford; 2002.
27. Kabat-Zinn J. Full catastrophe living. New York, NY: Delta; 1990.
28. Lovas DA, Barsky AJ. Mindfulness-based cognitive therapy for hypochondriasis, or severe health anxiety: a pilot study. J Anxiety Disord. 2010;24(8):931–5.
29. McManus F, Surawy C, Muse K, Vazquez-Montes M, Williams JMG. A randomized clinical trial of mindfulness-based cognitive therapy versus unrestricted services for health anxiety (hypochondriasis). J Consult Clin Psychol. 2012;80(5):817.
30. Noyes Jr R, Stuart SP, Langbehn DR, Happel RL, Longley SL, Muller BA, et al. Test of an interpersonal model of hypochondriasis. Psychosom Med. 2003; 65(2):292–300.
31. McManus F, Muse K, Surawy C, Hackmann A, Williams JM. Relating Differently to Intrusive Images: the Impact of Mindfulness-Based Cognitive Therapy (MBCT) on Intrusive Images in Patients with Severe Health Anxiety (Hypochondriasis). Mindfulness. 2015 Aug 1;6(4):788–96.

Self-Help Mindfulness-Based Cognitive Therapy

10

Fergal W. Jones, Clara Strauss, and Kate Cavanagh

Abbreviations

MBCT   Mindfulness-based cognitive therapy
MBSR   Mindfulness-based stress reduction
MMB   Mindful mood balance
RCT   Randomized controlled trial

In this chapter we examine how mindfulness-based cognitive therapy (MBCT) can be offered in self-help formats; namely online and in book form. We begin with some case examples that illustrate the need for such interventions.

F.W. Jones, Ph.D., Psych.D. (✉)
Salomons Centre for Applied Psychology,
Canterbury Christ Church University, Runcie Court,
Broomhill Road, Tunbridge Wells TN3 0TF, UK

Sussex Mindfulness Centre, Sussex Partnership NHS
Foundation Trust, Research and Development
Department, Sussex Education Centre, Mill View
Hospital Site, Neville Avenue, Hove BN3 7HZ, UK
e-mail: fergal.jones@canterbury.ac.uk

C. Strauss, D.Phil., Psych.D. • K. Cavanagh, D.Phil.,
D.Clin.Psych.
Sussex Mindfulness Centre, Sussex Partnership NHS
Foundation Trust, Research and Development
Department, Sussex Education Centre, Mill View
Hospital Site, Neville Avenue, Hove BN3 7HZ, UK

School of Psychology, University of Sussex,
Falmer, East Sussex BN1 9QH, UK
e-mail: c.y.strauss@sussex.ac.uk; kate.cavanagh@
sussex.ac.uk

Clinical Case Studies

As has been discussed in other parts of this book, MBCT has the potential to be helpful for people experiencing a range of difficulties, with arguably the strongest evidence for its efficacy to date being in relation to recurrent depression [1]. However, some people who might benefit from MBCT are either unable or unwilling to participate in it, at least in its traditional class-based format. To illustrate, consider the following examples of people who have previously experienced recurrent episodes of depression.

Julia, a 29-year-old single mother, had been on antidepressants for several years following three bouts of major depressive disorder. She had become concerned that, while the antidepressants had helped prevent further episodes of major depression, they were also somewhat numbing her emotional experience and reducing her ability to enjoy time with her children. On the basis of recent research [2], her family doctor recommended that she attend an MBCT course, with a view to tapering her antidepressants following this. However, the nearest available course was a 2 h drive away, and she was unable to afford the 6 h additional childcare per week, for 8 weeks, that would have been required to attend this. Therefore, she did not attend, but hoped that a more local MBCT course would become available soon.

© Springer International Publishing Switzerland 2016
S.J. Eisendrath (ed.), *Mindfulness-Based Cognitive Therapy*, DOI 10.1007/978-3-319-29866-5_10

Similarly, Tim, a 55-year-old who had experienced multiple episodes of depression over many years, had MBCT recommended to him by his primary care physician. In contrast to Julia, there was a local MBCT course that Tim could access and he had the resources to pay for it. However, Tim felt particularly ashamed of his experiences of depression, and believed that they were an indication of his person failings and weakness. Consequently, he had concealed these experiences from all but his closest friends and family members, and did not wish to disclose them to others. This meant he was very reluctant to attend a group-based intervention such as MBCT, and ultimately chose not to, both because he feared that its class-based format would mean he would have to let others in the class know about his depression and because he feared that friends or work colleagues might see him visiting the community mental health center where the course was held.

For both Tim and Julia, a self-help version of MBCT has the potential to provide a viable alternative to the traditional class-based format and could enable them to engage in MBCT when they otherwise would not.

The Need for Self-Help MBCT

The above case examples point towards some of the challenges of making MBCT widely available in its traditional class-based format. One challenge is posed by the fact that MBCT is a relatively recently developed therapy compared to other psychological interventions, such as cognitive therapy and behavioral therapy [3]. Therefore, there is a need for growth in the number of people who are qualified to teach MBCT, which has started from a relatively small base (cf. [4]). It seems likely that the rate of this growth will be constrained by the limited availability of MBCT teacher-training courses and experienced MBCT teachers who can act as supervisors. Moreover, the pool from which potential MBCT teachers can be drawn is likely narrowed by the need for MBCT teachers to have an established mindfulness practice and commitment to ongoing practice

(e.g., [5]). The problem of MBCT teacher availability should reduce as more new teachers are trained, existing teachers become more experienced and able to offer supervision, and more MBCT teacher-training courses become established. However, it seems likely to remain an issue for several years to come.

Arguably, the relative newness of MBCT also contributes to the variation in the extent to which health care and similar organizations are aware of, interested in, and able to introduce MBCT as one of the interventions they provide. For example, Crane and Kuyken [6] found that in the UK it was rare for mental health services to have a strategy to fully implement the national guidance that recommends the provision of MBCT for people who have experienced three or more previous episodes of depression but are currently in remission [7].

Furthermore, even when MBCT is locally available, there are practical reasons why potential participants may not be able to access it. Specifically, in countries where health care is not free at the point of delivery, some people may not be able to afford to pay for it nor have insurance that will. Alternatively, they may not be able to meet the time commitment of attending weekly 2-h classes for 8 weeks, with 30–60 min daily homework. The class-based format of MBCT may also act as a deterrent to participation for some, for instance people who experience social anxiety or self-stigma in relation to their difficulties (c.f. [8]). In relation to these points, it is interesting to note that in a recent MBCT research trial 644 participants who were eligible to participate declined to do so [2].

Taken together, these challenges suggest that participation in class-based MBCT is likely to fall short of the need for MBCT. Offering MBCT in a self-help format has the potential to overcome a number of these challenges. Specifically, self-help MBCT can be provided in the absence of trained MBCT teachers, can cost health care organizations and participants substantially less than class-based MBCT, can be accessed at times and in locations that are convenient to the user, and can provide a potential solution for people reluctant to attend a class-based intervention. In addition, self-help MBCT might also be useful in enabling people to have a taste of MBCT before deciding whether to attend a class-based MBCT course, and some class-based MBCT "graduates" might find that self-help material helps them to maintain post-course mindfulness practice. However, a key question raised by offering MBCT through self-help is whether we may be increasing accessibility at the expense of quality and efficacy. We return to this issue later in the chapter.

The Theoretical Rationale for Self-Help MBCT

The theoretical foundations of self-help MBCT are largely the same as those of class-based MBCT, and a range of different theories can be drawn on to understand the possible, key mechanisms of action of MBCT in either format (e.g., [9–11]). However, arguably the foundational theory for MBCT is the doing and being modes model that Segal et al. [3, 12] drew on when they developed the approach.

According to this model, when people who have previously suffered from depression experience low mood, associated patterns of depressive thinking, feeling and bodily sensations reactivate. People often attempt to avoid these experiences by automatically entering a "doing-mode" of mind, in which they use verbal problem solving and rumination in an attempt to prevent their mood from worsening. However, Segal et al. [3] argue that this doing-mode has the reverse effect, not least because unrealistically negative thoughts are experienced as truths, as opposed to events in the mind. Therefore, ruminating about them leads to a lowering of mood and deepening reactivation of the well-established depressive patterns, perpetuating the downward spiral back into clinical depression.

By this account, the key reason why MBCT reduces relapse is that practising mindfulness enables people to become aware of when they are entering the doing-mode in response to emotional difficulties, and helps them to disengage from this and enter a "being-mode" of mind

(Segal et al. [3], p. 91). The being-mode is characterized by an awareness and nonjudgmental acceptance of present moment experience [13]. It is argued that in this mode thoughts are experienced as events in the mind rather than truths, and rumination is unnecessary as people let go of striving for a different state of mind. Therefore, a downward spiral into clinical depression is prevented.

Furthermore, this theory has the potential to be applied to human suffering more generally [13], and so can explain the potential benefits of MBCT to conditions beyond depression. For example, Germer [14] applies a similar approach to the understanding and treatment of anxiety states, and Kabat-Zinn's [15] description of how mindfulness can help reduce stress is compatible with the model. Moreover, in principle this theory applies just as well to the benefits of mindfulness learnt by self-help as to by class-based MBCT.

Turning to Segal et al.'s [3, 12] theorizing concerning the process of learning mindfulness during MBCT, both self-help and class-based MBCT are underpinned by the view that mindfulness needs to be learnt experientially through mindfulness practice. However, two potentially important differences between these formats also emerge. Specifically, building on the work of Kabat-Zinn (e.g., [15]), Segal et al. [3, 12] argue that in class-based MBCT the teacher should relate to participants, and their descriptions of their experiences during enquiry, in an open, curious, warm, and accepting manner, with a focus on direct experience. This way of relating by the teacher is thought to model the being-mode of mind to the participants and so help to build an understanding and internalization of what it means to be mindful. However, typically self-help MBCT is not supported by sessions with a mindfulness teacher. Therefore, as is detailed in the next section, self-help MBCT attempts to use alternative means to help participants understand and internalize the nature of mindfulness.

Another important theoretical difference between class-based and self-help MBCT is that during the former the participants are part of a group, whereas in the latter case they are likely learning mindfulness on their own. Theories of group processes (e.g., [16]) speak about the value of the group setting to learning and therapeutic change. For example, the sense of universality of human experience that can emerge in a group potentially plays an important role in class-based MBCT, and is something that mindfulness teachers can draw out during enquiry. As we shall see, in self-help MBCT other means are needed to achieve the same ends.

Modifications of MBCT for Delivery by Self-Help

There is a growing range of mindfulness-based self-help interventions that are either publically available or used in research trials (e.g., [15, 17–19]—see ref. [20] for a review). Broadly speaking, these fall into two classes: self-help books, in paper, electronic or audio-book format, and multimedia/Internet-based self-help interventions, whose delivery can be via the Internet or smartphone apps. It is worth noting that not all of these interventions closely follow or draw on the MBCT program, and so it is important that clinicians and consumers are aware of the nature of the self-help material they use and ensure that it is a good match to their expectations and needs. In this section we focus on five self-help interventions that are close to the original MBCT program [3], and consider how they have each modified class-based MBCT. Teams involving one or more of the original developers of MBCT (i.e., Zindel Segal, Mark Williams, and John Teasdale) have created all of these interventions.

Considering first Williams et al.'s [21] self-help book *The Mindful Way Through Depression: Freeing Yourself From Chronic Unhappiness*, as its title suggests, this is aimed at people who have experienced depression, with a recommendation that "it may be wise not to undertake the entire program while in the midst of an episode of clinical depression" (p. 8). The book begins with chapters describing the nature of depression and how mindfulness may be helpful. These chapters cover some of the taught components of the class-based MBCT curriculum [3],

and arguably aim to convey a sense that participants are not alone in their experiences of depression and that these can be understood and alleviated. The use of case examples and quotes from people struggling with depression add richness to the descriptions, and perhaps go some way to compensate for the absence of the group setting of class-based MBCT.

These opening chapters are followed by ones focusing on the different mindfulness practices found in MBCT, including the raison exercise, mindfulness of the breath, body scan, mindful yoga, mindfulness of sounds and thoughts, and mindfulness in everyday life together with the three-minute breathing space. The chapters interweave practice guidance with teaching, poetry and other MBCT participants' experiences, much as an MBCT class would. They are supported by a CD of guided mindfulness practices. Some of these practices tend to be shorter in length than those in class-based MBCT, though participants have the option of combining several tracks into a single longer meditation. The teacher-led enquiry into participants' experiences of mindfulness that forms a core part of class-based MBCT is clearly not possible to fully replicate in book form. However, examples of people's experiences during mindfulness practice are included, along with advice in relation to these. Towards the end of the book, the reader is provided with guidance as to how they can combine the ideas and practices detailed in earlier chapters into an 8-week program, should they so wish. The structure of this closely follows the homework that is set over the course of the 8-weeks of class-based MBCT, with a similar program of daily practices being recommended [3].

More recently, Teasdale et al. [22] have released *The Mindful Way Workbook: An 8-Week Program to Free Yourself from Depression and Emotional Distress*. This can be used in a number of different ways, including as a self-help workbook read in conjunction with *The Mindful Way Through Depression: Freeing Yourself From Chronic Unhappiness*. It provides a useful complement to the earlier book, because of its greater focus on the practicalities of following the MBCT program step by step, including chapters guiding readers through each week of the course, and because of the opportunities it provides for participants to reflect on their experiences. Following developments in the research literature since the publication of the earlier book, the intended audience is widened to also include people who are currently experiencing depression but whose concentration is not too impaired, and "anyone who wishes to take the 8-week MBCT program" (p. 6). As previously, mindfulness practice guidance is interweaved with teaching, poetry and quotes from MBCT participants, and audio tracks of guided meditation practices (via MP3 CD or download) are provided; the latter are very similar in length and content to those found in class-based MBCT programs [12]. Furthermore, excerpts of dialogue from class-based MBCT enquiry are included to provide participants with some sense of this. In fact, the overall similarity and compatibility of the workbook with the class-based program means that it can also be used by MBCT-teachers as a supplement to their class-based courses.

Turning to the self-help book *Mindfulness: A Practical Guide to Finding Peace in a Frantic World* [23], arguably this has been written for a somewhat more general audience; namely anyone suffering "from anxiety, stress, unhappiness and exhaustion" (p. 3). As previously, it is grounded in the 8-week class-based MBCT program and contains a mix of teaching, descriptions of relevant research, mindfulness practice guidance, activities, examples from previous MBCT participants, and homework. Similar to the above-mentioned workbook, after chapters providing introduction and background, one chapter is devoted to each week of the 8-week MBCT course. And, as usual, audio tracks are supplied to support the various mindfulness practices; in this case they tend to be somewhat shorter than the norm for class-based MBCT, which probably makes them more possible to engage with for a more general readership who are experiencing a "frantic world." Nevertheless, each week's homework recommends daily engagement in the mindfulness practice(s) relevant to the current week. Furthermore, in an addition to the usual MBCT program, for most weeks the reader is encouraged

to undertake a "habit releaser," which involves noticing habitual behaviors (such as watching whatever happens to be on television) and trying alternatives, in order to loosen habits.

The two remaining self-help versions of MBCT that are reviewed here are Internet-based. The first of these is the *Mindful Mood Balance* (MMB) course [4, 24]. A professionals' version of MMB is available for use by therapists and clinicians with an interest in experiencing and learning more about MBCT, and can be accessed at http://www.mindfulnoggin.com/mindful-mood-balance. In addition, a patient version is currently being evaluated in a research trial, to determine whether it can reduce residual symptoms of depression in people who have experienced at least one previous depressive episode (www.ClinicalTrials.gov). MMB covers the core MBCT curriculum over eight sessions that progress in a similar manner to the eight sessions of class-based MBCT, but which are somewhat shorter in length, lasting 60–90 min. During each session, participants are guided through mindfulness practice by video or audio instructions, are invited to watch video of relevant excerpts of periods of enquiry and teaching from an MBCT class, and complete an interactive learning module that helps them explore and reflect on their own experiences.

Cognitive therapy elements of MBCT are presented in a similar manner, and home practice is set each session and supported by downloadable audio files and handouts, an online homework record, and email reminders when relevant. As with class-based MBCT, there is an invitation to engage in the relevant mindfulness practice(s) for 6 days out of 7, every week of the course. Participants can review the MMB materials at times of their choosing and can revisit sessions if they wish. They are also able to post anonymous questions that are answered by a mindfulness teacher within 1 week, with the questions and answers forming part of a growing bank that can be shared with future participants. In the research thus far, participants have also been able to access phone and email support in relation to technical problems and other difficulties affecting their engagement with the course. The professionals' version of MMB also provides access to a community of fellow participants.

Turning to the final intervention considered in this chapter, the *Be Mindful* course is another online, self-help variant of MBCT [25]. This course also draws on the closely related mindfulness-based stress reduction (MBSR) program. It is available to the public at http://www.bemindfulonline.com, and is intended to be accessed by anyone who is interested, with the caveat that participation is not recommended when someone is experiencing severe depression or major life changes, or is unable to commit the necessary time. Similarly to MMB, *Be Mindful* uses audio and video guidance to teach mindfulness practice. In contrast to class-based MBCT, the course comprises ten 30-min sessions that can be completed at the participant's own pace and in a minimum of 4 weeks. However, it nevertheless covers the core components of MBCT, including the range of formal and informal mindfulness practices, and participants are invited to practice mindfulness and other activities daily for homework. Participants are not able to submit questions to a mindfulness teacher. However, technical support is available and automated emails form part of the program.

In summary, we have reviewed five book or Web-based self-help versions of MBCT. These are all grounded in the core curriculum and mindfulness practices of MBCT, but vary in terms of the audiences they are aimed at and the length of sessions and practices, with the self-help interventions targeting more general audiences tending to require less time commitment. All the courses use at least some form of audio or video guidance to support mindfulness practice. Furthermore, they find various means to attempt to compensate for the absence of the MBCT class and its teacher(s). These include providing extensive written, audio or video material that is prepared by experienced MBCT teachers, providing case vignettes of people experiencing similar difficulties, and sometimes providing written or videoed excerpts of teacher-led enquiry from class-based MBCT programs.

The Evidence-Base for Self-Help MBCT

As discussed earlier, there is a question as to whether the increased accessibility and flexibility of self-help versions of MBCT comes at a cost in terms of effectiveness, not least due to the absence of teacher-led enquiry into the participants' experiences, teacher modeling of a being mode, and group therapeutic processes. The evidence-base for self-help MBCT is still emerging. Therefore, at the time of writing, it is not possible to definitively answer the question of whether self-help MBCT is effective, in particular in clinical settings. Nevertheless, the following studies suggest that self-help MBCT may be of some value.

Starting with self-help MBCT books, we are only aware of one published evaluation. Specifically, in a relatively small-scale randomized controlled trial (RCT) conducted by our group, 80 self-selecting students, who were experiencing stress, anxiety or low mood, were randomized either to a group asked to read and follow the program outlined in *Mindfulness: A Practical Guide to Finding Peace in a Frantic World*, or to a waiting-list control arm [26]. The intervention participants showed significantly lower levels of post-intervention depression, anxiety and stress relative to controls, with medium effect sizes, and also significantly greater life satisfaction, mindfulness and self-compassion, with medium or large effect sizes. Moreover, the treatment gains appeared to be maintained at a 10-week follow-up assessment, and the level of engagement was high, with only 5% of participants dropping out.

Turning to the Web-based versions of MBCT, Dimidjian et al. [4] conducted an open trial in which 100 people with at least one previous episode of depression, but who were currently in remission, were invited to participate in MMB. They found that depressive symptoms were significantly lower immediately after the intervention compared to pretreatment, with a medium effect size, and that these symptoms remained significantly lower at a 6-month follow-up. Moreover, when the MMB group was compared with a propensity matched control group, who received treatment as usual, this pre to post treatment improvement in symptoms was found to significantly differ from the worsening of symptoms seen in the control group, with a large effect size. Also, 53 % of participants completed at least 50 % of the MMB course. As mentioned above, the efficacy of MMB at reducing residual symptoms of depression is being more definitively examined in a relatively large RCT, with results due in 2018 [27].

With regard to the *Be Mindful* Web-based intervention, Krusche et al. [28] ran an uncontrolled trial with 273 participants who had self-referred to this course, and who had elevated mean levels of perceived stress, anxiety and depression compared to the general population. They found significant pre to post intervention decreases in perceived stress, anxiety and depression, with large effect sizes, and further significant decreases in all three areas from post intervention to a 1-month follow-up. Moreover, the level of effect sizes observed was similar to that found in face-to-face mindfulness-based interventions. The absence of a control group means that regression to the mean cannot be ruled out however.

In summary, there is emerging evidence to support the efficacy of self-help MBCT, but this evidence is not yet of sufficient quality to recommend self-help MBCT for any clinical population. Well designed, fully powered RCTs are now required to establish whether self-help MBCT is effective and for whom, whether the format (book vs. online) impacts upon effectiveness, how its efficacy compares with class-based MBCT, and whether its mechanisms of action are consistent with the underpinning theory. At least one such trial, investigating MMB, is currently underway.

Practical Considerations

Many people independently choose to access self-help MBCT, having learnt about it from the media or elsewhere (cf. [28]). The self-help courses reviewed here provide guidance to people who access them via this route, to help them decide whether now is the right time to start such an intervention. In this section, therefore, we focus on some of the things that we think a clinician should consider if he or she is thinking about suggesting self-help MBCT to a patient/client.

Firstly, we would recommend that clinicians be both familiar with class-based MBCT, including who it can be helpful for, and with the forms of self-help MBCT that have been reviewed here. If the clinician is not a trained MBCT-teacher then we would also recommend that they receive supervision or consultation from a qualified MBCT-teacher who is familiar with self-help MBCT. Secondly, given that the evidence-base for self-help MBCT is in its infancy, arguably currently it is best to only consider self-help MBCT in circumstances when someone seems likely to benefit from MBCT, but is unable or unwilling to attend class-based MBCT and there are no alternative, suitable, well-evidenced interventions available. In such circumstances, it would seem helpful for the clinician to be open with their patient/client about the current state of the evidence-base, so that they can make an informed choice, and to come to a collaborative decision with the patient/client about the way forward. Issues worth considering with the patient/client include which of the self-help versions of MBCT appears to fit best with them and their needs, and whether it would seem helpful and possible to have some contact with an MBCT-teacher and/or periodic review meetings with the clinician, while they are embarking on the self-help program. When a patient/client is particularly vulnerable or distressed, we would be especially cautious about recommending self-help.

Hopefully, as research into self-help MBCT develops and broadens, it will become possible to offer more evidence-based guidance with regard to when to recommend self-help MBCT, and perhaps possible to encourage its integration into stepped-care intervention pathways offered by health care organizations.

Conclusions

There are a number of challenges to making class-based MBCT accessible to all those who could potentially benefit from it. These include a shortage of trained MBCT teachers, variable provision of MBCT by health care organizations, the cost to participants of MBCT courses in some countries, time constraints, and the reluctance of some people to take part in class-based interventions. Self-help MBCT has the potential to overcome many of these challenges, and so become a valuable complement to class-based MBCT. It is currently available in both book-based and multimedia/Internet-based formats. All of the self-help interventions that have been reviewed here use audio or video guidance to support mindfulness practice. They attempt to compensate for the absence of the MBCT class and its teacher(s) by using case vignettes, through written, audio or video presentations concerning key principles, and sometimes by written or videoed examples of teacher-led enquiry. The current evidence-base is insufficient to confidently recommend self-help MBCT for specific clinical populations, but the evidence thus far is promising and further research is underway.

References

1. Piet J, Hougaard E. The effect of mindfulness-based cognitive therapy for prevention of relapse in recurrent major depressive disorder: a systematic review and meta-analysis. Clin Psychol Rev. 2011;31:1032–40. doi:10.1016/j.cpr.2011.05.002.
2. Kuyken W, Hayes R, Barrett B, Byng R, Dalgleish T, Kessler D, et al. Effectiveness and cost-effectiveness of mindfulness-based cognitive therapy compared with maintenance antidepressant treatment in the prevention of depressive relapse or recurrence (PREVENT): a randomised controlled trial. Lancet. 2015;386(9988):63–73. doi:10.1016/S0140-6736(14)62222-4.
3. Segal ZV, Williams JMG, Teasdale JD. Mindfulness-based cognitive therapy for depression: a new approach to preventing relapse. New York, NY: Guilford; 2002.
4. Dimidjian S, Beck A, Felder JN, Boggs JM, Gallop R, Segal ZV. Web-based mindfulness-based cognitive therapy for reducing residual depressive symptoms: an open trial and quasi-experimental comparison to propensity score matched controls. Behav Res Ther. 2014;63:83–9. doi:10.1016/j.brat.2014.09.004.
5. UK Network for Mindfulness-Based Teacher Training Organisations. Good practice guidelines for teaching mindfulness-based courses. 2015. Accessed 31 Jul 2015 from http://www.mindfulnessteachersuk.org.uk.
6. Crane RS, Kuyken W. The implementation of mindfulness-based cognitive therapy: learning from the UK health service experience. Mindfulness. 2013;4:246–54. doi:10.1007/s12671-012-0121-6.
7. National Institute for Health and Clinical Excellence. Depression in adults: the treatment and management of depression in adults: NICE clinical guideline 90. Manchester, UK: National Institute for Health and Clinical Excellence; 2009.
8. Wahbeh H, Svalina MN, Oken BS. Group, one-on-one, or internet? Preferences for mindfulness meditation delivery format and their predictors. Open Med J. 2014;1:66–74. doi:10.2174/1874220301401010066.
9. Bishop SR, Lau M, Shapiro S, Carlson L, Anderson ND, Carmody J, et al. Mindfulness: a proposed operational definition. Clin Psychol Sci Pract. 2004;11:230–41. doi:10.1093/clipsy.bph077.
10. Brown KW, Ryan RM, Creswell JD. Mindfulness: theoretical foundations and evidence for its salutary effects. Psychol Inq. 2007;18:211–37. doi:10.1080/10478400701598298.
11. Shapiro SL, Carlson LE, Astin JA, Freedman B. Mechanisms of mindfulness. J Clin Psychol. 2006;62:373–86. doi:10.1002/jclp.20237.
12. Segal ZV, Williams JMG, Teasdale JD. Mindfulness-based cognitive therapy for depression. 2nd ed. New York, NY: Guilford; 2013.
13. Teasdale JD. Mindfulness-based cognitive therapy. In: Yiend J, editor. Cognition, emotion and psychopathology: theoretical, empirical and clinical directions. Cambridge, UK: Cambridge University Press; 2004. p. 270–89.
14. Germer CK. Anxiety disorders: befriending fear. In: Germer CK, Siegel RD, Fulton PR, editors. Mindfulness and psychotherapy. New York, NY: Guilford; 2005. p. 152–72.
15. Kabat-Zinn J. Full catastrophe living: using the wisdom of your body and mind to face stress, pain and illness. New York, NY: Delacorte; 1990.
16. Yalom ID, Leszcz M. The theory and practice of group psychotherapy. New York, NY: Basic Books; 2005.
17. Cavanagh K, Strauss C, Cicconi F, Griffiths N, Wyper A, Jones F. A randomised controlled trial of a brief online mindfulness-based intervention. Behav Res Ther. 2013;51:573–8. doi:10.1016/j.brat.2013.06.003.
18. Glück TM, Maercker A. A randomized controlled pilot study of a brief web-based mindfulness training. BMC Psychiatry. 2011;11:175. doi:10.1186/1471-244X-11-175.
19. Morledge TJ, Allexandre D, Fox E, Fu AZ, Higashi MK, Kruzikas DT, et al. Feasibility of an online mindfulness program for stress management -a randomized, controlled trial. Ann Behav Med. 2013;46:137–48. doi:10.1007/s12160-013-9490-x.
20. Cavanagh K, Strauss C, Forder L, Jones F. Can mindfulness and acceptance be learnt by self-help? A systematic review and meta-analysis of mindfulness and

acceptance-based self-help interventions. Clin Psychol Rev. 2014;34:118–29. doi:10.1016/j.cpr.2014.01.001.

21. Williams JMG, Teasdale JD, Segal ZV, Kabat-Zinn J. The mindful way through depression: freeing yourself from chronic unhappiness. New York, NY: Guilford; 2007.

22. Teasdale JD, Williams JMG, Segal ZV. The mindful way workbook: an 8-week program to free yourself from depression and emotional distress. New York, NY: Guilford; 2014.

23. Williams JMG, Penman D. Mindfulness: a practical guide to finding peace in a frantic world. London, UK: Piatkus; 2011.

24. Boggs JM, Beck A, Felder JN, Dimidjian S, Metcalf CA, Segal ZV. Web-based intervention in mindfulness meditation for reducing residual depressive symptoms and relapse prophylaxis: a qualitative study. J Med Intern Res. 2014;16(3):e87. doi:10.2196/jmir.3129.

25. Krusche A, Cyhlarova E, King S, Williams JMG. Mindfulness online: a preliminary evaluation of the feasibility of a web-based mindfulness course and the impact on stress. BMJ Open. 2012;2:e000803. doi:10.1136/bmjopen-2011-000803.

26. Lever Taylor L, Strauss C, Cavanagh K, Jones F. The effectiveness of self-help mindfulness-based cognitive therapy in a student sample: a randomised controlled trial. Behav Res Ther. 2014;63:63–9. doi:10.1016/j.brat.2014.09.007.

27. ClinicalTrials.gov [Internet]. Reducing residual depressive symptoms with web-based mindful mood balance. Bethesda, MD: National Library of Medicine; 2014. 2014 Jul 10 - ; Identifier NCT02190968; Accessed 25 Jul 2015 from https://clinicaltrials.gov/ct2/show/NCT02190968; [about 4 screens].

28. Krusche A, Cyhlarova E, Williams JMG. Mindfulness online: an evaluation of the feasibility of a web-based mindfulness course for stress, anxiety and depression. BMJ Open. 2013;3:e003498. doi:10.1136/bmjopen-2013-003498.

Mindfulness-Based Cognitive Therapy for Couples

11

Kim Griffiths and Marcus Averbeck

Introduction

There has been an exponential growth in research exploring mindfulness-based approaches in recent years. The application of mindfulness-based approaches to working with couples has received some attention in the published literature, but in comparison with other areas of clinical health or mental health, couple work is under-represented [1].

A number of studies have theorised on the impact of mindfulness on relating to others, or upon the couple/intimate relationship. There have also been several programmes piloted for clinical and non-clinical populations. Some of these studies have been based on the direct use of MBCT/MBSR and others following integration of mindfulness techniques or adaptations of the 8-week programme.

The next sections take a broad overview of some of these studies. Other than a qualitative paper examining participant experiences of MBCT as a couple [2], which interviewed participants from the groups described in this chapter,

no other MBCT group programme for couples focusing on relapse for clinical depression had been identified at the time of writing.

Case Example

Barry and Leslie (not their real names) had been married their whole adult life. Now in his mid-50s Barry had taken early retirement from his engineering job. This transition, alongside other contributing life events, had led Barry to become extremely low. He spent several weeks acutely depressed on an acute mental health ward. The stress had been significant for Leslie, and reminiscent of Barry's previous periods of depression when they were first married.

Barry was referred to the community mental health team having received an assessment from the inpatient based clinical psychologist. Leslie also attended the assessment, and it was evident how involved Leslie was in supporting Barry, as well as the emotional impact she had experienced as a result of his difficulties. Both were keen on exploring ways of managing difficulty in a different way and looking to maintain their emotional well-being for the future. This was both in terms of Barry's own depressive relapse, as well as Leslie's fears of going through the suffering again.

MBCT for couples was introduced to help support people presenting with these kinds of narratives. Barry and Leslie attended the first group run in the service. At the time of writing, it

K. Griffiths, PClin.Psych. (✉) • M. Averbeck, Ph.D.
Department of Adult Mental Health, Erith Center,
Park Crescent, London DA8 3EE, UK
e-mail: Kim.griffiths@oxleas.nhs.uk; Marcus.
averbeck@oxleas.nhs.uk

is pleasing to report that neither has been re-referred to the mental health team as Barry had remitted and not suffered a relapse.

Mindfulness and Relating to Others

A number of papers have explored the role mindfulness can play in relationships, many of which have focused on the couple dyad. Some of these studies have focused on trait mindfulness, i.e. the measurement of mindfulness in personality as opposed to the consequence of a direct intervention.

In a study of 30 married couples from a non-clinical population, Wachs and Cordova [3] found self-reported mindfulness was positively associated with relationship satisfaction. In a comparative quantitative study, couples were found to demonstrate associations between increased scores of trait mindfulness and emotional skill repertoires (e.g. identifying and communicating emotions, regulation of anger expression), which in turn were associated with increased marital quality.

Barnes et al. [4] used an experimental longitudinal design to explore the role of trait mindfulness in couple well-being amongst a group of university student relationships. Data indicated that mindfulness predicted higher relationship satisfaction and greater capacities to constructively respond to relationship stress. Mindfulness was also found to be related to better communication, including pre- and post-conflict discussions.

These links between mindfulness and relationship satisfaction have been replicated. Indications have been made that spousal attachment (the degree to which spouses are attached to each other) may be a mediating mechanism through which mindfulness contributes to greater marital satisfaction [5]. This may suggest that mindfulness may offer benefits to couple therapy and the fostering of spousal attachment, i.e. the relationship between spousal attachment and mindfulness may be reciprocal.

MBSR/MBCT and Relating to Others

Several papers have explored outcomes of the MBSR or MBCT programme on relationships. In a study exploring the impact of MBCT on emotional reactions to social stress, Britton et al. [6] introduced a social stress test to couples before and after the 8-week programme. MBCT was found to be significantly associated with reductions in emotional reactivity to the social stress and concurrent improvements in depressive symptoms. The indication that MBCT can have a positive effect on social stressors offers a suggestion of similar positive links between mindfulness and relating to others, or similar in reactivity to the stress that can come in relationships.

Following a qualitative methodology, Bihari and Mullan [7] interviewed participants after an MBCT programme to directly examine the impact of the intervention on their relationships. Participants identified a core construct of relating mindfully to their own experiences with consequential profound changes in their relationships with others. By mindfully being in the moment participants described being more aware of their own internal triggers and how this related to interactions with others. As with the study with university students this was also inclusive of an improved management of conflict, as well an increase in empathy and being able to see others' perspectives. MBCT was also seen to facilitate a greater appreciation of being with others, being in the moment with others as opposed to being elsewhere in one's thoughts.

Beyond the couple relationship there have been a variety of applications of MBSR/MBCT to caregivers with similarly beneficial outcomes. The concept of caregivers could include parents, teachers and health care professionals.

Positive associations between MBCT have been identified with parents who suffer from recurrent depression and their relationship with their children one year after the intervention [8]. Parents described themes of improved emotional reactivity, empathy and acceptance, involvement, emotional availability and comfort alongside an increased recognition of their own needs.

Parents and educators of children with special needs have also been found to demonstrate improved empathic concern and forgiveness, as well as an individualised reduced stress and anxiety [9]. In this case participants received an adapted version of the recognised 8-week programme reported to be 70% similar to the components of MBSR.

Other mindfulness training adaptations have also been reported in working with staff of adults with learning disability [10]. Positive outcomes following intensive 5-day mindfulness training included reduced incidents of service user aggression, hypothesised as being a consequence of an increase in empathy, compassion and awareness in the mindfulness trained staff. Similar use of mindfulness-based approaches, including the full 8-week programme has been called for in working with parenting couples of children with autistic spectrum disorders [11].

Mindfulness-Based Interventions with Couples

The work of Carson et al. [12] on mindfulness-based relationship enhancement (MBRE) has been well documented. MBRE takes a similar 8-week structure to MBSR with the inclusion of specific couple based exercises. The groups were conducted with non-clinical populations and indicated a range of positive benefits for the couples involved. Relationship satisfaction, autonomy, closeness and acceptance were just some of the observed outcomes. A dose–response relationship was also observed in terms of mindfulness practice, i.e. those who practised more had better outcomes and improved levels of relationship happiness, relationship stress and stress-coping efficacy observed in days following high degrees of practice.

MBRE has shown some positive outcomes for non-distressed couples; however, it may not be so easily applied to the clinical setting. Perhaps central to this is the concept of intention. Alongside attention and attitude, intention has been posited as one of the three fundamental components of mindfulness practice [13]. The intention within MBRE, as the name suggests, points towards relationship enhancement, and therefore, practices such as mindful touching or partner yoga would be appropriate. However, in a clinical setting the intention may be more focused upon relapse prevention for depression or stress, or perhaps carer stress management or health symptomatology. In these approaches MBSR or MBCT may be more appropriate. This is not to say that relationship enhancement may not be a consequence of MBSR or MBCT attendance; however, it would not necessarily be the primary intention.

There have been some published reports on the direct use of 8-week programme (MBSR or MBCT) with couples. There have also been some case study reports, and calls for, the integration of mindfulness into couple therapy [1, 14, 15].

Pilot studies have indicated beneficial outcomes for cancer patients and their partners participating in MBSR [16] and multiple sclerosis [17]. In the former, 21 couples attended MBSR and significant reductions in mood disturbance and stress for both patient and partner were observed. Post MBSR partners' mood disturbance scores were also significantly correlated with patients' symptoms of stress. As indicated previously, highlighting the interaction between condition management and carer/partner stress.

Following MBSR groups with couples facing Relapse Remitting Multiple Sclerosis quantitative self-measures were administered to 21 couples. Outcome data indicated reduced levels of anxiety and improved tolerance of uncertainty for both partners and patients, as well as improved relationship satisfaction [17].

In working with couples referred to a counselling centre in Iran, Chaghazardi et al. [18] reported on the use of MBCT for couples struggling with marital adjustment. Significant associations between marital satisfaction, dyadic cohesion, dyadic consensus and amour expression were observed when compared to controls.

In the aforementioned qualitative study on the groups detailed in this chapter, Smith et al. [2] found the process of engaging in MBCT as a partnership included shifts in the couple relationship and the dual management of depression. Participants described a sense of responsibility in managing each other's well-being, with MBCT a mechanism to facilitate this. They also described an increased sense of mutual support, empathy and understanding, reduced worry, improved reconnection with one another and sharing in relapse prevention.

MBCT Couples Groups for Recurrent Depression

Background

The couples programme has been running in our service for several years alongside the standard MBCT group programme for individuals referred for depression. We work in a mental health service for working age adults in the National Health Service (NHS) in the United Kingdom. MBCT is included in the NHS clinical provision guidelines as an efficacious intervention for recurrent depression [19, 20] and it is in this context that we have been providing groups to service users since 2008.

The provision of MBCT for couples developed through, as many things do, a few converging variables. Perhaps primarily, alongside our own mindfulness practice (personally and professionally), we also have a shared interest in systemic family therapy and had been working together in a family therapy team when we also started to provide MBCT in the service.

At the same time there was growing emphasis in the NHS to offer support to family members and caregivers of people with mental health problems who use our service. Given MBCT's focus on relapse prevention for depression and stress reduction there seemed validity in offering groups to couples for the benefit of both sides of the couple and perhaps facilitating well-being on a more systemic level to prevent future relapse.

One of us (MA) also drew on his experience of being a participant in his own 8-week MBCT class together with his wife, who is also a psychotherapist. Having known each other for almost three decades and having undergone many different psychotherapy trainings, the joint experience of discovering new mindfulness practices for life and novel ways of talking about internal experiences made this course life enhancing for our relationship. We began to have conversations about things we would otherwise never have had. We decided to eventually also train as mindfulness teachers. On the way we learned to support each other in keeping up with our formal and informal mindfulness practices.

Group Adaptations and Considerations

As mentioned the MBCT group for couples described here closely follows the recognised programme [21]. Certain adaptations were only included to accommodate a systemic emphasis. The adaptations and considerations for the programme we have been providing are outlined below.

- Attendance—it is preferential for both partners to attend every session. However, should one not be available (by illness or other commitments) and the other is, the partner who can attend is still encouraged to come as planned. It is then suggested details of the session would be discussed that evening. Therefore, couple communications about the class, including struggles, joys, barriers and how to support each other are encouraged. It would also be important for the group teacher to identify certain salient points for the partner to hand over. Thus, the conversation and some of the content can be further reinforced.
- Home practice—where possible it was promoted for home practice to be a joint experience. Eating a meal mindfully together, holding a conversation about it, noticing opportunities to record shared events on the pleasant/unpleasant events diaries, seeing if it's possible to do the formal practices together, and as before have a conversation about it and so on. This may offer avenues for having new types of conversations with each other and having new activities and interests

as a shared experience. It was also hoped that joint home practice could have an influence on the frequency and quality of home practice engagement.

- In-group discussions—pair discussions took place within the couple. Joining partners together and patients together for group discussions could be helpful depending on the participants involved. It could offer a chance to have role specific conversations. Conversely such separation could be divisive and labelling and it was generally viewed that any role specific points could also arise in the group enquiries and the maintenance of the couple dyad was felt to be more pertinent in the smaller discussions.

- Relapse Prevention—A specific focus in the relapse prevention sections of the programme would fall on what each other may notice at times of difficulty, thus drawing a systemic focus on relapse indicators and action plans. It is often the partner of the person with the identified difficulties who is more aware of triggers and signs of relapse when they occur. It is then also important for the teacher to address how the partner then lets the other partner know what they notice, as the mentioning of triggers can itself become a trigger for arguments in the relationship.

- Teacher embodiment and modelling—Having two group facilitators is recommended. Embodiment is an important skill domain in MBCT [22]. In the couples groups this is furthered by the modelling of two teachers as a *pseudo-couple*, whereby positive communication, reflection and flexibility can be demonstrated via the therapist dyad. The use of two facilitators can also be beneficial in terms of the increased complexity in dynamics with a group of couples compared to a group of individual attenders.

- Assessment and suitability—a little more is outlined on assessment in due course. Here it is prudent to return to the foundation of intention for the course. MBCT for couples would not be advised with couples in interpersonal conflict or if the therapeutic intention is upon repairing marital discourse. Other couple, systemic therapy or marriage guidance paradigms may be more appropriate in these instances. The latter could of course include elements of mindfulness-based interventions. It may also be prudent to explain at the point of assessment that the MBCT course may help people to also become more aware of patterns in their relationships, and that the programme may help to also deal with relational difficulties if they arise.

Local Context

The groups took place in a community mental health setting in South East London. Psychological therapies have been an established part of the service, and MBCT was available alongside other interventions such as CBT, systemic family therapy, cognitive analytic therapy, compassion-based therapies and psychodynamic psychotherapy. The teams would work with people referred with a range of emotional difficulties including depression, trauma, PTSD, bipolar disorder and interpersonal/personality issues.

Assessment

MBCT referrals often followed a psychological assessment where MBCT had been viewed as a possible treatment of choice. Referrals would then receive an individual MBCT assessment where their needs would be discussed and decisions made on suitability and readiness for MBCT. A preference or appropriateness for the couples group or individuals group would be a standard part of this meeting. It would be explained that the group is not exclusively for couples, and could involve relatives or friends. A further pre-group meeting for the couple would also be offered.

The availability of partners and whether participants had a significant other to invite would be the main influencing factors on choosing couples or individual MBCT programmes. Similarly for some people, therapy (and indeed, mindfulness development) can be a private process and in such cases some participants have a personal preference to attend on their own, so as to have their own personal journey.

Groups Run

At the time of writing seven MBCT groups for couples have been run in the service. 21 couples have completed the programme. Four have started but for various reasons could not complete the programme. There have been some attendance by friends and relatives but the majority of participants have been married or cohabiting partners.

The groups were facilitated by experienced mindfulness teachers, adhering to the UK Good Practice Guidelines for Mindfulness Teachers [23]. It is commonplace for MBCT to be co-facilitated by two teachers; however, this is not a practice guideline. In terms of couples MBCT, as discussed previously, all groups were co-run.

Participants

All of the index clients were referred for depression in some form. Some also had other primary or secondary diagnoses of borderline personality disorder, anxiety and bipolar affective disorders. Four participants had significant concurrent physical health problems, including multiple sclerosis and chronic pain. Many had previously received other forms of psychological therapy including CBT and systemic or psychodynamic psychotherapy. At the outset each group consisted of 3–5 couples.

Results

Quantitative clinical outcome measures were administered pre and post group to both partners. Measures for depression (Beck Depression Inventory, BDI-II), hopelessness (Beck Hopelessness Scale, BHS), general mental health/well-being (Clinical Outcome Routine Evaluation, CORE) and mindfulness (Mindfulness Awareness Acceptance Scale, MAAS).

A number of the measures were incomplete hence the discrepancy against the attendance number.

CORE scores for the referred persons (N=15) demonstrated reliable change for ten participants, with six moving out of the clinical range entirely. Four showed slight non-significant increases in their outcome scores, and one stayed the same.

Of the partners ($N=7$) three scored in the mild clinical range at pre intervention, one of whom remained in the same range but showed a decreased score. The other two moved into non-clinical range upon outcome. Six demonstrated reduced scores, one showed a slight non-significant increase within the non-clinical range.

BDI-II pre and post scores for the referred persons are shown in Fig. 11.1 ($N=16$). Thirteen participants showed clinical change in their scores, two changed from scores in the severe depression range to moderate, three from severe to mild, four from moderate to mild, four from mild to minimal. Three remained in the severe range from pre to post intervention. Two of those who remained in the same range showed slight non-significant increases in their scores at post intervention.

Of the partners ($N=9$), three showed clinical changes in their scores from mild depression range to minimal, six remained in the minimal range.

Figure 11.2 shows pre and post scores for BHS for referred persons ($N=16$). One participant moved from the severe range to moderate, two from severe to mild, three from moderate to mild, one from moderate to minimal, five from mild to minimal, and four remained in the same range (2=moderate range, 2=severe), all of whom showed slight non-significant increases in their outcome scores.

Of the partners ($N=9$) four remained in the same range (1=mild, 4=minimal). Two partners moved from moderate to mild ranges, two from mild to minimal.

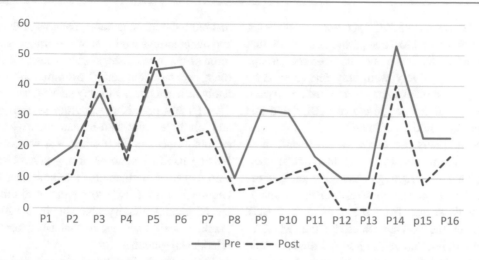

Fig. 11.1 BDI-II scores pre and post for referred persons

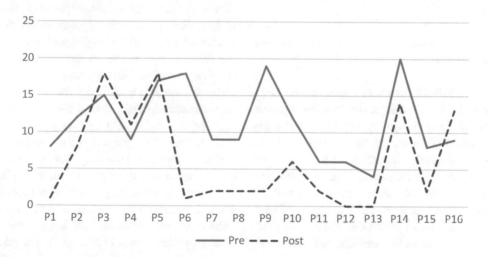

Fig. 11.2 BHS scores for pre and post for referred persons

On the MAAs ($N=14$), 13 referred persons showed increases on their scores, ten of which were significant. One reduced but the difference was not significant. Of the partners ($N=9$), all increased in scores.

Discussion

The preliminary data is encouraging. Though some slight increase in scores were found these were non-significant and did not change clinical ranges. The majority of service users demonstrated changes in clinical range, as did some of the partners. The latter showed a number of partners scoring in mild or moderate clinical ranges, further highlighting the impact of carer stress and the dual experience of managing depression.

Those who showed slight increases in scores may be a function of the difficulty in measuring outcome in MBCT. Similarly lower outcome scores could have been influenced by the ending of the group, rather than an increase in generalised distress. More research on the impact of the end of the group would be interesting to explore in terms of outcomes.

There appeared to be no correlation to outcome and diagnosis, including secondary diagnosis. This is interesting to note in terms of working with people with a diagnosis of emotionally unstable or borderline personality disorder. Certainly several of the participants with that psychiatric diagnosis in the current groups appeared to do very well, only one showed no reliable or clinical change at outcome. Again, further research into the use of MBCT and this population would be of interest.

The numbers are currently small and there were a significant amount of incomplete measures. This is something to pay attention to in the future. When the sample sizes increase comparisons with scores from the individual MBCT groups in the service would be interesting to explore. Follow-up or longitudinal studies would also be of use. It is interesting to note that at the time or writing only two have re-presented to the service.

Reflections

From a MBCT teachers perspective being involved in the couples groups have been powerful and at times moving experiences. The attendance has felt to be higher, as has the home practice, though this is nothing we have measured as yet. There is an aliveness in the room and people speak of transformative experiences both for themselves and as a couple. The depth of resonance and degree of positive expression we experience in the groups is something that is certainly hard to capture via quantitative measures.

Born out of interest, clinical need and service priorities the groups have developed from one to another. This, naturally, is an ongoing process and what is presented here is by no means a definitive programme for working with couples. Indeed following recent reflection into the exercises used in MBSR and the emphasis on stressful communications and insight dialogue, both of which offer things to consider for these groups as we move on.

Over the years, when teaching MBCT/MBSR classes and training clinicians in MBCT we noticed that many, if not most, difficulties that participants chose "to put onto the workbench of their mind" in session five of the 8-week programme, are relationship difficulties (e.g. an argument, a loss, a separation, a relational dilemma). It appears that our habitual behaviours, patterns of thoughts, and our emotions tend to show up primarily in and through our relationships with others; they have often become "automatic" overtime and consistently have a tendency to stay unexamined.

Arguably, practising mindfulness as a couple, and jointly learning to articulate the experiences of mindfulness to each other, is a way of challenging habitual patterns of any given relationship. For most partnerships a mindfulness-based enquiry is a novel way to interact, and thus, the act of mutual enquiry about their mindfulness practice itself becomes a "habit-breaker" of a relationship pattern.

One of the fruits of mindfulness practice, best described as "seeing the self and the world more clearly", also relates to interpersonal patterns which often appear rather opaque in our field of awareness as we are entangled and caught up in the relationship, unable to step outside. When couples in a MBCT/MBSR programme deliberately turn towards a difficulty that involves their partner/relative/friend, then there is an opportunity for this to be held in kindly awareness in such a way that the automatic reaction (e.g. avoiding, fighting, numbing) can be noticed as well as the intensity of the emotions and bodily sensations. Over time, patterns of reactions can become clearer. This practice of course can be done individually and in itself can be beneficial. The opportunity and challenge in the couples approach lies in the articulation of the relational difficulty and the holding of it in "joint awareness" without automatically slipping back into well-established reactive relational patterns. The mindfulness teacher's task then is to allow these difficulties to be present, to acknowledge the potential unease of the new way of interacting in the present moment, and to help the partners find a language through gentle enquiry.

It takes courage to turn towards a relational difficulty in the presence of the person who is part of the relationship. There is a degree of "relational risk-taking" [24] for the couple as well as the teacher and other participants that needs to be made explicit during the course of the MBCT/MBSR class. In this way the "relational risk-taking" is turned towards and seen more clearly. The context of the class with its clear structure and mindful attitudes, and the embodied non-judging awareness of the teacher, can provide a safe basis from which participants can take such relational risks. It is however important not to make relational difficulties the primary focus of attention during any guided practices as this is not the intended remit of the course. We merely highlight the importance of allowing relational difficulties to emerge so that they can be addressed in a mindful way, using the skills learned on the course.

Should it emerge during the course that such relational difficulties are extremely complex and entrenched, it may be useful to approach the couple outside the group session to see if some additional couple therapy or counselling sessions might be helpful. Again, dealing with the emergence of such difficulties in a mindful way means for the teacher to allow it to be present, notice his/her reactions, holding it in awareness, and opening the door towards wise action.

References

1. Gambrel LE, Keeling ML. Relational aspects of mindfulness: Implications for the practice of marriage and family therapy. Contemp Fam Ther. 2010;32:412–26.
2. Smith EL, Jones FW, Holttum S, Griffiths K. The process of engaging in mindfulness-based cognitive therapy as a partnership: a grounded theory study. Mindfulness. 2015;6:455–66.
3. Wachs K, Cordova JV. Mindful relating: exploring mindfulness and emotion repertoires in intimate relationships. J Marital Fam Ther. 2007;33:464–81.
4. Barnes S, Brown KW, Krusemark E, Campbell WK, Rogge RD. The role of mindfulness in romantic relationship satisfaction and responses to relationship stress. J Marital Fam Ther. 2007;33:482–500.
5. Jones KC, Welton SR, Oliver TC, Thoburn JW. Mindfulness, spousal attachment, and marital satisfaction: a mediate model. Fam J. 2011;19:357–61.
6. Britton WB, Shahar B, Szepsenwol O, Jacobs WJ. Mindfulness-based cognitive therapy improves emotional reactivity to social stress: results from a randomized control trial. Behav Ther. 2012;43:365–80.
7. Bihari JLN, Mullan EG. Relating mindfully: a qualitative exploration of changes in relationships through mindfulness-based cognitive therapy. Mindfulness. 2014;5:46–59.
8. Baillie C, Kuyken W, Sonnenberg S. The experiences of parents in mindfulness-based cognitive therapy. Clin Child Psychol Psych. 2012;17:103–19.

9. Benn R, Akiva T, Arel S, Roeser RW. Mindfulness training effects for parents and educators of children with special needs. Dev Psychol. 2012. doi:10.1037/a0027537.
10. Singh NN, Giulio E, Lancioni B, Winton ASW, Curtis J, Wahler RG, et al. Mindful staff increase learning and reduce aggression in adults with developmental disabilities. Res Dev Disabil. 2006;27:545–58.
11. Bluth K, Roberson PNE, Billen RM, Sams JM. A stress model for couples parenting children with autism spectrum disorders and the introduction of a mindfulness intervention. J Fam Theory Rev. 2013;5:194–213.
12. Carson JW, Carson KM, Gil KM, Baucom DH. Mindfulness-based relationship enhancement. Behav Ther. 2004;35:471–94.
13. Shapiro SL, Carlson LE. The art and science of mindfulness: Integrating mindfulness into psychology and the helping professions. Washington, DC: American Psychological Association; 2009. p. 3–14.
14. Averbeck M. Couples therapy: emotionally focused and mindfulness-based. Context. 2013;128:10–2.
15. O'Kelly M, Collard J. Using mindfulness with couples: theory and practice. In: Vernon A, editor. Cognitive and rational-emotive behaviour therapy with couples: theory and practice. New York, NY: Springer; 2012.
16. Birnie K, Garland SN, Carlson LE. Psychological benefits for cancer patients and their partners participating in mindfulness-based stress reduction (MBSR). Psychooncology. 2010;19:1004–9.
17. Hankin VM. Mindfulness based stress reduction in couples facing multiple sclerosis: impact on self reported anxiety and uncertainty. 2009. Accessed 27 July 2015 from http://gradworks.umi.com/33/78/3378573.html.
18. Chaghazardi FK, Mami S, Kaikhavani S. Effectiveness of mindfulness-based cognitive therapy on marital adjustment. J Appl Environ Biol Sci. 2015;5:86–8.
19. Kuyken W, Byford S, Taylor RS, Barrett B, Evans A, et al. Mindfulness-based cognitive therapy to prevent relapse in recurrent depression. J Consult Clin Psychol. 2012;76:966–78.
20. National Institute for Clinical Excellence. Depression: management of depression in primary and secondary care (Clinical Guideline No. 23). 2004. Accessed from www.nice.org.uk/CG023NICEguideline.
21. Segal ZV, Williams JMG, Teasdale JD. Mindfulness-based cognitive therapy for depression: a new approach to preventing relapse. New York, NY: Guilford; 2002.
22. Crabe RS, Eames C, Kuyken W, Hastings RP, Williams MG et al. Development and validation of the Mindfulness-Based Interventions – Teaching Assessment Criteria (MBI:TAC). 2015. Accessed 2 Aug 2015 from http://asm.sagepub.com/content/20/6/681.full.pdf.
23. UK Network for Mindfulness-Based Teachers. Good practice guidelines for teaching mindfulness-based courses. Accessed 2 Aug 2015 from http://mindfulnessteachersuk.org.uk/pdf/teacher-guidelines.pdf.
24. Mason B. Relational risk taking and the therapeutic relationship. In: Mason B, Perlesz A, Flaskas C, editors. The space between: experience, context and process in the therapeutic relationship. London, UK: Karnac; 2005.

Mindfulness-Based Cognitive Therapy for Treatment-Resistant Depression

12

Serina Deen, Walter Sipe, and Stuart J. Eisendrath

The Case of Sofia

Sofia is a 54-year-old married woman who has been suffering from depressive symptoms to varying degrees since her adolescence. She was adopted at an early age and experienced sexual abuse by her adoptive father from the ages of 8–12. Despite persistent low mood and poor energy, Sofia was able to maintain steady work as a massage therapist until she experienced a worsening of her depressive symptoms 2 years ago. She is now on disability and spends her day watching TV. Her current symptoms include dysphoric mood, poor energy, difficulty concentrating, poor sleep, guilty ruminations, and passive suicidal ideation of "I wish I wouldn't wake up tomorrow."

Through the course of her treatment, Sofia has had at least 8 week trials of three mechanistically different antidepressants at therapeutic doses without remission of her symptoms. She discontinued several other antidepressants early due to sexual side effects, increased irritability, and fears of weight gain. She also suffers from chronic back pain of unknown etiology, and suffers from intermittent panic attacks. She has tried psychodynamic psychotherapy and CBT in the past but did not find them helpful. Specifically, she felt "no need to delve into the past" with psychodynamic psychotherapy, and felt like a "bad student" in CBT because she could not change her negative thoughts and often did not do the homework.

The Problem of Treatment-Resistant Depression

Sofia's struggle with depression is unfortunately quite common. Depression is the number three cause of disability worldwide and the number one cause of disability in high-income countries [1]. Although definitions vary, the commonly held definition of treatment-resistant depression (TRD) is a failure to fully remit from depressive symptoms after two or more antidepressant trials [2, 3]. Thirty-five to fifty percent of all patients with depression may be treatment-resistant [4, 5]. TRD is associated with greater disability, morbidity,

S. Deen, M.D., M.P.H.
Department of Psychiatry, University of California, San Francisco, 401 Parnassus Avenue, San Francisco, CA 94143, USA
e-mail: serinadeen@ucsf.edu

W. Sipe
University of California, San Francisco, San Francisco, CA 94143, USA

S.J. Eisendrath, M.D. (✉)
The UCSF Depression Center, Langley Porter Psychiatric Institute, University of California, San Francisco, San Francisco, CA, USA
e-mail: stuart.eisendrath@ucsf.edu

© Springer International Publishing Switzerland 2016
S.J. Eisendrath (ed.), *Mindfulness-Based Cognitive Therapy*, DOI 10.1007/978-3-319-29866-5_12

mortality, and health care costs than non-resistant depression [6, 7]. As such, it is a major public health concern.

Adding or switching medications is the strategy most commonly used for TRD. As illustrated in the STAR*D trial, this strategy has limited effectiveness, with only half of patients remitting after two full antidepressant trial, and lower remission rates for each subsequent treatment step [5]. After patients fail to remit using first-line medications, medications with higher side effect burden or risk may be used (such as tricyclic antidepressants and monoamine oxidase inhibitors), or more stigmatized and/or invasive treatment options may be utilized such as electroconvulsive therapy and vagal nerve stimulation.

Clearly, alternative approaches to treating TRD are needed. MBCT may be a low-cost, minimally invasive, and well-tolerated option for those with TRD.

Theoretical Rationale of MBCT for Treatment Resistant Depression

Use of MBCT for Prevention of Depressive Relapse

MBCT was originally designed to prevent depressive relapse in people who had recovered from a major depressive episode and were at risk of relapsing [8]. In this section, we review mechanisms by which MBCT may prevent depressive relapse, and then outline the rationale for using MBCT as an active treatment for people with TRD such as Sofia.

Numerous studies have found MBCT to be efficacious in relapse prevention [9–11]. A meta-analysis of six randomized-controlled trials (RCTs) with 593 total participants found that MBCT reduced the risk of relapse for patients with recurrent MDD by 34% compared to treatment-as-usual (TAU) or placebo control, and the risk reduction increased to 43% for patients with three or more previous episodes [12]. MBCT appears to be equivalent to maintenance medication for relapse prevention [13–15]. Gains from MBCT treatment

were maintained over a 34-month follow-up period in one study [16] and 5-year follow-up period in another [17].

How does MBCT produce these results? The developers of MBCT postulated that people who had suffered from depression may react differently to sad mood states than people who had never been depressed, and then built the intervention based on this assumption. Teasdale [18] hypothesized that sad moods reactivate thinking styles associated with previous sad moods. This puts people who have been depressed in the past at risk of spiraling downward into another depressive episode. Several studies confirmed that when people who have experienced depression in the past feel sad, they are more likely to endorse dysfunctional thinking than those who have never been depressed [19, 20], and that people who display this reactivated dysfunctional thinking in response to sad mood are more likely to relapse into another depressive episode in the future [21, 22].

Mindfulness has been defined as the awareness that arises through paying attention on purpose in the present moment and nonjudgmentally [23]. Studies have confirmed that MBCT does in fact increase mindfulness, and that mindfulness skills may be the mediator of MBCT's treatment effect [24, 25]. One study using EEG found that MBCT improved participants' ability to shift their attention toward current moment experience and away from distracting stimuli during mild dysphoric states [26]. Another study with previously depressed participants found that after MBCT, participants showed less negative attentional bias; they showed a reduced facilitation of attention for negative information and a reduced inhibition of attention for positive information [27]. Mindfulness also encourages people to see the negative thoughts they experience as passing events of the mind that do not necessarily reflect reality. People may become less vulnerable to depressive relapse by being able to disengage from or "decenter" from negative thoughts and feelings [28, 29]. Mindfulness could thus lead to using less avoidance coping strategies [30], and could function as an exposure procedure to previously avoided aversive thoughts [31].

Applying MBCT to Treatment Resistant Depression

People with treatment-resistant depression may be maintaining their depression via a similar cognitive style that renders people who have recovered from depression vulnerable to relapse. Thus, several of the mechanisms that are thought to help prevent relapse may also help people who are actively depressed.

MBCT helps to decrease *rumination* [17, 32]. Nolen-Hoeksema defined ruminative responses to depression as "thoughts and behaviors that focus one's attention on one's depressive symptoms and the meaning of those symptoms" [33]. People often believe that ruminating about their symptoms will help them understand the causes of the depression better, and thus enable them to "fix" their mood. However, the depressive rumination often ends up paradoxically increasing sad mood [34]. Martin and Tesser [35] suggested that rumination is the result of discrepancies between an individual's goals and the actual state of things. MBCT may decrease rumination by encouraging participants to adopt a more accepting mode of being, one that does not need to evaluate experience in order to reduce discrepancies [8, 36]. This increased acceptance could be particularly useful for people with treatment-resistant depression, who might be mired in depressive ruminations as treatment after treatment has failed to alleviate their symptoms.

Mindfulness may also enhance *emotion regulation* [37, 38]. Chiesa and collaborators [38] suggest that one of the ways that mindfulness training enhances emotion regulation is by modifying how "higher" brain regions such as the prefrontal cortex modulate the input to the "lower" emotion-generative system (such as the amygdala) by actively reinterpreting emotional stimuli in a way that modifies their emotional impact [39]. This is similar to how cognitive behavioral therapy (CBT) has been postulated to exert its effect [40]. Mindfulness may also enhance emotion regulation by a direct reduction of reactivity in "lower" emotion-generative brain regions such as the amygdala, especially in long-term practitioners of mindfulness [41].

Self-compassion may be another mechanism by which MBCT treats active depression. Neff defines self-compassion as, "extending kindness and understanding to oneself rather than harsh self-criticism and judgment, seeing one's experiences as part of the larger human experience rather than as separating and isolating, and holding one's painful thoughts and feelings in balanced awareness rather than over-identifying with them" [42]. Kuyken and colleagues [43] found that increased self-compassion mediated MBCT's ability to successfully prevent depressive relapse and also mediated the effect of MBCT on post-treatment symptoms of depression.

Going back to our case example of Sofia, she had failed many change-based strategies and her providers felt it would be beneficial for her to try an intervention focused on acceptance. Sofia did not like talking about her trauma history, and liked that the intervention would be present-focused and not necessitate delving into her painful past. Sofia also liked that while group participation was encouraged, if she were feeling particularly depressed or anxious, she could participate silently in the meditations without needing to speak about her experience. She also had positive associations with the concept of mindfulness. Sofia knew friends who had a meditation practice who were not "sick" and thus found the concept of going to the group less stigmatizing. However she was skeptical that she'd be able to be "calm enough" to meditate. She was also concerned that her chronic pain would interfere with her ability to sit for long periods of time, and very worried that she would not be able to learn to meditate correctly.

Modifications of MBCT for Treatment-Resistant Depression

Despite the many indications that MBCT would be helpful in TRD, there are also unique challenges in treating this population [8, 44]. For one, it could be difficult to engage people with active depression. They may feel hopeless and may have low motivation to participate in group and do homework. They may have decreased ability to concentrate and attend to the teachings and exercises. Their negative thinking styles and self-criticism may make them believe they are "not meditating correctly" rather than being open to learning the new material. And given that they are actively depressed, the content of the present moment that they are being asked to focus on may be extremely painful. Accepting and allowing these negative thoughts and feelings could be a foreign and overwhelming concept. And finally, like Sofia, people with TRD are more likely to have comorbidities such as anxiety and physical pain [45, 46] that may interfere with their work in the group.

Eisendrath and colleagues [47, 48] have made several modifications to the MBCT manual developed by Segal et al. [8] to address these challenges. A summary of the modifications is listed in Table 12.1. Specific modifications are illustrated in detail using our case example of Sophia.

Table 12.1 Summary of MBCT for TRD modifications

Challenge with TRD	Modifications
Increased restlessness, decreased attentional control	–Shorter sitting meditation –Increased emphasis on mindful movement/yoga, walking meditation –Increased emphasis on brief breathing spaces
Difficulty with motivation and engagement	–Increased emphasis and time spent on identifying barriers to practice each week
Negative thinking styles, focus on "meditating the right way"	–Use of negative thinking examples to illustrate depressive symptomatology and "doing" versus "being" mode
Difficulty with acceptance and allowance of negative experience	–Incorporation of metaphors and exercises to convey teaching points
Comorbidities such as anxiety and chronic pain	–Demonstration of MBCT techniques with comorbidities as other examples of negative states

Illustration of MBCT modifications using the case of Sophia

General Modifications

Throughout the 8 weeks of the group, the length of several group sitting meditations were reduced from 30 min to 10–15 min to address the decreased attentional control and restlessness that is often experienced in depression. In addition, greater emphasis was placed on walking meditations and mindful movement/yoga. If participants suffered from physical limitations such as pain, instructors gave them suggestions for modification, for example sitting in a chair during the body scan instead of lying down. Given that several participants had a history of trauma, participants were given the choice of allowing their eyes to gently close or gazing softly a few feet in front of them if they were not comfortable closing their eyes in guided meditations. Similarly sitting in a chair rather than lying supine for a body scan may be preferred as less vulnerable.

The language instructors used was modified to address the change in focus from relapse prevention to treatment of active depression. For example, phrases like "when you become depressed," were replaced with "the experience of depression for you right now." The language was also modified from using commands like "close your eyes" to the present participle "closing your eyes" to help participants who might have difficulty with a more authoritative stance. See Table 12.2.

Going into MBCT, Sophia was of the mindset that if she actually let herself feel the full extent of her depression, she would sink further in it. Given that this is a natural and common way to think about depression, two exercises derived from Acceptance and Commitment Therapy (ACT) were added to the first session of MBCT to illustrate how and why people might want to relate differently to their depression. The ACT exercises helped to illustrate to participants why avoiding negative emotions and feelings may be counterproductive.

The Chinese Finger Cuff Exercise gave participants a physical metaphor for their psychological experience of depression [49]. Sophia and the other participants were given Chinese finger cuffs, asked to put their index fingers in them,

Table 12.2 Specific modifications in MBCT for TRD

Name of Modification	Session #	Goal of modification
Chinese finger cuff exercise	1	Illustrate drawbacks of experiential avoidance and benefits of a mindful approach to depression
Quicksand metaphor	1	Illustrate drawbacks of experiential avoidance and benefits of mindful approach to depression
Your mind is not your friend discussion	2	Discuss rumination; encourage decentering from negative thoughts
Black dog metaphor	2	Illustrate reactions to depression other than aversion
Empty boat metaphor	3	Illustrate using mindfulness to cope with anger
Suffering equation	4	Illustrate drawbacks of experiential avoidance
Donkey standoff exercise	5	Introduce moving forward in life while still depressed
Frankenstein exercise	7	Illustrate moving forward in life while still depressed
Self esteem equation	8	Illustrate the benefit of realistic expectations

and then asked to try to get out of the cuffs. When Sophia tried to pull her fingers out, the cuff tightened. She was then asked to try even harder, which made the cuff even tighter. She was then invited to push her fingers closer together, and she observed that the cuffs loosened up. This experience was then related to her depression. The perfectly natural method of trying to pull away from (or avoid) her depression had not worked in the past, and may have tightened depression's grip on her. Somewhat counterintuitively, allowing herself to get in close with the depression may give her some "wiggle room" to live her life.

Another modification derived from ACT is the **Quicksand Metaphor** [49]. The group was asked what happens when people in quicksand struggle to get out. From watching movies, a group member responded that people sink even deeper when they struggle. We discussed how the best strategy when someone is in quicksand is actually to come into full contact with the quicksand by leaning back and floating in it.

In session 2, the standard Thoughts and Feelings exercise was paired with an added ACT exercise entitled **Your Mind is Not Always Your Friend** [50] to promote decentering from negative thoughts. Participants observed their own negative thoughts in the Thoughts and Feelings exercise, and were then invited to explore how the mind sometimes may not be helpful by (1) creating problems to worry about when there is nothing to worry about, (2) trying to solve problems that cannot be solved, (3) assigning blame, often to oneself, when a problem is detected. Sophia was invited to explore how actually engaging with her mind, and the negative thoughts it produces (as all minds do) may sidetrack her from doing what she values in life.

Another modification in Session 2 was the **Black Dog Analogy** that invited participants to think about their depression as something that they could react to in a number of different ways. Winston Churchill referred to his depressive states as the "black dog," [51] and a depressed day as a day in which "the black dog has returned." Participants were asked what their reaction to a black dog may be. Some people may be scared of a large black dog, but others may be curious about it. The exercise encouraged participants to consider different reactions to their depression, for example, recognizing that it may be a signal that something was not working in their lives that needed tending to. Sophia recognized that her "black dog" often returned when she was ignoring problems with her husband and consequently feeling more isolated from him.

In Session 3, while reviewing the home practice, Sophia talked about how angry she became when someone left their shopping cart haphazardly in the supermarket parking lot, and it rolled down and hit her car. She said that she could not stop thinking about how inconsiderate that person who left the cart was, and it ruined the rest of her day. This was a perfect lead-in to the **Empty**

Boat Analogy. The group was told the story about a man on his boat who is awakened by the sound of another boat hitting his boat. When he comes up to the deck he is angry at the other boatman who hit him. When he looks more carefully at the other boat, he realizes that the other boat is empty and has merely drifted into his. The group discussed what impact this had on the boatman's anger. Sophia saw how if she regarded the shopping cart incident as more neutral, versus being aimed at her, it diminished some of her anger. But she wondered how she could possibly view it that way in the heat of the moment. When the group was asked what Sophia might do, another group member suggested using a three minute breathing space the next time something like this occurred.

In Session 4, the **Suffering Equation** was used to continue to illustrate the drawbacks of experiential avoidance. The equation SUFFERING = RESISTANCE X PAIN was written on the board, where pain was described as physical or emotional pain such as depression [52]. Sophia and the other participants were told that pain is inevitable in life, which leads to a certain amount of suffering. But resisting the pain actually increases suffering. The group was asked if anyone could think of a situation in which resisting or avoiding something made the situation worse. Sophia said that she watched a lot of TV when she felt depressed to distract herself and avoid self-loathing feelings, and so that she would not "inflict" herself upon her loved ones. However in group discussion, she realized that this further isolated her, and admitted that watching TV all day made her feel even more worthless.

At this point, while Sophia was starting to be curious about what it would be like to relate to her depression differently, she wondered if not resisting her depression would be akin to giving up. This invited a discussion about acceptance versus resignation. Sophia found it helpful to think about how in Alcoholics Anonymous, members must first accept that they are "alcoholics" before they can change their actions. In a similar manner, relinquishing the struggle to escape depression may set the path for recovery.

The **Donkey Standoff Exercise** [53] was used in Session 5 to illustrate the concept of moving forward in life while still having symptoms of depression. Sophia was told of the difficulty of pulling a donkey by a rope directly in front of it, because the donkey will resist mightily. Instead, the way to get the donkey moving is to move alongside the donkey and look in the direction that you want to go. The group discussed the concept of moving forward in life alongside the depression, instead of resisting the depression fruitlessly or standing still in life waiting for the depression to completely disappear.

In Session 7, another modification that built on the black dog metaphor was used called the **Frankenstein Exercise**. This exercise was originally observed in a mindfulness-based stress reduction class. All the participants, including Sophia, were paired with other group members. Sophia played the role of "Frankenstein monster" in several scenarios, and then switched with her partner to take the role of "victim." Frankenstein would come toward the victim, and then the victim could react to Frankenstein in several ways, just as participants could react to depression coming toward them in several ways. Sophia was asked what it felt like when she were instructed to freeze and cower in front of Frankenstein (submissive), sidestep Frankenstein (avoidant), forcefully hold Frankenstein at a distance (resistant), or come close to Frankenstein, hold his arm, and lead him in the direction she wanted to go (mindfully assertive). These scenarios were used to discuss how the mindfully assertive stance did not change the monster (depression), but allowed Sophia to start to take back control and direction in her life without needing to avoid or fight the depression. She did not need to wait for the depression to resolve before doing things in her life that she found meaningful.

Finally, in Session 8, the **Self-Esteem Equation** [54] was used to help participants understand the relationship between expectations, self-esteem, and depression. The equation "Self-Esteem = Achievements/Expectations" was written on the board and discussed. Sophia realized that she had unrealistic, unachievable expectations of herself. She had always thought that setting impossibly high goals of herself would be motivating. This equation helped her to understand that these impossible expectations actually undermined her self-esteem and caused her to sink further into depression, which then decreased her motivation to accomplish things. She was interested in coming up with more realistic goals for herself, such as finding part-time work in medical records and being more open about her feelings with her husband.

When sharing her overall experience with the group in Session 8, Sofia said she still found it hard to do sitting meditations, but was taking mindful walks and found the 3-min breathing spaces to be very helpful throughout the day. She said that she was starting to see how some of the negative things she thought about herself may just be "thoughts" and not "facts." When she approached her self-talk this manner, she found it easier to not get stuck in these thoughts. As a result, she was spending more time with her husband and less time in front of the TV. Group members gave Sofia the feedback that she looked "lighter," and Sofia acknowledged that she felt less depressed and more hopeful about the future.

Evidence of MBCT for TRD

There is a growing body of evidence that MBCT is an effective treatment for active depression [44, 55]. MBCT was better than Treatment As Usual (TAU) in patients with three or more episodes of depression [32], including those with a history of suicidal ideation [56]. When compared to active competitors, MBCT was shown to be equally effective to CBT [57, 58] and superior to a psychoeducational control group designed to be structurally equivalent to MBCT but excluding mindfulness meditation practice [25]. Improvements in depressive symptoms persisted through the 26-week follow-up period of one study [25] and for up to 5 years of follow-up in another [17].

There are fewer studies of MBCT's efficacy on TRD in particular. Kenny and Williams [59] studied the effects of MBCT on participants with continuing symptoms of depression despite treatment with antidepressant medication or CBT or both in

a small sample of 50 participants. They reported a mean pre-MBCT Beck Depression Inventory (BDI) score of 24, versus a post-MBCT score of 14. In another small study, Eisendrath and colleagues [60] reported the results of MBCT augmentation of psychotherapy and medication treatment for 51 participants who were currently depressed and had failed to remit with at least two antidepressant trials. They reported a similar drop in BDI from 24 to 15.

Eisendrath and colleagues [61] recently presented the results of a large randomized controlled trial (n=173) of MBCT versus a manualized active control for people with TRD. The control condition was the Health Enhancement Program (HEP) that includes physical activity, nutritional education, and music therapy [62]. They reported a significantly greater mean percent reduction in HAM-D in MBCT versus HEP (37 % versus 25 %, $p = .01$) and a significantly greater number of treatment responders (30 % versus 17 %, $p = .029$).

Mechanism of Change

As discussed earlier, many of the same mechanisms of change may be at play in the reduction in active depressive symptoms versus relapse prevention. Unfortunately, few studies have been done to study the mechanism of change in active depression. We can look to studies that reported on MBCT's effect on residual symptoms of depression to provide some illumination on the topic.

Kuyken and colleagues [43] found that enhanced mindfulness and increased self-compassion mediated the effect of MBCT on post-treatment symptoms of depression in a population of patients with three or more depressive episodes who were in full or partial remission. A small RCT done with recurrently depressed patients, the majority of them in partial remission, showed that reductions in brooding (an aspect of rumination) and increases in mindfulness mediated the effects of MBCT on depressive symptoms [63]. Another RCT with patients with three or more previous depressive episodes, with and without a current depressive episode, found that effect on depressive symptoms were mediated by a decrease in worry and rumination, and an increase in the mindfulness skill "accept without judgment" [32]. Batink and colleagues [64] found that the effects of MBCT on residual symptoms of depression were mediated by changes in mindfulness skills and worry, but did not find rumination to be a mediator.

Another mechanism by which MBCT may reduce depressive symptoms is through increasing momentary positive emotions, which could lead to an "upward spiral" in affect and cognition [65]. In support of this theory, Geschwind and colleagues [66] found that MBCT compared to a waitlist control increased momentary positive emotions and reward from pleasant daily life activities for people with a history of MDD and current residual depressive symptoms. Batink and colleagues [64] found that changes in positive affect mediated 61 % of the effect of MBCT on residual depressive symptoms. And Garland and colleagues [65] found that MBCT enhanced momentary positive cognition, and appeared to strengthen the relationship between current positive affect and positive cognition the next day.

In terms of brain changes associated with MBCT, Eisendrath and colleagues [61] recently presented fMRI data regarding the effects of MBCT training compared to the aforementioned HEP control condition in a TRD population. Relative to HEP, during a working memory (WM) task, MBCT was associated with increased dorsolateral prefrontal cortex activation during WM encoding and maintenance and decreased ventrolateral activation during WM maintenance. In addition, in MBCT, but not in HEP, Hamilton Depression Rating Scale-17 improvement at 8 weeks was associated with enhanced regulation of amygdala activity during WM performance. Taken as a whole, these fMRI findings suggest MBCT has significant effects on brain circuitry that is associated with enhanced dorsolateral executive control mechanisms relative to ventral affective processing regions.

Practical Considerations of MBCT for TRD

Patient Selection

Overall, studies of MBCT have reported high adherence, low attrition rates, and no serious adverse events related to MBCT interventions [55]. Participants would be best served if they are able to tolerate a group format, can attend all eight weekly sessions, and are willing and able to do home practice.

Early studies suggested that MBCT was only effective in preventing depressive relapse for those with three or more episodes of depression [9, 67]. However a more recent study, albeit an open study, found that the number of previous episodes did not impact result when treating active depression, nor did the severity of depression [17]. Patients who have concurrent suicidal ideation may benefit from MBCT, in that their BDI scores have been shown to decrease with treatment [59]. However they may not experience a decrease in their suicidal ideation [56], and those with a history of suicide attempt were shown to have a higher dropout rate in MBCT trials [13].

MBCT may be particularly useful for depressed patients with psychiatric and physical comorbidities. For example, although results are mixed, many studies suggest MBCT may decrease anxiety [17, 24, 68, 69], making it an appealing treatment for TRD patients with comorbid anxiety. Patients with a history of childhood adversity may benefit more from MBCT than those who did not have childhood adversity [67, 70]. In addition, mindfulness in general has been linked to better physical and emotional functioning in those with chronic pain [71, 72].

Home Practice

Home Practice closely follows the MBCT manual recommendations [73]. Participants receive CDs or audio downloads of guided meditations (available through www.guilford.com/MBCT_ materials) to practice with at home. Participants are encouraged to practice 6 days per week, approximately 45 min per day. In the TRD population, participants may find this amount of home practice especially daunting. Given that no clear relationship between total time of practice and clinical outcomes has been established in mindfulness-based interventions [17, 74], more emphasis may be placed on practicing shorter meditations, and utilizing 3 min breathing spaces throughout the day. Shortening the home practice to 30 min/day may be sufficient to sustain positive effects [17] and even 15 min a day may be effective for participants with mild to moderate depression [24] .

Group Size

The developers of MBCT created groups of around 12 people in their research [73]. Group size can vary depending on resources available, but generally should be no larger than 16 people.

Format

Groups run for 8 consecutive weeks, with 2.25 h per session. There are usually 2–3 facilitators per group. Of note, Pots and colleagues [24] adapted the intervention to run for 11 sessions with 1.5 h per session for people with mild to moderate depressive symptomatology.

Facilitator training: Facilitators should have training in psychotherapy, treatment of mood disorders, and have a familiarity with cognitive behavioral therapy. They should also have some familiarity with running groups. In addition, the developers of MBCT firmly believe that facilitators should have their own, ongoing mindfulness practice [73]. Their own practice helps facilitators to demonstrate and embody mindfulness for the group members, and clarifies facilitators' own conceptions about pain, suffering, and acceptance [48]. Given that MBCT is asking participants with TRD to pay direct attention to experiences they would much rather avoid, the facilitators own familiarity and embodiment of this process is a key element to group success.

Summary/Conclusions

In summary, MBCT appears to be a safe and promising treatment for TRD with a growing evidence base. There are several challenges in treating patients with TRD, such as potential motivational and attentional deficits and multiple comorbidities. These challenges can be addressed with modifications to the original format, as outlined in this chapter and elsewhere [47, 48]. Despite the challenges, people with TRD may particularly benefit from this type of intervention, given that they are often ruminative with persistent self-critical thoughts [75].

The mechanisms by which MBCT may exert its effect are still being investigated. However several potential mediators such as increased self-compassion, decreased rumination, increased emotion regulation, and increased positive affect have been identified. It may be that several of these mediators contribute to the overall effect of the intervention. Globally, Chiesa [25] suggests that the benefits of mindfulness may be related to a "radical shift" in an individual's attitude toward his or her own experience that leads him/her to "reperceive" in a more adaptive and less reactive way.

Identifying further neural correlates of MBCT treatment would be illuminating, especially given recent evidence that MBCT may exert its effects via circuitry involving regions such as the prefrontal cortex and the amgydala [38, 61]. So far, two EEG studies have yielded contradictory findings on MBCT's effect on prefrontal alpha-asymmetry [26, 76]. If we better understand how MBCT affects brain circuitry, we might be able to predict which patients would benefit from the intervention the most. We also may be able to predict patient response based on genetics, although we are in the infancy of this research now. A recent study of patients with residual depressive symptoms suggested that gene variation (of an acetylcholine receptor and an opioid receptor) may moderate how MBCT boosts positive affect [77].

There are several areas of investigation that would help to clarify the potential mediators of MBCT's effect, and could help target the intervention to those who would benefit the most from it. However, there is already a sound theoretical rationale for applying MBCT to TRD as well as a growing evidence base to support its use.

References

1. UN World Health Organization. World Report on Disability [Internet]. 2011. Accessed 15 Jun 2015. Available from http://www.who.int/disabilities/world_report/2011/report.pdf.
2. Trivedi MH, Rush AJ, Crismon ML, Kashner TM, Toprac MG, Carmody TJ, et al. Clinical results for patients with major depressive disorder in the Texas Medication Algorithm Project. Arch Gen Psychiatry. 2004;61(7):669–80.
3. Souery D, Papakostas GI, Trivedi MH. Treatment-resistant depression. J Clin Psychiatry. 2006;67:16–22.
4. Nemeroff CB. Prevalence and management of treatment-resistant depression. J Clin Psychiatry. 2007;68(8):17–25.
5. Rush A, Trivedi M, Wisniewski S, Nierenberg A, Stewart J, Warden D, et al. Acute and longer-term outcomes in depressed outpatients requiring one or several treatment steps: a STAR* D report. Am J Psychiatr. 2006;163(11):1905–17.
6. Crown WH, Finkelstein S, Berndt ER, Ling D, Poret AW, Rush AJ, et al. The impact of treatment-resistant depression on health care utilization and costs. J Clin Psychiatry. 2002;63(11):963–71.
7. Greden JF. The burden of disease for treatment-resistant depression. J Clin Psychiatry. 2001;62 Suppl 16:26–31.
8. Segal Z, Williams JM, Teasdale J. Mindfulness-based cognitive therapy for depression: a new approach to preventing relapse. 1st ed. New York, NY: Guilford; 2002.
9. Teasdale JD, Segal ZV, Williams JM, Ridgeway VA, Soulsby JM, Lau MA. Prevention of relapse/recurrence in major depression by mindfulness-based cognitive therapy. J Consult Clin Psychol. 2000;68(4):615–23.
10. Bondolfi G, Jermann F, der Linden MV, Gex-Fabry M, Bizzini L, Rouget BW, et al. Depression relapse prophylaxis with Mindfulness-Based Cognitive Therapy: replication and extension in the Swiss health care system. J Affect Disord. 2010;122(3):224–31.
11. Godfrin KA, van Heeringen C. The effects of mindfulness-based cognitive therapy on recurrence of depressive episodes, mental health and quality of life: a randomized controlled study. Behav Res Ther. 2010;48(8):738–46.
12. Piet J, Hougaard E. The effect of mindfulness-based cognitive therapy for prevention of relapse in recurrent major depressive disorder: a systematic review and meta-analysis. Clin Psychol Rev. 2011;31(6):1032–40.
13. Kuyken W, Byford S, Taylor RS, Watkins E, Holden E, White K, et al. Mindfulness-based cognitive therapy to prevent relapse in recurrent depression. J Consult Clin Psychol. 2008;76(6):966–78.
14. Segal ZV, Bieling P, Young T, MacQueen G, Cooke R, Martin L, et al. Antidepressant monotherapy vs sequential pharmacotherapy and mindfulness-based cognitive therapy, or placebo, for relapse prophylaxis in recurrent depression. Arch Gen Psychiatry. 2010;67(12):1256–64.
15. Kuyken W, Hayes R, Barrett B, Byng R, Dalgleish T, Kessler D, et al. Effectiveness and cost-effectiveness of mindfulness-based cognitive therapy compared with maintenance antidepressant treatment in the prevention of depressive relapse or recurrence (PREVENT): a randomised controlled trial. Lancet. 2015;S0140–6736(14):62222–4. Internet article cited Jun 15 2015.
16. Mathew KL, Whitford HS, Kenny MA, Denson LA. The long-term effects of mindfulness-based cognitive therapy as a relapse prevention treatment for major depressive disorder. Behav Cogn Psychother. 2010;38(05):561–76.
17. Munshi K, Eisendrath S, Delucchi K. Preliminary long-term follow-up of mindfulness-based cognitive therapy-induced remission of depression. Mindfulness. 2013;4(4):354–61.
18. Teasdale JD. Cognitive vulnerability to persistent depression. Cognit Emot. 1988;2(3):247–74.
19. Miranda J, Persons JB. Dysfunctional attitudes are mood-state dependent. J Abnorm Psychol. 1988;97(1):76–9.
20. Miranda J, Persons JB, Byers CN. Endorsement of dysfunctional beliefs depends on current mood state. J Abnorm Psychol. 1990;99(3):237–41.
21. Segal ZV, Kennedy S, Gemar M, Hood K, Pedersen R, Buis T. Cognitive reactivity to sad mood provocation and the prediction of depressive relapse. Arch Gen Psychiatry. 2006;63(7):749–55.
22. Segal ZV, Gemar M, Williams S. Differential cognitive response to a mood challenge following successful cognitive therapy or pharmacotherapy for unipolar depression. J Abnorm Psychol. 1999;108(1):3–10.
23. Kabat-Zinn J. Mindfulness for beginners: reclaiming the present moment – and your life. Boulder, CO: Sounds True; 2011.
24. Pots WT, Meulenbeek PA, Veehof MM, Klungers J, Bohlmeijer ET. The efficacy of mindfulness-based cognitive therapy as a public mental health intervention for adults with mild to moderate depressive symptomatology: a randomized controlled trial. PLoS One. 2014;9(10):e109789.
25. Chiesa A, Castagner V, Andrisano C, Serretti A, Mandelli L, Porcelli S, et al. Mindfulness-based cognitive therapy vs. psycho-education for patients with major depression who did not achieve remission following antidepressant treatment. Psychiatry Res. 2015;226(2):474–83.
26. Bostanov V, Keune PM, Kotchoubey B, Hautzinger M. Event-related brain potentials reflect increased concentration ability after mindfulness-based cognitive therapy for depression: a randomized clinical trial. Psychiatry Res. 2012;199(3):174–80.
27. De Raedt R, Baert S, Demeyer I, Goeleven E, Raes A, Visser A, et al. Changes in attentional processing of emotional information following mindfulness-based cognitive therapy in people with a history of depression: Towards an open attention for all emotional experiences. Cogn Ther Res. 2012;36(6):612–20.

28. Fresco DM, Segal ZV, Buis T, Kennedy S. Relationship of posttreatment decentering and cognitive reactivity to relapse in major depression. J Consult Clin Psychol. 2007;75(3):447.

29. van der Velden A, Kuyken W, Wattar U, Crane C, Pallesen KJ, Dahlgaard J, et al. A systematic review of mechanisms of change in mindfulness-based cognitive therapy in the treatment of recurrent major depressive disorder. Clin Psychol Rev. 2015;37:26–39.

30. Chiesa A, Anselmi R, Serretti A. Psychological mechanisms of mindfulness-based interventions: what do we know? Holist Nurs Pract. 2014;28(2):124–48.

31. Baer RA. Mindfulness training as a clinical intervention: a conceptual and empirical review. Clin Psychol Sci Pract. 2003;10(2):125–43.

32. Van Aalderen J, Donders A, Giommi F, Spinhoven P, Barendregt H, Speckens A. The efficacy of mindfulness-based cognitive therapy in recurrent depressed patients with and without a current depressive episode: a randomized controlled trial. Psychol Med. 2012;42(05):989–1001.

33. Nolen-Hoeksema S. Responses to depression and their effects on the duration of depressive episodes. J Abnorm Psychol. 1991;100(4):569–82.

34. Nolen-Hoeksema S, Morrow J. Effects of rumination and distraction on naturally occurring depressed mood. Cognit Emot. 1993;7(6):561–70.

35. Martin LL, Tesser A. Some ruminative thoughts. Adv Soc Cognit. 1996;9:1–47.

36. Crane C, Winder R, Hargus E, Amarasinghe M, Barnhofer T. Effects of mindfulness-based cognitive therapy on specificity of life goals. Cogn Ther Res. 2012;36(3):182–9.

37. Arch JJ, Craske MG. Mechanisms of mindfulness: emotion regulation following a focused breathing induction. Behav Res Ther. 2006;44(12):1849–58.

38. Chiesa A, Serretti A, Jakobsen JC. Mindfulness: top–down or bottom–up emotion regulation strategy? Clin Psychol Rev. 2013;33(1):82–96.

39. Quirk GJ, Beer JS. Prefrontal involvement in the regulation of emotion: convergence of rat and human studies. Curr Opin Neurobiol. 2006;16:723–7.

40. Goldapple K, Segal Z, Garson C, Lau M, Bieling P, Kennedy S, et al. Modulation of cortical-limbic pathways in major depression: treatment-specific effects of cognitive behavior therapy. Arch Gen Psychiatry. 2004;61(1):34–41.

41. van den Hurk PAM, Janssen BH, Giommi F, Barendregt HP, Gielen SC. Mindfulness meditation associated with alterations in bottom-up processing: psychophysiological evidence for reduced reactivity. Int J Psychophysiol. 2010;78(2):151–7.

42. Neff KD. The development and validation of a scale to measure self-compassion. Self Identity. 2003;2(3):223–50.

43. Kuyken W, Watkins E, Holden E, White K, Taylor RS, Byford S, et al. How does mindfulness-based cognitive therapy work? Behav Res Ther. 2010;48(11):1105–12.

44. Strauss C, Cavanagh K, Oliver A, Pettman D. Mindfulness-based interventions for people diagnosed with a current episode of an anxiety or depressive disorder: a meta-analysis of randomised controlled trials. PLoS One. 2014;9(4):e96110.

45. Kornstein SG, Schneider RK. Clinical features of treatment-resistant depression. J Clin Psychiatry. 2001;62:18–25.

46. Bair MJ, Robinson RL, Eckert GJ, Stang PE, Croghan TW, Kroenke K. Impact of pain on depression treatment response in primary care. Psychosom Med. 2004;66(1):17–22.

47. Eisendrath S, Chartier M, McLane M. Adapting mindfulness-based cognitive therapy for treatment-resistant depression: a clinical case study. Cogn Behav Pract. 2011;18(3):362–70.

48. Sipe WE, Eisendrath SJ. Mindfulness-based cognitive therapy for treatment-resistant depression. In: Baer R, editor. Mindfulness-based treatment approaches: clinician's guide to evidence base and applications. 2nd edn. Elsevier; 2014. p. 61–76.

49. Hayes SC, Strosahl KD, Wilson KG. Acceptance and commitment therapy: an experiential approach to behavior change. New York: Guilford; 1999.

50. Zettle RD. ACT for depression: a clinician's guide to using acceptance & commitment therapy in treating depression. Oakland, CA: New Harbinger; 2007.

51. Johnstone M. Living with a black dog: his name is depression. Kansas City: Andrews McMeel; 2006.

52. Young S. Break through pain: a step-by-step mindfulness meditation program for transforming chronic and acute pain. Boulder, CO: Sounds True; 2004.

53. Luoma JB, Hayes SC, Walser RD. Learning ACT: an acceptance and commitment therapy skills-training manual for therapists. Oakland, CA: New Harbinger; 2007.

54. Eisendrath SJ. Psychiatric problems. In: Bongard F, Sue D, editors. Current critical care diagnosis and treatment. New York, NY: Lange Medical Books/McGraw Hill; 2002.

55. Chiesa A, Serretti A. Mindfulness based cognitive therapy for psychiatric disorders: a systematic review and meta-analysis. Psychiatry Res. 2011;187(3):441–53.

56. Barnhofer T, Crane C, Hargus E, Amarasinghe M, Winder R, Williams JM. Mindfulness-based cognitive therapy as a treatment for chronic depression: a preliminary study. Behav Res Ther. 2009;47(5):366–73.

57. Manicavasagar V, Perich T, Parker G. Cognitive predictors of change in cognitive behaviour therapy and mindfulness-based cognitive therapy for depression. Behav Cogn Psychother. 2012;40(02):227–32.

58. Omidi A, Mohammadkhani P, Mohammadi A, Zargar F. Comparing mindfulness based cognitive therapy and traditional cognitive behavior therapy with treatments as usual on reduction of major depressive disorder symptoms. Iran Red Crescent Med J. 2013;15(2):142–6.

59. Kenny M, Williams J. Treatment-resistant depressed patients show a good response to mindfulness-based cognitive therapy. Behav Res Ther. 2007;45(3):617–25.

60. Eisendrath SJ, Delucchi K, Bitner R, Fenimore P, Smit M, McLane M. Mindfulness-based cognitive

therapy for treatment-resistant depression: a pilot study. Psychother Psychosom. 2008;77(5):319–20.

61. Eisendrath SJ. The practicing alternative techniques to heal depression study: a randomized controlled trial of mindfulness-based cognitive therapy for treatment-resistant depression with clinical and fmri effects. Findings presented at American Psychiatric Association Annual Meeting; Toronto; May 2015.

62. MacCoon DG, MacLean KA, Davidson RJ, Saron CD, Lutz A. No sustained attention differences in a longitudinal randomized trial comparing mindfulness based stress reduction versus active control. PLoS One. 2014;9(6):e97551.

63. Shahar B, Britton WB, Sbarra DA, Figueredo AJ, Bootzin RR. Mechanisms of change in mindfulness-based cognitive therapy for depression: preliminary evidence from a randomized controlled trial. Int J Cognit Ther. 2010;3(4):402–18.

64. Batink T, Peeters F, Geschwind N, van Os J, Wichers M. How does MBCT for depression work? Studying cognitive and affective mediation pathways. PLoS One. 2013;8(8):e72778.

65. Garland EL, Geschwind N, Peeters F, Wichers M. Mindfulness training promotes upward spirals of positive affect and cognition: multilevel and autoregressive latent trajectory modeling analysis. Front Psychol. 2015;6:15. Internet article accessed 15 Jun 2015.

66. Geschwind N, Peeters F, Drukker M, van Os J, Wichers M. Mindfulness training increases momentary positive emotions and reward experience in adults vulnerable to depression: a randomized controlled trial. J Consult Clin Psychol. 2011;79(5):618–28.

67. Ma SH, Teasdale JD. Mindfulness-based cognitive therapy for depression: replication and exploration of differential relapse prevention effects. J Consult Clin Psychol. 2004;72(1):31–40.

68. Kim YW, Lee SH, Choi TK, Suh SY, Kim B, Kim CM, et al. Effectiveness of mindfulness-based cognitive therapy as an adjuvant to pharmacotherapy in patients with panic disorder or generalized anxiety disorder. Depress Anxiety. 2009;26(7):601–6.

69. Piet J, Hougaard E, Hecksher MS, Rosenberg NK. A randomized pilot study of mindfulness-based cognitive therapy and group cognitive-behavioral therapy for young adults with social phobia. Scand J Psychol. 2010;51(5):403–10.

70. Williams JMG, Crane C, Barnhofer T, Brennan K, Duggan DS, Fennell MJ, et al. Mindfulness-based cognitive therapy for preventing relapse in recurrent depression: a randomized dismantling trial. J Consult Clin Psychol. 2014;82(2):275.

71. McCracken LM, Gauntlett-Gilbert J, Vowles KE. The role of mindfulness in a contextual cognitive-behavioral analysis of chronic pain-related suffering and disability. Pain. 2007;131(1):63–9.

72. Rosenzweig S, Greeson JM, Reibel DK, Green JS, Jasser SA, Beasley D. Mindfulness-based stress reduction for chronic pain conditions: variation in treatment outcomes and role of home meditation practice. J Psychosom Res. 2010;68(1):29–36.

73. Segal Z, Williams JM, Teasdale J. Mindfulness-based cognitive therapy for depression. 2nd ed. New York, Ny: Guilford; 2013.

74. Carmody J, Baer RA. How long does a mindfulness-based stress reduction program need to be? A review of class contact hours and effect sizes for psychological distress. J Clin Psychol. 2009;65(6):627–38.

75. Moore RG, Garland A. Cognitive therapy for chronic and persistent depression. England, UK: John Wiley & Sons; 2003.

76. Barnhofer T, Duggan D, Crane C, Hepburn S, Fennell MJ, Williams JM. Effects of meditation on frontal alpha-asymmetry in previously suicidal individuals. Neuroreport. 2007;18(7):709–12.

77. Bakker J, Lieverse R, Menne-Lothmann C, Viechtbauer W, Pishva E, Kenis G, et al. Therapygenetics in mindfulness-based cognitive therapy: do genes have an impact on therapy-induced change in real-life positive affective experiences? Transl Psychiatry. 2014;4(4):e384.

Mindfulness-Based Cognitive Therapy for Generalized Anxiety Disorder

13

Susan Evans

Brief Description of Generalized Anxiety Disorder

Generalized anxiety disorder (GAD), characterized by long term, intense, and excessive worry is a chronic, relatively common disorder with high rates of comorbidity [1]. The estimated lifetime prevalence rate for GAD is 5.7 % [2] and the diagnosis is associated with considerable distress and impairment in social and occupational functioning [3]. Females are twice as likely as males to experience GAD.

According to the Diagnostic and Statistical Manual of Mental Disorders Fifth Edition DSM-V [4] the criteria for GAD are the following:

A. Excessive anxiety and worry (apprehension expectation), occurring more days than not for at least 6 months, about a number of events of activities (such as work or school performance).
B. The individual finds it difficult to control the worry.
C. The anxiety and worry are associated with three (or more) of the following six symptoms (with at least some of the symptoms having been present for more days than not for the past 6 months):
   1. Restlessness or feeling keyed up or on edge.
   2. Being easily fatigued.
   3. Difficulty concentrating or mind going blank.
   4. Irritability.
   5. Muscle tension.
   6. Sleep disturbance.

Additionally, the anxiety, worry, or physical symptoms cause clinically significant distress or impairment. The disturbance is not attributable to the physiological effects of a substance or explained better by another mental disorder.

Treatment Approaches and Key Features

Case Example

Sarah is a 38-year-old single woman with hypertension working in finance who identifies herself as a chronic, life-long worrier. She is a high achiever, having attained a strong academic record and regular promotions throughout her successful career. She reports being in a very stressful job with enormous performance expectations and frequent deadlines. Sarah has expe-

S. Evans, Ph.D. (✉)
Weill Cornell Medical College,
525 East 68th Street, Box 147, New York, NY
10065, USA
e-mail: sue2002@med.cornell.edu

© Springer International Publishing Switzerland 2016
S.J. Eisendrath (ed.), *Mindfulness-Based Cognitive Therapy*, DOI 10.1007/978-3-319-29866-5_13

rienced some recent losses including the breakup of a 5-year relationship. Although she reports being sad about the breakup, her affect is restricted and she has difficulty expressing emotion. Sarah was interested in pursuing a course of mindfulness-based cognitive therapy (MBCT) to learn ways to manage her constant worrying so that "I can begin to enjoy my life." Sarah's worries often centered on work, for example, "What if I don't make the deadline?" "What if my boss is disappointed in my work?" "What if I get so stressed out I won't be able to function?" Sarah was aware that her worry covers a whole range of topics from her own health, her parent's health, to whether she would make a big enough bonus to maintain her standard of living. It is apparent that most of Sarah's thinking and experience is somewhere in the future with only rare moments of being present. Additionally, Sarah often finds that she worries about worrying, "I'm so stressed out I could have a stroke." Despite recognizing that her worry is both unrealistic and unhelpful, Sarah holds both positive and negative beliefs about her worry: "I can't help myself from worrying," "I worry so much I'm going to have a heart attack," "I'll be better prepared when bad things happen if I've worried about them." Sarah notes that she feels extremely anxious if she senses she is not in control of all aspects of her life and readily admits that worrying provides her with the illusion of control over her work, health, and relationships.

Cognitive behavior therapy (CBT) has been found to be efficacious in the treatment of GAD [5–8]. Borkovec and Ruscio [5] point out the typical CBT approach for GAD involves training clients to detect internal and external anxiety cues and to employ coping strategies to manage the psychological and somatic symptoms. While CBT is effective in treating the disorder, GAD nonetheless remains the least successfully treated of the anxiety disorders [9]. Ninan [10] points out that nearly twice as many patients in treatment for GAD achieve partial remission as those who achieve full remission and indicates the persistence of

residual symptoms in many who respond to treatment. One rationale for testing new treatments for GAD is the fact that despite effective therapies, the persistence of GAD symptoms in treatment responders is a problem.

Mindfulness training, with its focus on attentional control, may be a particularly helpful approach due to some specific characteristics of GAD. These include the temporal nature of worry, which tends to be future or past directed, as well as the individual's perceived need for control and difficulty tolerating uncertainty. As Barlow [11] pointed out nearly 40 years ago, the primary problem with GAD is "intense, excessive, chronic anxiety, with its strong sense of loss of control and inappropriate attentional focus." People with GAD are often preoccupied with potentially threatening events and typically engage in a "what if" scenario (i.e., "what if I get sick"). Consider Sarah who worries about the potential for some negative event or even catastrophe in the future. She is highly vigilant towards somatosensory cues and frequently misinterprets benign sensations as life-threatening; for example she may assume that a headache means that she is experiencing the early signs of a stroke.

There is growing evidence of the negative effects of not living in the present moment. Killingsworth and Gilbert [12] at Harvard investigated the emotional consequences of mind wandering in everyday life in the general population and found that people were less happy when their mind wandered than when they were engaged in the present moment. Individuals with GAD may be particularly vulnerable to suffering the emotional toll of such mind wandering. GAD worriers often complain that they are exhausted from worrying and therefore cannot fully enjoy their lives: "I'm always somewhere else and never appreciate what's happening," "I wish I could just shut off my brain; it's constantly running and wearing me down." Sarah, for example, sought MBCT to "rid myself" of worry so she could lead a more "productive and happy life."

Since worry is a key feature of GAD, it is important to consider the function it serves.

Borkovec [13] has conceptualized worry as a form of experiential avoidance. Worry involves significant cognitive effort and resources and may play a role in warding off unpleasant and distressing emotional experiences. The GAD worrier is so entangled in their thoughts that there is no space to process emotions or other experiences. Roemer and Orsillo [14] have pointed out that the conceptualization that worry serves an experiential avoidance function fits well with Ladoucer et al.'s [8] findings that individuals with GAD are more likely than individuals suffering from other anxiety disorders to express difficulty tolerating or accepting uncertainty.

Further exploring the functional nature of emotions, Mennin et al. [15] have proposed an emotional regulation deficit model of GAD in which individuals with GAD have difficulty understanding their emotional experience and also lack the skills to manage their emotions. Based on a number of laboratory experiments, the authors found that worry is a "cognitive control strategy" used to avoid strong emotional experiences. The authors suggest that emotion regulation approaches that include acceptance and mindfulness may be beneficial in patients with GAD.

Neurobiology of GAD

New research into the neurobiology of GAD using neuroimaging is providing valuable information for understanding the cognitive and behavioral presentation of individuals with GAD and may help to inform novel therapeutic approaches, including mindfulness training. There is compelling evidence [16,17] to suggest that there may be a dysfunction in the connectivity between important brain regions in patients with GAD including the prefrontal cortex, responsible for executive function, and the amygdala, a component of the brain's fear circuitry. In a systematic review conducted by Mochocovitch et al. [18], the authors concluded that emotion dysregulation appeared to be an important cognitive dysfunction in patients with GAD and the fMRI data suggested that the dysfunction is related to prefrontal cortex (PFC) and anterior cingulate cortex (ACC) hypofunction. Results from this review also found impairment in the connectivity between the cortex and the amygdala.

A recent study conducted by Holzel et al. [19] sought to investigate potential neural mechanisms of symptom improvement in GAD following mindfulness training. The authors randomized 26 patients with GAD to an 8-week mindfulness-based stress reduction program (MBSR) ($N=15$) or to a stress management education program ($N=11$). The authors measured brain activity with fMRI during the explicit labeling of angry and neutral facial expressions before and after treatment. The authors found ambiguous stimuli produces greater amygdala activation in subjects with GAD ambiguous compared to normal controls.

The authors also found increases in connectivity between the amygdala and several regions of the PFC after the MBSR course but not the stress education program. The authors concluded that mindfulness training is associated with enhanced activation in connectivity between brain areas that are associated with healthy emotion regulation.

Integration of Mindfulness to Traditional Approaches

Mindfulness, moment-to-moment nonjudgmental awareness, is cultivated through the regular practice of mindfulness meditation and emphasizes an open awareness to the contents of the mind [20]. Astin [21] suggests that the techniques of mindfulness meditation help the person to develop a stance of detached observation towards the contents of consciousness and may be a useful cognitive behavioral coping strategy. Sarah, for example, began to notice and label her worried thoughts and to note to herself, "that is an unproductive worry, let me come back to my breath, to the present moment."

Mindfulness training makes sense as an augmentation strategy to standard CBT because it targets the key characteristics that are salient in GAD including the temporal nature of worry, avoidance of one's internal experience, difficulty tolerating uncertainty, and a perceived need for control. As Roemer and Orsillo [14] point out, since the nature of worry is future directed, training in present-moment mindful awareness may provide a useful alternative way of responding for individuals with GAD. With repeated practice, the GAD worrier becomes skilled in bringing his/her mind back to the present moment rather than being on automatic pilot and caught up into the contents of the worried thoughts, fantasies, and images. The GAD practitioner learns to observe the "here and now" versus worrying about the past or the future. Roemer et al. [22] point out that the relationship between mindfulness and GAD may be "bidirectional" in that worry may be associated with decreasing present moment awareness, acceptance, and self-compassion and these reductions reinforce worry and other GAD symptoms. Cultivating mindfulness may therefore lead to beneficial effects in that with practice, individuals with GAD learn to observe the here and now rather than focusing on the past or the future. For example, with practice, Sarah was able to take her mindfulness practice off the cushion and mat and to recognize when she got ensnared in negative thinking about the future. Rather than getting involved in the worry, i.e., "Sam (boss) will be disappointed in my presentation to the client," Sarah was able to notice the thought, label it as a worry, and then let it go.

Furthermore, individuals with GAD often experience a need to control many aspects of their lives which may relate in part to their difficulty experiencing unpleasant emotions and uncertain outcomes. Sarah readily admits that she is a "control freak" and noted that a lot of her thinking and behavior, ranging from reassurance seeking to avoidance, is motivated by a strong urge to feel that she is in control over all aspects of her life.

Another key aspect of mindfulness practice is training in acceptance. Bishop et al. [23] discuss a definition of mindfulness developed by a consensus of experts in the field who posit that mindfulness involves self-regulation of attention to the present moment as well as cultivating an attitude of openness, curiosity, and acceptance towards one's experience.

The MBCT practitioner learns to observe their thoughts and emotions without over-identifying with them and at the same time develop an attitude of acceptance towards whatever experience they may be having in the present moment. Cultivating acceptance requires regular contact with the contents of consciousness. Rather than distract, ignore, and avoid difficult emotional experiences, GAD worriers learn to accept and practice tolerating whatever experience they may be having in the moment (e.g., a sense of sadness, loss, guilt, distress), as well as learning to let go of judgments and expectations. Kabat-Zinn [24] refers to this skill in a chapter entitled, "Letting go" in his book, *Wherever you go, there you are*. He notes that letting go is "an invitation to cease clinging to anything—whether it be an idea, a thing, an event, a particular time, or view, or desire."

Mindfulness-Based Cognitive Therapy (MBCT) for GAD

There have been relatively few studies examining the effectiveness of MBCT for GAD. In an open trial of acceptance-based behavior therapy for GAD, Roemer and Orsillo [25] found that patients who received a treatment combining CBT and learning and practicing mindfulness and acceptance-based strategies experienced significant reductions in symptoms and improvement in quality of life. Evans et al. [26], in a small open pilot study, adapted Segal et al.'s [27] MBCT protocol for depression to target GAD (described below) and found that there were significant reductions in anxiety following the 8-week course. Importantly, it appears that the treatment was both feasible and acceptable in this subject pool since all 12 subjects accepted into study completed the 8-week protocol. One subject's data was excluded from the final analysis due to suffering a fracture during the trial. Despite experiencing pain and some disability, the patient specifically requested to be allowed to participate and complete the program. Kim et al. [28] further compared the relative effectiveness of MBCT versus an anxiety education program for patients with panic disorder or generalized anxiety and found that MBCT was superior in reducing symptoms of anxiety and depressive symptoms in both types of anxiety disorders.

In a meta-analytic review of mindfulness-based therapy on anxiety and depression, Hofmann et al. [29] concluded that mindfulness-based therapy was moderately effective for improving anxiety. The authors also noted however that there were relatively few clinical trials specifically examining MBTs for anxiety. In fact, a report published by the Cochrane Collaboration [30] raised a question regarding the feasibility and acceptability of meditation based treatments for GAD. The report focused only on randomized clinical trials investigating the effectiveness of meditation for anxiety disorders. Only 2 of 50 studies, one involving transcendental meditation and the other utilizing Kundalini yoga, met the rigorous inclusion criteria. The drop-out rate was quite high in both studies and the authors suggested that adherence to practicing regular meditation in those formats for individuals suffering from anxiety disorders may be of significant consideration. The authors concluded that the small number of studies did not permit conclusions to be drawn on the effectiveness of meditation for anxiety disorders and suggested that more trials are needed.

Despite the small number of randomized trials of mindfulness for anxiety it would seem that individuals with GAD would benefit from mindfulness training. As Brown and Ryan [31] note, a mindful state of being captures a quality of consciousness that is characterized by a clarity and vividness of current experience. Nonetheless, the practice of mindfulness medi-

tation is demanding for anyone and may present particular challenges to individuals with GAD whose contents of mental consciousness are for most of the time oriented anywhere but in the present moment.

A Proposed Format for MBCT for GAD

The following is a proposed format for GAD. The program is based on MBCT developed by Segal et al. [27]:

Sessions 1–3:

The focus is on developing a formal mindfulness practice that includes the body scan meditation, sitting meditation, gentle hatha yoga. Sitting meditation and the body scan meditation are introduced in session 1 and 2. Gentle hatha yoga, walking meditation, and the three minute breathing space are introduced in the third session. Each session is structured and includes formal meditation practice (i.e., sitting meditation, body scan, and gentle hatha yoga). Practitioners also learn to practice mindfulness in everyday life including mindful eating and paying attention to pleasant and unpleasant events. Group discussions initially focus on potential barriers to starting a meditation practice including the time, personal commitment, and having an adequate setting for practice. Some discussion may address the role that anxiety and worry has played on the lives of the participants. The role of home practice is emphasized throughout and participants practice approximately 45 min a day of formal meditation.

Session 4–7

The practice continues with the body scan, sitting meditation, and gentle hatha yoga in the classroom and for daily homework. The group leader provides psycho-education about the symptoms and key characteristics of GAD, including the temporal nature of worry, need for control, and intolerance of uncertainty. Participants learn to identify their own positive and negative beliefs by completing the metacognition questionnaire developed by Adrian Wells [32]. The questionnaire helps patients identify both positive beliefs about worry: "Worrying helps me to avoid problems in the future," "I need to worry to remain organized" as well as negative beliefs about worry might, "I could make myself sick with worrying," "Worrying puts my body under a lot of stress."

Case Example

Bill, for example, a successful young banker with a promising career, reported that while he leaves the office each evening, he never puts work aside as he worries he may miss some new piece of information. He has gotten into the habit of checking his phone all evening and has developed mid-insomnia since anytime he wakes up in the middle of the night he immediately looks at his phone. In fact, without being aware of it, his checking behavior has served to reinforce his anxiety and contributed to the worsening of his sleep disturbance. Upon examination, Bill expresses the positive belief that worrying gives him an edge: "If I worry and think about work all the time I'll be successful." He acknowledges: "If I don't worry I may lose my advantage." Bill has implicitly developed a positive belief about worry, "Worry is good for success" and he is operating from a rule or principle, "I must worry."

Group members also learn that they may be vulnerable to interpreting information in a threatening manner thus leading to cognitive biases. Bill, for example, received an email from his boss one evening requesting that they meet early the next morning to discuss an investment they were working on together. Bill's automatic thought was that he must have missed communicating something important to their client. Bill learned to notice and record his thoughts using a worry diary.

Worry Diary

At this stage in the course, homework includes maintaining a worry diary. The worry diary is a record that includes worry thoughts, what effect the worry has on the person, when and where the worry occurs. This homework encourages the individual to step back and observe the contents of consciousness with an attitude of detached observation. The skill involves identifying the worry without getting caught up in rumination.

To help participants develop awareness around their cognitive processes participants are given the list of common cognitive distortions [33] and asked to observe if they may be using any of the cognitive distortions as they review their worry diary.

Some examples of cognitive distortions that may particularly apply to individuals with GAD include:

- Overgeneralization—Seeing a single negative event as something that will keep repeating.
- Mental Filter—Focusing on a single negative event and dwelling on it.
- Jumping to Conclusions—Making a negative interpretation about something when there are no facts to back it up.
- Catastrophizing—Exaggerating the significance of things: over-reacting.

Here is an example of Sarah's worry diary:

Day/time	Trigger	Worry thought	Level of anxiety	Behavior	Cognitive distortion
Tuesday	Meeting with boss	He's disappointed in my report	80	Apologetic	Mental filter
Wed	Headache	Maybe I have a brain tumor	100	Internet search	Catastrophizing
				Reassurance seeking	

Unproductive Vs. Productive Worry

Another useful tool that group members learn is to distinguish between productive and unproductive worry. Leahy [34] devotes an entire chapter to this subject in his popular book, *The Worry Cure*. Unproductive worry is about thinking of situations that may or may not happen and does not involve taking any action; in other words ruminating and obsessing about possible future events or situations that occurred in the past. Productive worry is about events that are more likely to occur and involves taking some specific, concrete action. For example, Sarah noticed a lot of unproductive worry: "What if I get really nervous on the conference call and my boss notices?" "What if my boss thinks I'm doing a bad job?"

Having observed this thought and recognized that it was unproductive worry, Sarah was able to practice productive worry: "Is there anything I can do about this now?" This shift in thinking contributed to her taking action: "I can review my notes and be really prepared."

Bill also learned to employ productive worry rather than get caught up in ruminating about missing some critical piece of information. He shared the example of feeling stressed out that his sleep disturbance would affect his ability to make the most effective decisions at work, "what if I am so tired I mess up a transaction and lose the client?" Bill found that he was literally spinning his wheels and perseverating on this worry. As he began to apply his mindfulness practice to everyday life, Bill was able to identify the unproductive nature of these thoughts. He eventually identified a productive response to his worry, "I can focus on improving my sleep hygiene by not checking my phone in the middle of the night."

Cultivating Acceptance

For patients suffering from GAD cultivating acceptance of one's internal experience is a useful skill that may be reinforced over and over again. Ruminating and worrying are primary strategies that individuals with GAD rely on. People with GAD often seek reassurance to alleviate their discomfort only to find that they still feel anxious and often end up frustrating/tiring those around them. Learning to sit with the discomfort of unwanted emotions or other experiences is a challenging but an important part of the therapeutic process for individuals with GAD. Class participants may reject the idea of cultivating an attitude of acceptance in that they may view it as a form of resignation or giving up. The group leader will point out to the class that acceptance is an active process that allows one to fully engage in the present moment experience.

MBCT employs the use of carefully selected poems to capture the essence of mindfulness practice. Rumi's Guest House Poem (see Moyne & Barks [35] for reference), which is read and discussed in Class 5, illustrates the concept of acceptance that is developed in mindfulness training. The poem suggests that as humans we open ourselves, each day, to all our emotions and thoughts whether they be negative or positive (i.e., a joy, a depression, the dark thought). The poem often generates a lot of discussion from the group. Some may express confusion and question: "Why would we welcome bad thoughts and feelings?" With further processing, participants may recognize that they, in fact, hold certain core beliefs around their emotions such as "feeling sad is a weakness." Acknowledging that all emotions are worth attending to can alleviate a certain burden that individuals with GAD carry with them. Bill, for example, learned to sit with the anxiety and discomfort that he felt when he resisted the urge of checking his phone and experienced the thought that he was missing something important. As one patient commented, "learning to drop the rope in the tug of war I was having with myself to always feel like I was in control of everything felt like such a relief."

Sessions 7–8

In sessions 7 and 8 the practical mindfulness skills (using thought record, worry diary, unproductive/productive worry) related to anxiety and worry are reviewed and reinforced as well the formal meditation practice. In class 8 participants are asked to record what they have learned: strategies that have been particularly helpful to them, and ones that they are willing to commit to practicing when the class is over. Group members share their experiences and discuss how they plan to extend what they've taken from the class to their "next steps."

Challenges Implementing MBCT for GAD

With the significant increase in the dissemination of MBCT programs, there is a growing need to identify and learn to manage some of the challenges and obstacles that both practitioners and participants experience. Edwards et al. [36] note that these may include participant expectations, difficulty carving out time for practice, the presence of comorbid medical and psychiatric differences, and complex group dynamics.

Individuals seeking MBCT understandably present with goals and expectations of feeling less depressed or anxious and more satisfied and fulfilled in their lives. Many equate meditation with relaxation and may be disturbed when they experience negative or unwanted internal stimuli during their meditation practice. Others may express the attitude that one "should" be able to "just clear my mind" and "not think about anything." Often times, these sets of assumptions and rules lead to a sense of frustration and disappointment. It is important, at the very beginning, that the group leader educates the group around the goals of mindfulness including the willingness to cultivate being fully open to all experiences: pleasant, unpleasant, or neutral. Providing some bibliotherapy can be very helpful. For example, encouraging the group to read *Full Catastrophe Living* [20] and *Wherever you go, there you are* [24]. Group members often need to be reminded of the goals of mindfulness training; for example meditation is not synonymous with relaxation or being in a zen-like state. Rather, the group leader encourages members to cultivate the goal of practicing the skill of mindfulness, that is, to simply practice coming back to the present moment when their mind has drifted off.

Another issue that comes up is the difficulty of starting and maintaining a daily practice. Group members often talk about the challenges of carving out time from their busy daily lives and may get discouraged if they see themselves as "failing" their homework. Spending time during the first few sessions to address the challenges of finding time, making the commitment, and addressing practical issues such as the setting for practice can be very helpful to group members. For example, from the beginning the group may wonder if there is a best time to meditate or if there are other particular conditions that are necessary to have in place. Group members may ask, for example, if it is ok to meditate on the commute to work or whether they can practice while exercising. Having ample opportunity to discuss the question of when, where, and how to meditate is enormously helpful.

The group leader may expect to find their own set of challenges that they will need to manage over the 8-week course. Group dynamics, for example, may pose some interesting issues. The group may include a monopolizer who dominates the discussions. There may also be some members who are reticent and have difficulty expressing themselves in a group setting. Socializing the group early on to practice mindful listening and speaking may help in regard to the group dynamic. Despite these efforts, the leader may need to gently interrupt the monopolizer and redirect the discussion. Likewise, the leader may encourage participation from the quiet members by calling on them for their thoughts and opinions.

Letting the group know at the beginning that everyone's input is important, helpful, and an expectation for everyone. The leader may suggest: "Over the next 8 weeks each of you will have a set of observations that will be notable and worth sharing with everyone in the group. The group thrives when everyone participates by sharing their experience."

Practical Considerations for Training

Cognitive behavioral practitioners who are interested in integrating mindfulness into standard CBT treatment for GAD can begin by developing their own daily mindfulness practice. It is helpful if the group leader learns meditation from personal contact with an experienced meditation teacher. A daily meditation practice should be considered a requisite experience for any MBCT leader. Kabat-Zinn [37] notes that the instructor's relationship to mindfulness in terms of being grounded in an extensive personal practice is key to bringing authenticity and relevance to the group participants. The MBCT leaders themselves must be experienced in meditation in order to be prepared to address the kinds of questions and issues the group members bring up in discussion and to be equipped to guide the group appropriately. Group members will also be interested in the leaders' practice and how the leader has been able to integrate their mindfulness practice into their everyday lives.

In addition to a personal mindfulness practice, formal MBCT trainings are offered throughout the USA and abroad. The Center for Mindfulness Studies http://www.mindfulnessstudies.com/ in Toronto provides professional MBCT training.

MBCT.Com (http://mbct.com/) provides information on training and resources such as online therapist training, meditation retreat centers, and articles about MBCT.

References

1. Brown TA, Barlow DH. Comorbidity among anxiety disorders: implications for treatment and DSM-IV. J Consult Clin Psychol. 1992;60:835–44.
2. Kessler RC, Berglund P, Demler O, Jin R, Walters EE. Lifetime prevalence and age-of-onset distributions of DSM-IV disorders in the National Comorbidity Survey Replication. Arch Gen Psychiatry. 2005;62: 593–602.
3. Maier W, Gansicke M, Freyberger HJ, Linz M, Huen R, Lecrubier Y. Generalized anxiety disorder (ICD-10) in primary care from a cross-cultural perspective: a valid diagnostic entity? Acta Psychiatr Scand. 2000;101:29–36.
4. American Psychiatric Association. Diagnostic and statistical manual of mental disorders fifth edition DSM-5. Washington, DC: American Psychiatric Publishing; 2013. p. 222–6.
5. Borkovec TD, Ruscio AM. Psychotherapy for generalized anxiety disorder. J Clin Psychiatry. 2001;62 Suppl 11:37–42.
6. Borkovec TD, Newman MG, Lytle R, Pincus A. A component analysis of cognitive behavioral therapy for generalized anxiety disorder and the role of interpersonal problems. J Consult Clin Psychol. 2002; 70:288–98.
7. Butler G, Fennell M, Robson P, Gelder M. Comparison of behavior therapy and cognitive behavior therapy in the treatment of generalized anxiety disorder. J Consult Clin Psychol. 1991;59:167–75.
8. Ladouceur R, Dugas MJ, Freeston MH, Leger E, Gagnon F, Thibeau N. Efficacy of a new cognitive-behavioral treatment for generalized anxiety disorder: evaluation in a controlled clinical trial. J Consult Clin Psychol. 2000;68:957–64.
9. Brown TA, Barlow DH, Lebowitz MR. The empirical basis of generalized anxiety disorder. Am J Psychiatry. 1994;151:1272–80.
10. Ninan PT. General anxiety disorder: why are we failing our patients? J Clin Psychiatry. 2001;62 Suppl 19:3–4.
11. Barlow DH. Anxiety and its disorders: the nature and treatment of anxiety and panic. New York, NY: Guilford; 1988. p. 579.
12. Killingsworth MA, Gilbert DT. A wandering mind is an unhappy mind. Sci Mag. 2010;330:932.
13. Borkovec TD. The nature, functions, and origins of worry. In: Davey GCL, Tallis F, editors. Worrying: perspectives on theory, assessment, and treatment. New York, NY: Wiley; 1994.
14. Roemer L, Orsillo SM. Expanding our conceptualization of and treatment for generalized anxiety disorder: integrating mindfulness/acceptance-based approaches with existing cognitive-behavioral models. Clin Psychol Sci Pract. 2002;9(1):54–68.
15. Mennin DS, Heimberg RG, Turk CL, Fresco DM. Applying an emotion regulation framework to integrative approaches to generalized anxiety disorder. Clin Psychol Sci Pract. 2002;9(1):85–90.
16. Kim MJ, Loucks RA, Palmer AL, Brown AC, Solomon KM, Marchante AN, et al. The structural and functional connectivity of the amygdala: from normal emotion to pathological anxiety. Behav Brain Res. 2011;223(2):403–10.
17. Tromp DP, Grupe DW, Oathes DJ, McFarlin DR, Herandez PJ, Krai TR, et al. Reduced structural connectivity of a major frontolimbic pathway in generalized anxiety disorder. Arch Gen Psychiatry. 2012;69(9):925–34.
18. Mochcovitch MD, da Rocha FR, Ferreira R, Nardi GA. A systematic review of fMRI studies in generalized anxiety disorder: evaluation its neural and cognitive basis. J Affect Disord. 2014;167(10):336–42.
19. Holzel BK, Hoge EA, Greve DN, Gard T, Creswell JD, Brown KW, et al. Neural mechanisms of symptom improvements in generalized anxiety disorder following mindfulness training. Neuroimage Clin. 2013;2:448–58.
20. Kabat-Zinn J. Full catastrophe living: Using the wisdom of your body and mind to face stress, pain, and illness. New York, NY: Dell; 1990.
21. Astin JA. Stress reduction through mindfulness meditation. Effects on psychological symptomatology,

sense of control and spiritual experiences. Psychother Psychosom. 1997;66:97–106.

22. Roemer L, Lee JK, Salters-Pedneault K, Erisman SM, Orsillo SM, Mennin DS. Mindfulness and emotion regulation difficulties in generalized anxiety disorder: preliminary evidence for independent and overlapping contributions. Behav Ther. 2009;40:142–54.

23. Bishop SR, Lau M, Shapiro S, Carlson L, Anderson ND, Carmody J, et al. Mindfulness: a proposed operational definition. Clin Psychol Sci Prac. 2004;11:230–41.

24. Kabat-Zinn J. Wherever you go there you are: mindfulness meditation in everyday life. New York, NY: Hyperion; 1994. p. 53.

25. Roemer L, Orsillo SM. An open trial of an acceptance-based behavior therapy for generalized anxiety disorder. Behav Ther. 2007;38:72–85.

26. Evans S, Ferrando S, Findler M, Stowell C, Smart C, Haglin D. Mindfulness-based cognitive therapy for generalized anxiety disorder. J Anxiety Disord. 2008;22:716–21.

27. Segal ZV, Williams JMG, Teasdale JD. Mindfulness-based cognitive therapy for depression: a new approach to preventing relapse. New York, NY: Guilford; 2002.

28. Kim YW, Lee S-H, Choi TK, et al. Effectiveness of mindfulness-based cognitive therapy as an adjuvant to pharmacotherapy in patients with panic disorder of generalized anxiety disorder. Depress Anxiety. 2009;26:601–6.

29. Hofmann S, Sawyer AT, Witt AA, Oh D. The effect of mindfulness-based therapy on anxiety and depression: a meta-analytic review. J Consult Clin Psychol. 2010;78(2):169–83.

30. Krisanaprakornkit T, Krisanaprakornkit W, Piyavhatkul N, Loapaiboon M. Meditation therapy for anxiety disorders (review). The Cochrane Collaboration. New York, NY: Wiley; 2006.

31. Brown KW, Ryan RM. The benefits of being present: the role of mindfulness in psychological well-being. Am J Psychiatry. 2003;151:1272–80.

32. Wells A. Emotional disorders & Metacognition: Innovative cognitive therapy. New York, NY: Wiley; 2000.

33. Burns D. Feeling good: the new mood therapy. New York, NY: Avon Books; 1999.

34. Leahy RL. The worry cure. New York, NY: Harmony Books; 2005.

35. Moyne J, Barks C. Say I am you. Poems of Rumi. Maypop; 1994.

36. Edwards AR, Evans S, Aldao A, Haglin D, Ferrando SJ. Implementing a mindfulness–based stress reduction program in the community: lessons learned and suggestions for the future. Behav Ther. 2014; 37(1):13–7.

37. Kabat-Zinn J. Mindfulness-based interventions in context: past, present & future. Clin Psychol Sci Pract. 2003;10:144–56.

The Effects of Mindfulness-Based Cognitive Therapy in Bipolar Disorder

14

Victoria L. Ives-Deliperi, Fleur Howells, and Neil Horn

Case Study

Maria suffered several severe bouts of depression as a teenager and young adult. These came without clear stressors and did not respond to medication with antidepressants, which she decided not to take after the second episode. Psychological therapy did not seem to help, and the family was referred to a family therapist who did not feel that the family would benefit from a specific intervention. There was a family history of suicide in that the maternal grandmother had died by suicide, but no one had spoken about this with Maria as it was felt that she was too young to understand. The depression felt like a dark cloud that came quickly and settled after a couple of days. She felt cold and slow, and no energy for activities and as if colors had turned to grey. She lost her appetite for food and fun. She tried to take alcohol to lighten up once she was old enough. She often felt like there was no point in living through these days but eventually learnt they would go away after a few weeks.

When she was 21 she tried taking alcohol and cocaine to relieve the feelings of dullness and emptiness. She became euphoric, and disinhibited, hardly slept for a week, and had multiple sexual partners in the space of a few days. After a week her family insisted she see a doctor but she refused to go to a clinic and ran into the traffic—the police were called and she was admitted in hospital, against her will. This manic state lasted for a month, and she was heavily sedated for the first week. She felt that there was nothing wrong with her and said she felt better than she had for years and that the doctors and hospital team were cruel and vowed never to have anything to do with them or her family since they had called the Police after she escaped.

Three years and three manic episodes later, she understands that she has bipolar disorder, and that her symptoms do respond to mood stabilizer medication, and that she needs to reduce stress and abstain form alcohol and drug use, as these trigger manic episodes. She misses the manic and euphoric feelings and the energy that comes with them but understands how costly a manic episode can be having had to terminate a pregnancy following a sexual indiscretion while manic. She remains an anxious person and her self-confidence has been damaged.

V.L. Ives-Deliperi, Ph.D. (✉)
Department of Neurology, University of Cape Town, 209B Mediclinic Constantiaberg, Burnham Road, Plumstead, Cape Town, South Africa
e-mail: vives@mweb.co.za

F. Howells, Ph.D. • N. Horn, M.B.Ch.B., UCT, M.R.C.(Psych.)
Department of Psychiatry, University of Cape Town, Cape Town, South Africa

The Problem

Bipolar disorder (BD) is a cyclic disorder of mood, characterized by alternating states of mania and depression. There are two types of bipolar disorder; bipolar disorder I is characterized by episodes of both depression and mania and bipolar disorder II is defined by episodes of depression and hypomania. Mania includes persistent elevated mood and also high levels of irritability, while depression involves periods of persistent feelings of sadness, futility, and worthlessness (DSM-5).

The incidence of comorbid psychiatric and medical conditions in patients with bipolar disorder is extremely high with anxiety disorders, alcohol or drug dependence, diabetes, cardiovascular disease, obesity, migraine, and hepatitis C frequently reported. Symptoms of bipolar disorder typically begin in adolescence or early adulthood and chronicity develops with associated disability leading to compromised quality of life and overall functioning.

Bipolar disorder affects 3.9 % of the US population [1], with comparable prevalence internationally [2]. The disorder is also among the most costly of all mental health conditions to manage [3]. The rate of suicide among patients is reported to be 20 times greater than in the general US population.

Emotional dysregulation and executive dysfunction are the core clinical and psychological features of bipolar disorder [4–6]. Dysregulation of emotional responses is considered a consequence of inappropriate coping strategies within the environment and related to dysfunction in neural circuitry between the frontal cortex and limbic structures [6, 7]. It has been shown that the amygdala is activated during the observation of fearful facial expressions and fearful scenes [8, 9] while the ventral lateral prefrontal cortex (VLPFC) modulates limbic activity, specifically the amygdala, when executive tasks are undertaken [10]. Such modulation of the amygdala through activation of the VLPFC has been shown to be defective in patients with bipolar disorder patients [11, 12].

Pharmacological management is considered the treatment of choice for bipolar disorder but relapse rates are still very high with 73 % of patients relapsing within a 5-year period [13]. Despite developments in psychopharmacology, a high percentage of patients develop chronicity with related disability and burden of disease on families and society [14, 15]. Medication non-adherence is arguably the most significant contributor to poor outcomes in this patient population. It is reported that more than 75 % of patients take their medication less than 75 % of the time. One remedy to this problem is evidence-based accessible, affordable, and effective adjunctive therapeutic interventions. A number of studies have been undertaken over the last decade to investigate the efficacy of a range of interventions. The current literature on the efficacy of psychotherapeutic interventions as adjunctive therapies in bipolar disorder has primarily centered on psychoeducation, interpersonal and social rhythm therapy (IPSRT), family therapy, cognitive behavioral therapy (CBT), and more recently mindfulness-based cognitive therapy (MBCT).

Pychoeducation involves informing patients about the disorder, adherence to treatment, and early detection of new episodes. Group psychoeducation programs have been shown to have better benefited those in the early stages of the disorder who have previously relapsed but generally show a long-term prophylactic benefit, particularly regarding the relapse of manic episodes [16]. IPSRT is based on the premise that vulnerable individuals are offset by stressful events and disrupted routines and therapy is designed to encourage adherence to treatment and stabilizing social routines and dealing with interpersonal conflict [17]. This form of therapy applied in the early stages of the acute phase in bipolar disorder has been shown to prolong the time to relapse [16]. Family therapy tailored to patients with bipolar disorder involves elements of psychoeducation and enhancing problem-solving and communication skills in the family unit. Although findings from studies investigating the efficacy of family therapy in bipolar disorder offer missed results, there appears to be beneficial effects for family members. Cognitive remediation and functional remediation interventions educating patients on neurocognitive, communications, and stress management appear to offer some benefit to patients with less severe cognitive deficits, particularly in terms of alleviating depressive symptoms [18].

Next to psychoeducation, CBT is the most frequent therapy to have been studied in this group of patients. CBT in bipolar disorder focuses on recognizing early promodal symptoms and using behavioral regulation strategies to prevent relapse. There is some evidence that CBT may be beneficial as adjuncts to pharmacological maintenance treatments for the prevention of relapse in stable patients and those in the early stages of the disease [19, 20]. The current body of literature shows less optimistic outcomes related to CBT during the acute phase of bipolar depression and in the maintenance phase [16].

Theoretical Rationale of MBCT for Bipolar Disorder

The technique of noticing and observing mood fluctuations and changes in symtomatology, and responding in a regulated and skilled way to these signals, is a common feature of numerous psychotherapeutic interventions and geared to nurturing emotion regulation. This technique is also adopted in mindfulness-based interventions. Since mindfulness training has shown to effectively alleviate anxiety and mood disorders, and increase positive affect and reduce cognitive vulnerability to stress and emotional distress in clinical and non-clinical populations [21], it is fitting that related training may benefit patients with bipolar disorder. The efficacy of MBCT in preventing relapse in these patients is of particular interest given the literature as it has been shown to reduce relapse in major depression [22]. These group interventions incorporate mindfulness practices designed to cultivate nonjudgmental observation of thoughts, emotions, and bodily sensations, highlighting these events as transient in nature and separate from the self. This process is said to embrace the cognitive therapy technique of decentering, which may be described as a learnt meta-cognitive skill in which emotional experiences are considered ephemeral events,

disparate to the self, and is so believed to prevent the escalation of negative thoughts into ruminative patterns [22]. In this way, MBCT has been shown to bring about improved emotion regulation [23] and that higher levels of dispositional mindfulness are related to enhanced modulation of the amygdala by the VLPFC [24], which lies at the heart of pathophysiology of bipolar disorder.

Evidence of MBCT for Bipolar Disorder

A number of studies have been conducted to investigate the efficacy of MBCT as an adjunctive therapy in bipolar disorder. These investigations have explored cognitive, behavioral, and neural changes in response to the standard 8-week intervention. A preliminary evaluation of the immediate effects of MBCT in bipolar disorder was conducted with a specific focus on between-episode anxiety and depressive symptoms [25]. The study used data from pilot randomized wait list trail of MBCT for people with bipolar disorder in remission and it was shown that the intervention leads to improved immediate outcomes of anxiety and depressive symptoms. The study was limited by the small sample size and the prohibition of recruitment of patients with suicidal ideation.

In a subsequent wait list control study, significant improvements were reported following the 8-week MBCT intervention, in anxiety, emotional regulation, working memory, spatial memory, and verbal fluency [26]. In this study 23 patients with bipolar disorder underwent neuropsychological testing and functional MRI. Sixteen of these patients were tested before and after an 8-week MBCT intervention, and seven were wait-listed for training and tested at the same intervals and the results were compared with ten healthy controls. Prior to MBCT, bipolar patients reported significantly higher levels of anxiety and symptoms of stress, scored significantly lower on a test of working memory, and showed significant BOLD signal decrease in the medial PFC during a mindfulness task, compared to healthy controls. This finding is consistent with previous research in which significant signal decreases have been observed in the medial PFC, and other PFC regions in bipolar patients [27]. Following MBCT, there was significant improvements in the bipolar treatment group, in measures of mindfulness, anxiety, and emotion regulation, and in tests of working memory, spatial memory, and verbal fluency compared to the bipolar wait list group. BOLD signal increases were noted in the medial PFC and posterior parietal lobe, in a repeat mindfulness task. A region-of-interest analysis revealed strong correlation between signal changes in medial PFC and increases in mindfulness. In a similar trend Strakowski et al. [27] reported signal increases in the medial PFC following pharmacological treatment. These data suggest that MBCT improves mindfulness and emotion regulation and reduces anxiety in bipolar disorder, corresponding to increased activations in the medial PFC, a region associated with cognitive flexibility and previously proposed as a key area of pathophysiology in the disorder.

Further, improved emotional regulation of brain circuitry was found after 8-week course of MBCT, using electroencephalography (EEG) [28]. This study assessed the N170 event-related potential (ERP) wave component during the completion of affect-matching task, with the presentation of a visual image of a face that was scared, happy, or angry. The participant was required to match the face's emotion with one of similar emotion or apply a label with matched emotion displayed in the image. The task has been described in detial elsewhere [29]. Before the course of MBCT the individuals with bipolar disorder showed a significantly exaggerated response to the affect matching of images, and increased N170 amplitude, over frontal, central, and parietal electrodes. After 8-week course of MBCT that individuals with bipolar disorder showed a complete attenuation of the N170 to that similar of healthy participants. The N170 peak is known to peak with both the presentation of faces—specifically the structural encoding of faces [30, 31], sometimes referred to as the "face potential"—and the process of matching [32]. The findings from this paper support altered emotional processing

in bipolar disorder and with MBCT this altered emotional processing can be attenuated [28].

A second EEG study addressed cortical arousal, EEG frequency band activity, and attentional processing, and ERPs during a continuous performance task, in bipolar disorder before and after 8 weeks of MBCT [28]. Cortical arousal in bipolar disorder during a resting condition suggested decreased attentional readiness over frontal and central electrodes, as theta band power was decreased, and beta band power was increased, and this resulted in a decreased theta/beta ratio. At the 8-week MBCT intervention cortical arousal improved to that reported for the healthy controls [28]. In attentional processing during a continuous performance task (A–X, where A was the cue, and X was the target), individuals with bipolar disorder showed increased cortical processing over frontal cortex, as seen by their P300 ERP wave component amplitude, of the cue compared to controls, and a tendency was evident for the target. With 8 weeks of MBCT this enhanced P300 attenuated, we suggested that in bipolar disorder MBCT, we suggested that this attenuation was related to MBCT reducing the activation of non-relevant information processing during attentional processes; that is, in bipolar disorder there is additional recruitment of neural pathways that are not necessary to complete the task at hand [28].

In a recent randomized controlled trial 95 bipolar patients were randomly assigned an MBCT intervention and treatment as usual with TAU arm ($N = 48$) and TAU-only arm ($N = 47$) and tested them at intervals over 12 months [33]. There were no differences between the groups in terms of relapse and recurrent rates of any mood episodes but there was some beneficial effect of MBCT on anxiety symptoms. This finding suggests a potential role of MBCT in reducing anxiety comorbid with bipolar disorder. Additional analyses in the same cohort of patient showed that a greater number of days meditated during the 8-week MBCT program was related to lower depression scores at a 12-month follow-up, and there was evidence to suggest that three or more mindfulness meditation practices a week during the intervention were associated with improvements in depression and anxiety symptoms.

Proposed Mechanisms of Change

Emotion dysregulation and executive dysfunction are cited as two core domains of pathology in the disorder and represent possible endophenotypes of the condition [5, 6]. The findings of the studies discussed in this chapter suggest that mindfulness training may target the key deficits underlying bipolar disorder. A core skill taught in mindfulness-based interventions is cultivating a quality of awareness in which thoughts and emotions are acknowledged without judgment and considered passing mental events and individuals with bipolar disorder have been shown to improve on measure of anxiety and emotion regulation, as well as attention following training in these skills. Cognitive and psychological changes have been accompanied by changes in brain activity, which may present the underlying mechanism for improved outcomes.

A large body of literature has been amassed on the functional neuroanatomy of disturbed emotion processing in patients with bipolar disorder. More specifically, a relative hypoactivity of dorsal brain structures, including the dorsolateral PFC, the dorsal anterior cingulate, and the posterior cingulate cortex, has been reported in bipolar patients. This imbalance between the networks has been proposed to underlie deficient emotion regulation in bipolar disorder. Prior to mindfulness training, BOLD signal increases have been observed in the ACC and PFC in bipolar group compared to healthy subjects during the viewing of faces displaying emotion, suggesting that bipolar patients need to work harder to modulate their response to emotional stimuli, compared to those without the illness. Following MBCT training significant signal increases have been observed in patients with bipolar disorder in the medial PFC in a meditation task [26]. The medial PFC is believed to play a critical role in generating self-referential thought during conscious appraisal of threatening stimuli, as well as

in behavioral flexibility during tasks of inhibition [27]. The medial PFC, together with the ACC, plays a key role in regulating emotional responses to engage effectively in executive functioning. As already discussed, and based on previous neuroimaging findings, the medial PFC is considered a key region of pathophysiology in bipolar disorder. Specifically, during the regulation of emotion, the medial PFC is proposed to mediate the inhibition of the amygdala by the ventrolateral PFC through its dense projections between these two regions [34]. This neuroimaging finding may present a mechanism through which MBCT facilitates improved emotion regulation.

From the few EEG papers on MBCT in bipolar disorder, prior to MBCT individuals with bipolar disorder activate emotion-related frontal cortical networks (ERP N170) and attention-related frontal cortical networks (ERP P300) with greater intensity, as seen by the exaggerated ERP wave components. Further cortical arousal during rest suggests deficits in attentional readiness again over frontal cortex. However with MBCT these deficits are improved towards that of health controls, suggesting improved cortical arousal and cortical activation.

Summary and Conclusions

Most notably findings from studies on the efficacy of MBCT in patients with bipolar disorder show improvements in symptoms of anxiety but also emotion regulation and attention. These finding suggest a potential role of MBCT in reducing anxiety comorbid with bipolar disorder. There is also evidence to show that the greater the number of days meditated during the intervention period, the greater the impact on symptoms of depression 12 months later.

These data suggest that MBCT improves mindfulness and emotion regulation and reduces anxiety in bipolar disorder, corresponding to increased activations in the medial PFC, a region associated with cognitive flexibility and previously proposed as a key area of pathophysiology in the disorder.

References

1. National Institutes of Health. National Institute of Mental Health. Statistics. Accessed 1 Dec 2014 from www.nimh.nih.gov/health/statistics/prevalence/ bipolar-disorder-among-adults.shtml.
2. Merikangas KR, Jin R, He J-P, et al. Prevalence and correlates of bipolar spectrum disorder in the World Mental Health Survey Initiative. Arch Gen Psychiatry. 2011;68(3):241–51.   doi:10.1001/ archgenpsychiatry.2011.12.
3. Williams MD, Shah ND, Wagie AE, et al. Direct costs of bipolar disorder versus other chronic conditions: an employer-based health plan analysis. Psychiatr Serv. 2011;62:1073–8.
4. Bearden CE, Hoffman KM, Cannon TD. The neuropsychology and neuroanatomy of bipolar affective disorder: a critical review. Bipolar Disord. 2001;3:106–50. doi:10.1034/j.1399-5618.2001.030302.x.
5. Green MJ, Cahill CM, Malhi GS. The cognitive and neurophysiological basis of emotion dysregulation in bipolar disorder. J Affect Disord. 2007;103:29–42.
6. Phillips ML, Ladouceur CD, Drevets WC. A neural model of voluntary and automatic emotion regulation: implications for understanding the pathophysiology and neurodevelopment of bipolar disorder. Mol Psychiatry. 2008;13:833–57.
7. Le Doux JE. Emotion circuits in the brain. Annu Rev Neurosci. 2000;23:155–84.
8. Hariri AR, Tessitore A, Mattay VS, Fera F, Weinberger DR. The amygdala response to emotional stimuli: a comparison of faces and scenes. NeuroImage. 2002;17(1):317–23.
9. Hariri AR, Mattay VS, Tessitore A, Fera F, Weinberger DR. Neocortical modulation of the amygdala response to fearful stimuli. Biol Psychiatry. 2003;53:494–501.
10. Wager TD, Davidson ML, Hughes BL, Lindquist MA, Ochsner KN. Prefrontal-subcortical pathways mediating successful emotion regulation. Neuron. 2008;59(6):1037–50.
11. Foland LC, Altshuler LL, Bookheimer SY, Eisenberger N, Townsend J, Thompson PM. Evidence for deficient modulation of amygdala response by prefrontal cortex in bipolar mania. Psychiatry Res. 2008;162(1):27–37.
12. Malhi GS, Lagopoulos J, Sachdev PS, Ivanovski B, Shnier R. An emotional Stroop functional MRI study of euthymic bipolar disorder. Bipolar Disord. 2005;7(s5):58–69.
13. Gitlin MJ, Swendsen J, Heller TL, Hammen C. Relapse and impairment in bipolar disorder. Am J Psychiatry. 1995;152:1635–40.
14. Murray CJ, Vos T, Lozano R, Naghavi M, Flaxman AD, Michaud C, et al. Disability-adjusted life years (DALYs) for 291 diseases and injuries in 21 regions, 1990-2010: a systematic analysis for the Global Burden of Disease Study 2010. Lancet. 2012;380 (9859):2197–223.
15. Rosa AR, Reinares M, Michalak EE, Bonnin CM, Sole B, Franco C, et al. Functional impairment and disability across mood states in bipolar disorder. Value Health. 2010;13(8):984–8.
16. Miziou S, Tsitsipa E, Moysidou S, et al. Psychosocial treatment and interventions for bipolar disorder: a systematic review. Ann Gen Psychiatry. 2015;14:19. doi:10.1186/s12991-015-0057-z.
17. Reinares M, Sanchez-Moreno J, Fountoulakis KN. Psychosocial interventions in bipolar disorder: what, for whom, and when. J Affect Disord. 2014;156:46–55.
18. Deckersbach T, Nierenberg AA, Kessler R, Lund HG, Ametrano RM, Sachs G, et al. RESEARCH: cognitive rehabilitation for bipolar disorder: an open trial for employed patients with residual depressive symptoms. CNS Neurosci Ther. 2010;16(5): 298–307.
19. Beyon S, Soares-Weiser K, Woolacott N, Duffy S. Psychosocial interventions for the prevention of relapse in bipolar disorder: systematic review of controlled trials. Br J Psychiatry. 2008;192:5–11.
20. Scott J, Colom F, Vieta E. Ameta-analysis of relapserates with adjunctive psychological therapies compared to usual psychiatric treatment for bipolar disorders. Inter J Neuro psychopharmaco. 2007;10: 123–129.
21. Grossman P, Niemann L, Schmidt S, Walach H. Mindfulness-based stress reduction and health benefits: a meta-analysis. J Psychosom Res. 2004;57(1):35–43.
22. Teasdale J, Segal S, Williams J. How does cognitive therapy prevent depressive relapse and why should attention control mindfulness training help? Behav Res Ther. 1995;33(1):25–39.
23. Farb NAS, Anderson AK, Segal ZV. The mindful brain and emotion regulation in mood disorders. Can J Psychiatry. 2012;57(2):70–7.
24. Creswell J, Baldwin M, Eisenberger N, Lieberman M. Neural correlates of dispositional mindfulness during affect labeling. Psychosom Med. 2007;69(6):560–5.
25. Williams J, Alatiq Y, Crane C, Barnhofer T, Fennell M, Duggan D, et al. Mindfulness-based Cognitive Therapy (MBCT) in bipolar disorder: preliminary evaluation of immediate effects on between-episode functioning. J Affect Disord. 2008;107(1–3):275–9.
26. Ives-Deliperi VL, Howells F, Stein DJ, Meintjes EM, Horn N. The effects of mindfulness-based cognitive therapy in patients with bipolar disorder: a controlled functional MRI investigation. J Affect Disord. 2013;150(3):1152–7.
27. Strakiowski SM, Adler CM, Holland SK, Mills NP, DelBello MP, Eliassen JC. Abnormal FMRI brain activation in euthymic bipolar disorder pateints during a counting Strrop interference task. Am J Psychiatr. 2005;162(9):1697–705.
28. Howells FM, Ives-Deliperi VL, Horn NR, Stein DJ. Mindfulness based cognitive therapy improves frontal control in bipolar disorder: a pilot EEG study. BMC Psychiatry. 2012;12:15. doi:10.1186/1471-244X-12-1.
29. Hariri AR, Bookheimer SY, Mazziotta JC. Modulating emotional response: effects of a neocortical network on the limbic system. NeuroReport. 2000;11:43–8.

30. Bentin S, Allison T, Puce A, Perez E, McCarthy G. Electrophysiological studies of face perception in humans. J Cogn Neurosci 1996;8:551–565.

31. Eimer M, Kiss M, Nicholas S. Response profile of the facesensitive N170 component: a rapid adaptation study. Cereb Cortex. 2010;20:2442–2452.

32. Rossion B, Joyce CA, Cottrell GW, Tarr MJ. Early lateralization and orientation tuning for face, word, and object processing in the visual cortex. Neuroimage. 2003;20:1609–1624.

33. Perich T, Manicavasagar V, Mitchell PB, Ball JR, Hadzi-Pavlovic D. A randomized controlled trial of mindfulness-based cognitive therapy for bipolar disorder. Acta Psychiatrica Scandinavica, Online publication date: 1-Dec-2012.

34. Ghashghaei HT, Barbas H. Pathways for emotions: Interactions of prefrontal and anterior temporal pathways in the amygdala of the rhesus monkey. Neuroscience. 2002;115:1261–1279.

Mindfulness-Based Cognitive Therapy for Combat-Related Posttraumatic Stress Disorder

Anthony P. King and Todd K. Favorite

A.P. King, Ph.D. (✉)
Department of Psychiatry and University
Psychological Clinic, University of Michigan,
Ann Arbor, MI 48105, USA

Research Service, VA Ann Arbor Health System,
Ann Arbor, MI, USA
e-mail: Samadhi@med.umich.edu

T.K. Favorite, Ph.D., A.B.P.P.
Department of Psychiatry and University
Psychological Clinic, University of Michigan,
Ann Arbor, MI 48105, USA

PTSD Clinic, Mental Health Service, VA Ann Arbor
Health System, Ann Arbor, MI, USA

Over the past 8 years we have used 8-week MBCT groups adapted for PTSD, as well as longer PTSD exposure-based groups incorporating MBCT techniques and "curriculum" with combat veterans seeking treatment for PTSD of various ages who served in a number of combat deployments. We have provided MBCT with veterans who served in Korea, Vietnam, Somalia, Kuwait, and Iraq ("Operation Desert Storm," 1991), Afghanistan ("Operation Enduring Freedom/OEF," 2001–2015), and Iraq ("Operation Iraqi Freedom, OIF," 2003–2010, "Operation New Dawn, OND," 2010–2015). Many of these veterans also had major depression and/or chronic pain issues in addition to PTSD. We have been very interested that the majority of veterans who participated said they found the groups and the mindfulness techniques useful, and most report they often enjoy doing the mindfulness exercises. Most have also shown a high level of engagement, and the dropout rate from MBCT in younger OEF/OIF veterans has tended to be lower than is usual for this population.

A Case Study of Using MBCT with Combat PTSD

"Sam" (not his actual name) was a 32-year-old Army veteran who was seeking treatment for PTSD in our clinic. He had served a 15-month deployment to Iraq, which he completed 2 years before he came to us for treatment. Although his "military operational specialty" was in transportation, his convoy came under fire from automatic weapons (and occasionally RPGs) "more times than I can recall." In his intake evaluation, he shared that he had witnessed several explosions from IEDs, one of these, recorded as his "index trauma," had instantly killed a close friend of his who was driving a different truck. His base came under mortar and rocket attack regularly, for periods almost every night, and although people on his base were killed in these attacks, he said "strangely, you got used to it." He initially declined first-line trauma-focused individual treatment at the clinic, but was already taking an SSRI, and agreed to do the mindfulness group because "it sounded interesting" and reminded him somewhat of the approach in his martial arts.

Sam was friendly and talkative, and quickly bonded with other members of the group, and openly discussed his PTSD symptoms. He was active in discussions in the group, and shared with the group about some of the details of deployment in Iraq, the smells and sometimes horrific stench, the trash and dead bodies of people and animals that were often on the side of the roads, and the sound of the rocket attacks, etc. but we had agreed ahead of time that we would not discuss specific traumatic events in the group. Sam shared that he found things such as eating out at restaurants and going to movie theaters extremely anxiety-provoking, even though he "knew" intellectually there was little or no danger of attack or bombing. He could not tolerate people sitting or walking behind him. Shopping in a crowded grocery store was "out of the question," and the few times he had tried to go shopping with his wife and two small children, he became panicked and angry, and they had to leave the store. He felt intensely ashamed about this, as he felt about regularly "blowing up" at his wife, and sometimes his kids. "I can go from zero to 100 in less than a second, and its like I can't control it. And I get so angry over such stupid, trivial stuff." All of this was taking a big toll on his marriage and family.

Sam liked his job and the people he worked with and was happy to have work in a time many were out of work. He also noticed in general feeling "amped up" most of the day, and needing to keep himself "absolutely busy" as a way to feel safer. Driving was "exhausting," as he was constantly scanning overpasses for snipers and becoming anxious about trash on the side of the road, and often became very angry and aggressive when driving. (Although he said "it's a lot better now than it used to be!") He would come home from work exhausted, but also feeling profoundly "out of place" with his wife and kids, and often would spend time watching TV by himself, isolating himself because he did not

want to get angry and blow up at his children. Each night before bed, he did an extensive "perimeter sweep" of the house, and checking locks on windows and doors. Although he felt "beyond exhausted" at bedtime, he usually found he could not sleep, that his mind was racing with anxious ruminations, and after his wife fell asleep he would be up watching TV alone again. He averaged about 3–4 h of sleep, often while sitting in his chair with the TV on.

Sam greatly enjoyed the MBCT Raisin Exercise, and shared with the group an experience when his unit had just gotten to Kuwait for the first time after a year in Iraq, and he had gone to eat at a Burger King. "It was surreal – it was like the first time I had ever had a Whopper, it was just amazing," and he was intrigued he could recreate such feelings of expansiveness and intensity of sensory experience on purpose using mindfulness.

Sam also really liked the body scan. The first time we did it in class, we locked the door and made it optional to lie on a mat or sit. Sam chose to lie down; and he fell asleep by the time we got to the right leg. Sam used the body scan every night as a sleep aid, and said he would listen to the audio in bed on his phone (wearing ear buds) and this was very helpful for him to be able to fall asleep in bed. He said he often stayed asleep for 2–5 h, and when he woke, he sometimes would do the body scan again. Although of course this was not the initial intent of the body scan as a mindfulness exercise, Sam said "it really helped me to be able to have my body as an anchor for my awareness, and helped me to not have all these crazy thoughts and worries running out of control. Then I could actually sleep!" This experience was shared by many other PTSD patients.

Sam also actively engaged in the "Pleasant Event" calendar, even though he initially seemed doubtful there would be *any* pleasant events to report. He seemed rather bemused that he noticed squirrels and chipmunks playing in his backyard, and was surprised by the peaceful feelings this set upon him. In the "Unpleasant Event Calendar," Sam like many other veterans noted experience of PTSD symptoms, including "road rage," feeling anxious and panicked, and sudden anger at his wife, followed by shame and sadness. He said exploring (and documenting) the physical sensations, the feelings, and the thoughts associated with these events helped him to "move into" his experiences rather than trying to distract himself and quickly and shamefully try to banish these upsetting experiences out of his awareness. Doing this he also came to acknowledge that it was helpful for him to be able to feel more compassion and kindness towards himself about his PTSD symptoms. Sam practiced formal mindfulness exercises nearly every day, using his mobile "smart phone." He also picked up the "3-minute Breathing Space" quickly, and used it regularly. "It's a great 'attitude adjuster' and you can do it anywhere" and said this also helped him feel more confidence that he would blow up less at his young kids.

Sam's level of PTSD at intake, assessed by the clinician-administered PTSD scale was in the moderate to severe range (~80). At the conclusion of the group, Sam no longer met DSM-IV criteria for PTSD, and his CAPS score was less than 50. Sam was among our "strong responders"; while not everyone had as large a decrease in PTSD symptoms as Sam, many shared Sam's sentiments that the experience of doing the mindfulness exercises had enhanced many aspects of their lives, in addition to helping him cope better with PTSD. Sam said he planned to continue his nearly daily mindfulness practice for the foreseeable future.

The Problem of Posttraumatic Stress Disorder

Posttraumatic stress disorder (PTSD) is highly prevalent psychiatric disorder that is associated with considerable human suffering, disability, and economic costs. The National Comorbidity Survey Replication study [1], a nationally representative sample of over 10,000 adults in the USA found the lifetime prevalence of PTSD was over 7 %, and the 12 month prevalence (percent of people who had met criteria for PTSD over the past year was 4 %). This makes PTSD the third most prevalent disorder in the USA, after major depres-

sion (17 % lifetime) and social anxiety disorder (12 % lifetime). Furthermore, PTSD is twice as common in women (11 % lifetime) than in men (5 %). PTSD is a major clinical issue for the Armed Services and the Veterans Administration [2–6], associated with suffering, disruption of families, and often leading to significant loss of productivity, unemployment, and high economic costs to patients and to society [7]. Military service-connected PTSD is a common disorder (estimates as high as 30 % lifetime incidence in combat veterans [3, 5, 6], chronic disorder that can lead to substantial disability lasting for decades [3, 5, 6, 8, 9]. Over 10 % of all Desert Storm veterans (>20 % of combat-exposed veterans) were diagnosed with PTSD 6 years after deployment [5, 8].

Studies of soldiers and Marines serving in "Operation Iraqi Freedom" (OIF) found nearly 30 % had some form of clinically significant psychiatric symptoms, and ~20 % had clinically significant PTSD symptoms [2, 3]. In a subsequent study of US infantry soldiers given diagnostic assessments in 2013 [4], infantry combat veterans deployed to OIF had rates of PTSD of nearly 20 % (using ether DSM-IV or DSM-5 criteria), compared to about 13 % of all infantry soldiers; and this compares to about 6 % of overall military personnel. PTSD is frequently associated with psychiatric comorbidity such as depression, alcohol and substance abuse, and related anxiety disorders. It is also associated with chronic medical problems such as cancer, cardiovascular disease, arthritis, pulmonary disorders, and all forms of mortality in epidemiological studies [10–12]

Definition of PTSD

While severe psychological disruptions associated with the experience of psychological trauma has been documented in the historical literature since ancient times (and descriptions of PTSD, and in particular combat-related PTSD, can be found in Homer, Herodotus, the Bible, the Mahabharata, and Shakespeare) the formal diagnostic category of "Posttraumatic Stress Disorder" did not appear in the Western psychiatric/medical nosological system until the publication of the third edition of the Diagnostic and Statistical Manual (DSM-III-R) by the American Psychiatric Association in 1980. The specific definition of what constitutes a "trauma" and the diagnostic criteria of PTSD have continued to be refined since that time.

DSM-IV defined trauma as an aversive event in which both of the following were present: (1) The person experienced, witnessed, or was confronted with an event or events that involved actual or threatened death or serious injury, or a threat to the physical integrity of self or others (i.e., through sexual assault), and (2) The person's response involved intense fear, helplessness, or horror. In its latest revision, DSM-5, the types of events which qualify as potential traumas was further defined, and the requirement of a reaction of fear, helplessness, or horror occurring right after the trauma has been removed, as it did not improve diagnostic accuracy for the disorder. In addition to the experience of a traumatic event, a specific constellation of symptoms must be present for at least 1 month. DSM-IV had three symptom clusters of: (A) reexperiencing (e.g., intrusive, upsetting memories, getting upset to reminders of the trauma, nightmares), (B) avoidance (e.g., avoiding trauma reminders, emotional numbing), and (C) hyperarousal (e.g., hypervigilance, exaggerated startle, concentration problems, irritability, sleep disturbance). In DSM-5 the clusters of Reexperiencing (now called Intrusion symptoms, Criterion A) and Hyperarousal (now called Alterations in Arousal and Reactivity, Criterion B) remain. Avoidance and numbing are separated into two clusters, Avoidance (Criterion C), and a new cluster called Negative Alterations in Cognitions and Mood (Criterion D).

There is evidence that psychotropic medications can be helpful in reducing symptoms for a portion of people struggling with PTSD, but the great majority of patients taking medications tend to retain their PTSD diagnosis. Selective serotonin reuptake inhibitors (SSRIs) are considered evidence-based pharmacological treatment for PTSD. Sertraline (Zoloft) and paroxetine (Paxil) show a slightly greater effect over pla-

cebo in randomized controlled trials (RCT) and are approved by the FDA for treatment of PTSD. However, there is considerable variability in therapeutic response to SSRIs, with about 60 % of PTSD patients having any clinically significant response, and only 20–30 % of PTSD patients treated with effective doses of SSRIs achieve complete remission of symptoms [13]. There is limited evidence that other "off label" medications, including other antidepressants (e.g., mirtazapine (Remeron) and trazodone (Oleptro), some anticonvulsants (e.g., topiramate (Topamax)), and alpha-adrenergic agents (e.g., prazocin (Minipress)) may also have efficacy for PTSD and may be alternatives to SSRI "nonresponders." However, the overall effectiveness of most medications has been low [13].

A number of psychosocial treatments for PTSD have been shown to be highly effective for many patients with PTSD, Therapies that focus on the memories and experiences related to the trauma (often called "trauma-focused" or "exposure based" psychotherapies) have had particularly significant results. Several psychotherapeutic interventions which include explicit processing of traumatic material (e.g., memories of the trauma itself), including Prolonged Exposure (PE), Eye-Movement Desensitization and Reprogramming (EMDR), Trauma Focused-Cognitive Behavioral Therapy (TF-CBT), and Cognitive Processing Therapy (CPT), now have considerable empirical support [14, 15]. A relatively large number of well-designed RCTs with both civilian and military veteran populations have found PE, CPT, and EMDR to all have considerable efficacy for treatment of PTSD, and they have come to be regarded as "first line" treatment in the fields of both civilian and combat-related PTSD. Currently, exposure therapy is the only treatment for PTSD that has been judged by the Institute of Medicine (IoM) to have adequate evidence supporting efficacy [16], and is often referred to as "the gold-standard" by PE therapists and researchers. The effect of these psychotherapies in reducing PTSD symptoms measured before and after treatment (pre-post therapy effect sizes, expressed as the statistic Cohen's d) are consistently in the 1.0–2.0 range

(Cohen's *d* values of greater than 0.80 are considered "large"). While most of the studies to date use waitlist or "treatment as usual" as comparison groups, some studies have also reported statistically significant improvement over active comparison psychotherapies. Although these treatments are effective for many PTSD patients seeking relief, they do not appear to work with every person struggling with PTSD, which has led some within the VA to feel that a "one-size-fits-all" approach to PTSD treatment is not supported by the actual evidence, and is not the best way to serve the substantial needs of veterans struggling with PTSD [17].

The Veterans Administration (VA) has invested considerable resource into training and dissemination of the PE and CPT as "first-line treatments," and has embarked on an impressive training and roll-out of these psychotherapies nation-wide [18–21]. VA guidelines now require that all veterans with PTSD be offered one of these treatments. Even with the strong evidence of efficacy of PE and CPT for PTSD, many veterans do not to engage in these treatments and drop out of them early [22, 23]. A substantial proportion of those that complete these "first line treatments" continue to evidence PTSD symptoms [15, 22]. The reported dropout rates in both RCT trials [24–26],and clinic-based studies [22, 27, 28], range from 30 % to over 40 %. Available data suggests that from 30 % to as high as 50 % of veterans who complete these treatments do not show clinically meaningful improvement in their PTSD symptoms [24, 25, 29], and approximately two-thirds (62–70%) of veterans with PTSD who make the considerable personal investment to engage in treatment with PE or CPT retain their PTSD diagnosis at the end of the treatment [15].

Patient reluctance and/or avoidance of engaging in trauma-focused treatments, as well as difficulty tolerating or engaging in the trauma-focused treatments, are contributing to problems in patients access to effective treatments [22]. This has been highlighted in recent high-profile cases of veterans having particularly difficult reactions to prolonged exposure [30], and the ensuing public debate among veterans, chairs of psychiatry, and directors of

PTSD treatment centers that has recently played out publicly in the New York Times [31]. Given this reluctance to engage and high rates of dropout in trauma-focused approaches, it becomes important to determine if alternate forms of evidence-based treatments can be better tolerated by patients with PTSD.

While the greatest amount of evidence and empirical support currently supports trauma-focused, exposure-based therapies, there is also emerging evidence that psychotherapeutic approaches that do not contain explicit trauma processing and exposure also demonstrate comparable effectiveness for PTSD, including "Present Centered Therapy" (CPT) [32] and "Interpersonal Therapy" (IPT) [33]. Interestingly, both of these therapies were initially designed for use in RCTs as "nonspecific, control therapies," a sort of scientific straw man designed to control for "common factors" in psychotherapy (e.g., relationship with a therapist, talking about one's problems) but lacking the presumed "active principle" of trauma exposure. Yet recent studies suggest they may actually be as effective as the most rigorous "trauma exposure based" therapies, but without needing to engage in any "trauma exposure," which a substantial portion of both clients and therapists find difficult [34].

Mindfulness-based approaches are often delivered in a group format, which strongly engages patients in work concerning patterns of emotional reactivity, but not specific "trauma narratives." Group psychotherapies are a common and well accepted format in VA settings, including PTSD clinics. Group interventions allow therapists to reach more patients in a cost-effective fashion, and may also have additional therapeutic benefits (e.g., enhancing adherence, social support). Yet while group therapies are among the most common interventions available to returning combat veterans, existing group therapies for combat PTSD have limited empirical support at this time, (exceptions to this are Present-centered and Trauma-focused Group Therapy [35], and the group version of Cognitive Processing Therapy, CPT [36]). However, effect sizes reported for group therapies have generally been smaller than for trauma-focused individual therapies. Development of new empirically supported therapeutic interventions that can be delivered efficiently and effectively within existing venues is crucial, and we feel that approaches like mindfulness meditation could be helpful for patient engagement, and may be an important alternative for patient-centered personalized treatment.

Theoretical Rationale of MBCT for PTSD

As described in more detail in other chapters, MBCT as an intervention for depression relapse prevention is highly effective and durable, decreasing depression relapse by >50% at 12 month follow-up in randomized controlled trials [37, 38]. These are among the largest and most clinically meaningful effects of any meditation training studied to date, demonstrating effectiveness comparable to continuous antidepressant medication [39, 40]. While MBCT was initially designed for remitted MDD patients, subsequent studies have provided evidence that MBCT has potential effectiveness in the treatment of active psychiatric disorders [41]. There is now considerable evidence that MBCT (and MBSR) are acceptable and efficacious for patients with persistent depressive disorder during a depressive episode [42–46]. MBCT is also showing effectiveness with anxiety disorders [47–49], bipolar disorder [50], patients with suicidal ideation [51, 52], and borderline personality disorder [53].

Given the evidence for potential efficacy in anxiety and depression, including severe depression, it seems reasonable to suggest that MBCT might also be helpful for patient with PTSD. There is a considerable symptom overlap between PTSD and major depression, and PTSD and depression are frequently comorbid psychiatric disorders. There is evidence that MBCT decreases rumination, which is thought to be a maintenance factor in both PTSD and depression. There is also evidence that MBCT alters a patient's "relationship" to negative cognitions, rather than altering the belief in the content of the cognition [54], which may make it particu-

larly useful for a range of traumatic experiences. There is evidence that a substantial portion of veterans who utilize VA healthcare services with are interested in mindfulness and mind-body approaches, for treatment of somatic and mental health issues, as well as for the promotion of wellness. A recent systematic review by the VA Evidence-Based Synthesis Program [55] which examined the effectiveness of mindfulness interventions for a number of somatic and mental health problems, found that the most consistent beneficial effect of mindfulness interventions was seen in major depression. This review also saw evidence for beneficial effects on overall health and psychological outcomes, in particular in chronic illness and somatization disorders.

Mindfulness practices through the use of MBCT or MBSR provide a strategy diametrically opposed to thought suppression (i.e., nonjudgmental acknowledging of trauma memories, threat assessments, and ruminative worry). Cognitive processes engaged by mindfulness training (i.e., sustained, nonjudgmental attention to sensations, memories, thoughts, and emotions that are evocative, or even painful), can be conceptualized of as a form of "*exposure*." Mindfulness appears to engage and strengthen *emotional regulation*, and may strengthen the ability to engage other active coping strategies. Mindfulness meditation focusing on the breath alone may have positive effects in relation to PTSD symptoms,, particularly if the mindfulness practice "targets" PTSD symptoms and trauma related memories, images, and cognitions. Mindfulness practices may also facilitate the change mechanisms found in both exposure based and cognitive psychotherapies by reducing experiential avoidance negative attributions and maladaptive behavioral patterns.

Both theoretical [56–61] and empirical reviews [56, 62–66] outline potential mechanisms of mindfulness-based interventions. A number of psychological constructs have been proposed based on this work, including self-regulation, cognitive-behavioral flexibility, exposure, relaxation, decreased rumination and worry. Additionally, concepts such as de-centering, metacognition, mindfulness, self-compassion, and values clarification have been suggested as potential mechanisms for the positive outcomes of mindfulness-based interventions.

How these specific theoretical constructs and therapeutic mechanisms may influence outcomes in PTSD continues to be an open question. While mindfulness practice might be nice for improving one's mood or attitude, it could seem quite controversial to some to propose that a mindfulness-based intervention could be considered for a severe psychopathology like PTSD, which is seen to require intensive, prolonged, and sometimes painful, trauma-focused exposure work. Perhaps even more controversial are questions of whether or not trauma exposure is actually needed to treat PTSD. This could have seemed almost "heretical" in some circles until very recently, as does the consideration of "common" factors as potential "active" mechanisms of a psychotherapeutic intervention for PTSD. Interventions that do not have a specific trauma-focused component, such as supportive therapy, relaxation training, and present-centered therapy (PCT), frequently demonstrate considerable efficacy for PTSD [14, 15, 67, 68]; however, many of the RCTs using these treatments indicate the effect size was not as strong as that for the active intervention using a trauma-focused protocol. However, there is now emerging evidence that psychotherapeutic approaches without explicit trauma exposure (e.g., PCT and IPT) might be as effective for PTSD as the most intensive trauma-based therapies [32, 33]. This intriguing emerging work, while as yet still preliminary, suggests that the "common factors" found in these so-called "nonspecific control" therapies may in fact be on par with "gold-standard" trauma focused treatments. However, it is as yet an open question whether the factors found in mindfulness and MBCT might also be "active" for treatment of PTSD?

Much of the research on etiology, neuroscience, and treatment of PTSD has focused on the phenomenon of "fear conditioning" (classical or Pavlovian conditioning) at the time of the trauma. Within this paradigm normal recovery or exposure-based cognitive-behavioral treatments operate as an "extinction trial" of the fear conditioning. These phenomena have extensive experimental documentation in the field of psychology dating back to the 1890s, and are integral theoretical components of trauma-focused treatments such as PE. Therefore, focus on the traumatic experiences and the techniques enlisted to help patients directly process it make considerable theoretical and practical sense. Given the dominance of these concepts in the PTSD treatment research, it is not surprising that trauma-focused interventions have the most empirical support, at this time. Although environmental factors such as stress, loss, social pressures, and trauma figure large in precipitating and/or exacerbating psychiatric disorders such as major depression, bipolar disorder, anxiety disorders, and even schizophrenia, PTSD is the only psychiatric disorder that specifically requires an environmental event (i.e., a trauma) as part of its diagnostic criteria.

Clearly the experience of the trauma and the impact of the trauma on the patient's life plays a central role in development of PTSD. However, it is important to recognize that there is incontrovertible evidence that the majority of people who are exposed to trauma, even to severe trauma, do not develop PTSD [3, 4, 9, 69, 70], Interestingly, there is evidence that the vast majority of people experience many or all of the symptoms of PTSD in the days following exposure to a trauma, but in most people these symptoms diminish within a few weeks, and people have "recovered" within a month, and thus do not meet criteria for PTSD. This has led many researchers to think of PTSD as a problem of being able to "recover" and psychologically metabolize the traumatic event. This is largely thought to reside in the way people respond to the trauma, and find ways to incorporate and/or "make sense" of the trauma in the context of their world and self-view. This is a different explanatory model than a problem of primarily of overactive fear conditioning.

This also suggests that specific cognitive, emotional, neurobiological, developmental, or even genetic vulnerability and/or resilience factors exist for PTSD. Therefore it might also be important for effective treatments to specifically engage with changeable vulnerability factors, especially if they play roles in maintenance of PTSD symptoms. Epidemiological studies have identified a history of childhood maltreatment and/or adversity and trait neuroticism as predictors of both PTSD and depression in adulthood. Other personality traits, cognitive styles, and maladaptive cognitions have also been associated with increased PTSD risk, and could also be involved in maintenance of PTSD. Experience of a trauma can lead to "shattered beliefs" about oneself as a good person and the world as safe, just, and benevolent world [71, 72]. A further phenomena has been described as "moral injury" when people or institutions that were once held in high esteem are now incongruous with our core beliefs. Thus, dysfunctional cognitions about oneself as incompetent, the world as dangerous, and beliefs of self-blame for the trauma are associated with PTSD (PTCI). Some forms of psychotherapy such as CPT focus on addressing dysfunctional cognitions on the basis of assimilation and/or accommodation of core belief systems [73].

Several psychological models for the development of PTSD have been posited that incorporate learning theory, information processing theory, and cognitive behavioral theory, that explain symptoms of PTSD, and suggest specific treatment rationale. A thorough description of these theories is beyond the scope of this chapter (several books are available [74, 75]. Given the dominance of "fear conditioning" models in the PTSD field, it is important to first review current theory about the etiology PTSD and potential therapeutic mechanisms when considering how MBCT may be useful for PTSD,. An early but still very relevant and influential model for development of anxiety disorders is the "Two-stage model" originally proposed by Mowrer [76] for the acquisition of specific phobias. This theory posits that an initial effect (first stage) of a traumatic exposure will also lead to classical (Pavolvian) "fear conditioning" of cues associated with the trauma (in this language, the "unconditioned stimulus"). In this model any stimuli associated with the trauma (e.g., for rape victims, the smell of the perpetrator's cologne or features of the site of the attack,

for combat veterans the sound of helicopters, smell of diesel, seeing people dressed in garb of the country of the combat zone, etc.) can become a "conditioned stimuli." Encountering these stimuli can later produce fear a "conditioned response" similar to that of the original trauma. Additional stimuli that are less directly associated with the trauma can also become "paired" or associated with the "conditioned stimuli" through higher order conditioning and/or "stimulus generalization" [87]. Thus, more and more types of cues or aspects of the victim's environment can become associated with the memory of the trauma event, and consequently trigger a fear response. Pavlov (citation?) observed that while "conditioned responses" can be powerful, they can also rapidly abate when the "conditioned stimulus" is repeatedly presented in the absence of the "unconditioned stimulus," a process labeled "extinction." Thus, conditioned fear responses to trauma-related cues are also expected to extinguish after multiple exposures; for example, the smell of the specific cologne or diesel fuel following the trauma that are not "paired" with a dangerous or frightening event, and this is part of the natural recovery process However, it is posited that in PTSD, the initial Pavlovian conditioned fear (and the avoidance behaviors associated with these conditioned fears), is maintained by Skinnerian, operant conditioning, in the form of negative reinforcement (i.e., the reduction of the fear response when trauma-related cues are avoided, such that avoidant behavior is reinforced, and the helpful exposure leading to extinction does not occur).

Thus, "two factor" Cognitive Behavioral/learning theories for the development of PTSD have invoked both classical conditionings to the traumatic exposure, as well as operant conditioning of learned avoidance behaviors that perpetuate symptoms by blocking opportunities for extinction [78]. Further elaboration of the two-stage model of PTSD, incorporates Lang's (1984) information processing theory of emotion, the "Emotional Processing Theory of PTSD" [77] posits that trauma exposure leads to the development of a semantic memory network (or "fear network") comprised of interconnected nodes of information. In addition to trauma-related stimuli these include informational elements about physiological and behavioral responses to the trauma, as well as semantic meanings of both the stimuli and conditioned responses. These "fear networks" are proposed to contain a particularly large number of "paired" elements, thus making the network highly sensitive and reactive to conditioned fear. Stimulus generalization and second-order conditioning can incorporate more and more associated elements that were previously neutral or safe into the "fear network," explaining how symptoms of PTSD can actually get worse over time rather than gradually habituating and resolving through the process of extinction.

One logical conclusion that could be drawn from this theory is that since avoidance to trauma cues drive PTSD symptoms, that the most powerful and efficient approach to stop this vicious cycle would be to address the avoidance "head-on." This is accomplished by therapeutic exposure to reminders of the trauma and avoided activities, by pushing back against the operant learning that allow them to maintain the classical fear conditioning. Prolonged Exposure therapy does just that, by engaging in repeated and prolonged exposure to the trauma memories themselves (called imaginal exposure), in a safe environment where nothing dangerous occurs (i.e., the therapists office). Foa (1994) asserts that PTSD results from distorted fear structures that need to be (re)activated for "corrective information" to be incorporated so that it reflects a more realistic perspective in the current context. In this way the person suffering from PTSD will "learn" that the trauma memories (while certainly painful) are not in and of themselves dangerous, and the automatic conditioned fear responses will diminish through the process of extinction. In addition, patients also complete a hierarchy of "in vivo" exposures (similar to CBT for panic disorder) for situations, or activities they are currently avoiding because they trigger fear responses. The purpose is to engage in the feared or avoided activity one at a time until the patient's Subjective Unit of Distress (SUD) decreases enough to move to the next exposure on the hierarchy. Emotional Processing Theory

also recognizes that PTSD is also often associated with negative emotions and distorted negative cognitions about the patient's incompetence, or that the trauma was one's own fault (self-blame) and the world at large as dangerous. Thus, PE also engages patients in discussions at the end of each exposure to help identify dysfunctional cognitions or attributions. This "trauma processing" component of the therapy provides ways to reframe the trauma memory similar in many ways to cognitive restructuring of cognitive therapy.

Each of the forms of existing psychotherapy for PTSD with the most empirical support (e.g., PE, EMDR, CPT) contains multiple components. A detailed description of these therapies is beyond the scope of this chapter, but several (but not all) of these basic principles are shared across the approaches, although these principles are approached with more or less emphasis within each of these treatments. These differences will be briefly discussed next. The components could be operationalized roughly as *psychoeducation* about PTSD and presentation of the therapy rationale, *relaxation* training, *exposure to the trauma memory*, *processing* of the trauma memory, the impact of the trauma on one's life, and working with *dysfunctional cognitions*, *affect modulation*/self-regulation skills, and in vivo *exposure*, or purposely engaging with feared or avoided (nondangerous) cues, activities, or situations.

In PE, EMDR, and CPT exposure to and "processing" of the trauma is done in somewhat different manners, but the idea that the trauma memory needs to be accessed and incorporated is common among most of the empirically supported therapies. As described, PE focuses heavily upon trauma exposure In the form of "imaginal exposure" during the therapy session, as well as in recordings of the session, which the patient listens to between sessions as "homework." EMDR in particular has theories about processing of trauma memories that are not shared with other theories or therapies, in particular the role of "bilateral stimulation" (usually with back-and-forth eye movements or other bilateral stimulation, e.g., tones and tapping, that are used as a "dual-attention" task or distractor within the procedure. EMDR also has other unique elements, such as "installation" of "resources" or positive memories and thoughts, and titration and moving between the trauma memory and the resource. A detailed presentation of that theory is beyond the current scope, but multiple presentations of that theory are available in the literature. Although approached in its own particular manner, EMDR does involve having the patient encounter with trauma memories with the therapist, as does PE, and thus could be thought in that way to have an "imaginal exposure" component, in that trauma memories are specifically accessed in the therapy session. In CPT, the patient is engaged in trauma exposure by helping them to create a "trauma narrative." This is accomplished by writing about the trauma in detail, and to focus on and refine the trauma narrative to build a story of how the trauma impacted the patient's life. CPT has the patient read and revise their trauma narrative between session on a daily basis while attending to the ways in which it is impacts current experiences. Emotion regulation is also utilized in order to enhance self-efficacy around fear stimuli as an alternative to avoidant or "safety behaviors."

All of the therapies provide some form of psychoeducational about PTSD, to normalize symptoms, and description of the rationale, to promote positive expectancies; common factors in psychotherapy. CPT is based on the processing of traumatic experiences by identifying rigid cognitive/affective patterns that stem from trauma memories, and impact current thoughts and behaviors. These rigid or "stuck thoughts" create distorted themes about oneself and the world. CPT works at the cognitive, affective and thematic level to enhance cognitive flexibility and adaptive functioning.

As can be seen, MBCT may in fact provide some therapeutic mechanisms already posited and in place in existing PTSD therapies. It is possible it could have novel mechanisms, or at least get at existing mechanisms through different techniques that may help with patient engagement. We briefly consider some of the previously proposed "mechanisms" of mindfulness-based interventions, and how they may play out in the particular case of PTSD therapy.

Relaxation

Whether or not relaxation training is properly considered meditation per se or not, relaxation techniques such as Progressive Muscular Relaxation (PMR) and autogenics have a long history for use in treatment of anxiety; a meta-analysis [79] of studies 1997–2007 (both RCT and uncontrolled) found a medium-high effects size (Cohen's $d = 0.57$) for reduction of trait anxiety, but also did not find differences in effects of various forms of relaxation or between relaxation and meditation. Interestingly, here are probably more RCT studies of relaxation training for the treatment of PTSD than any other "Mind-Body" treatment; albeit in all of these, the relaxation arm is included as a nonspecific or "inert" control condition, and not expected by the researchers to be effective. A recent meta-analysis [14] of RCTs of primary psychotherapies (e.g., PE, EMDR, CPT) for treatment of PTSD found pre-post effect sizes of relaxation of $d = 0.34 - d = 1.29$ in four RCTs consistent with previous findings [80], but in each case the primary therapies were superior to relaxation; however, "relaxation" attributed to doing mindfulness practices can be considered among the "common" factors (i.e., relatively nonspecific) in terms of psychosocial interventions for PTSD symptoms. Given that veterans report that they often find the mindfulness exercises relaxing and even enjoyable, and feel some forms of immediate benefit from relaxation, this can help with engagement and adherence.

Exposure

In mindfulness meditation, therapists encourage patients to keep their focus on the breath (or whatever the designated focus of the practice is), but also to acknowledge and try to engage a "nonjudgmental" or accepting stance toward whatever thoughts, sensations, or feelings arise during this practice. Even if the thought or feeling that is occurring at that moment should be fear or horror, the patient is encouraged to "engage" and "notice" the mental phenomenon, observe its features and acknowledge it as a mental phenomenon rather than a threat. As the exposure provided by mindfulness is to extemporaneously experienced thoughts and feelings, first within the confines of the formal mindfulness meditation session, and then throughout one's day, rather than to a specific trauma narrative, it might be thought of as "in vivo" exposure to avoided experiences (and thus lead to lessening of experiential avoidance). Exposure to avoided internal states (e.g., negative self-cognitions, frightening physiological sensations, traumatic memories) has good face validity for mindfulness training, which aims toward nonjudgmental acceptance of sensations, thoughts, and emotions, and is also a central feature of CBT treatment for anxiety disorders (phobias, panic) and PTSD. "Experiential avoidance" has been proposed by Hayes et al., and Roemer as playing a key role in the maintenance of PTSD and other psychopathologies as described in the two-stage model of anxiety related disorders.

for decreasing depression [86–88]. Furthermore, having a deficit in metacognitive capacity has also been posited as a risk and/ or maintenance factors for PTSD; metacognitive capacity is necessary for perspective taking, which helps us to make sense and integrate our representation of self, others, in the context of the trauma. "Making sense" of the trauma and one's reactions to it facilitates acceptance, integration, and eventually recovery from the trauma. Metacognition has been proposed to be a central aspect of resiliency by helping one to adaptively integrate the trauma into a larger context of their life experiences. There is interesting evidence that patients with chronic presentations of PTSD appear to have deficits in metacognition processing [89–92] which may contribute to difficultly in gaining a perspective of the trauma and ultimately interfering with recovery. There is emerging evidence that therapies that specifically teach trauma patients to enhance metacognitive skills (e.g., metacognitive therapy) [93] demonstrates substantial reduction of PTSD symptoms.

Decentering, Re-perceiving, or Metacognition

Mindfulness-based interventions strive to entrain sustained mindful attention to, and acknowledgment of, even unpleasant emotions or memories in a nonjudgmental manner. As previously suggested [81], such techniques stand diametrically opposed to the psychological processes of avoidance, suppression of painful emotions and memories, which are thought to contribute to symptom maintenance in PTSD [82]. Interestingly, in contrast to "refuting" or changing the content of negative cognitions which is typical of traditional cognitive-behavioral therapies, MBCT appears to alter one's relationship to negative cognitions [54].

Previous research has posited "de-centering" as a theoretical component in cognitive therapy [83, 84], as therapeutic mechanism of cognitive therapy for depression [85]. Mindfulness practice and MBCT central to the mechanism of action

Rumination

In addition to the dysfunctional cognitions themselves, there is thinking that trait rumination, or the tendency to "get stuck" in certain patterns of negative thoughts also contributes to the symptoms of PTSD, and there is considerable evidence that rumination is a maintenance factor for PTSD [94, 95]. Mindfulness practices is proposed to promote "decentering" which acts to reduce rumination [86–88] as therapeutic mechanism of cognitive therapy for depression [85]. There is evidence that MBCT leads to decreases in rumination, and that post-treatment levels of rumination predicted the risk of relapse [96].

Developing Self-Compassion/ Kindness Towards Oneself

Self-compassion and loving-kindness techniques have face validity for several features of PTSD, including guilt, irritability, and numbing. Not surprisingly, self-compassion measures (such as the Neff Self-compassion scale) are significantly lower in PTSD patients, and correlated with PTSD symptom severity [97, 98] and King and Favorite, unpublished data). Mindfulness interventions such as MBCT, even when not engaging in "overt" self-compassion or loving kindness meditations, are thought to engender a greater sense of acceptance and self-kindness [44, 99], and this may be an important therapeutic mechanism for PTSD, which like depression is associated with considerable guilt, shame, and self-blame (refs.). Interestingly, recent work with overt loving-kindness and self-compassion meditations have found these to be also be acceptable to veterans with PTSD [100, 101] and our experiences have been similar.

Contextual Processing

There have been interesting theoretical suggestions that addition to having problems with mis-identification of specific cues and "cue generalization," PTSD patients may fail to use safety signal [102], and/or may have deficits in processing "context" and being able to utilize contextual information in making assessments of relative threat and danger [103]. We have recently provided evidence that PTSD patients appear to have deficits in being able to identify safe vs dangerous "contexts" [104] in experimental fear conditioning and extinction paradigms, and that these deficits appear to be linked to altered hippocampal functioning. An intriguing possibility is that mindfulness techniques utilized in MBCT, in particular "informal mindfulness" and the 3-min Breathing Space, may be useful by helping patients to "contextualize" themselves in time, space, social milieu, etc., and that the perceptual and cognitive openness and engagement encouraged in MBCT may help PTSD patients to be able to better disambiguate safe from threatening cues, as well as better identify "safety context." We are actively pursuing these questions.

How Can MBCT "Fit in" to Effective PTSD Treatment?

When considering how MBCT may be helpful for PTSD, it is also important to factor in how MBCT can be incorporated into the PTSD patient's treatment vis-à-vis other interventions involving trauma processing and other forms of exposure. While we have discussed emerging evidence that treatments that do not contain explicit exposure to and processing of trauma material appear to nonetheless have efficacy for PTSD, a relatively brief 8-week group intervention that does not directly address PTSD symptoms and does not have an individual component, may not be sufficient treatment for many people with PTSD. An MBCT group might be considered to serve as an adjunctive "preparation" for an exposure-based treatment (especially for patients who decline trauma-focused treatments), that may be helpful for patients by increasing their ability to tolerate experiencing strong emotions. MBCT groups might also be a concurrent adjunctive to cognitive or exposure-based individual therapies by increasing engagement and developing cognitive skills, similar to the highly successful group-individual format of dialectical behavior therapy (DBT). MBCT groups of patients with PTSD who are also undergoing concurrent trauma exposure therapy could utilize separate trauma-focused therapists to process their trauma, or trauma processing could be done in "pull-out" individual sessions with the MBCT therapist. Alternately, MBCT or related therapies that incorporate the "curriculum" and techniques of MBCT could be crafted into a stand-alone intervention to modulate emotional reactivity, and/or into an extended group intervention that incorporates specific components effective in treating PTSD, such as "in vivo" exposure. The feasibility of combining MBCT with other cognitive-behavioral approaches, and interventions such as social skills training, IPT [105], and Cognitive Behavioral Analysis System of Psychotherapy (CBASP) that focus on developing and cultivating "perceived functionality" within interpersonal relationships [106], and area in which patients with PTSD often struggle, is of great interest to us. The authors are developing several of these approaches through ongoing work with veterans at a Veterans Administration PTSD clinic.

Modifications of MBCT for PTSD

We made several adaptations to the 8-week MBCT protocol we used in our research protocol, and have continued to make changes to best suit the needs of PTSD patients. In our opinion, the overarching interests in adapting the MBCT protocol is to be sensitive to the specific needs and concerns of patients struggling with PTSD. These are in terms of group members' sense of safety and comfort with the group, gearing the specific exercises and discussion towards topics relevant to people struggling with PTSD symptoms (including discussion of PTSD symptoms), and doing group exercises they can have a reasonable amount of comfort doing. Therapists working with people struggling with PTSD also need to be able to appropriately manage actual safety concerns (e.g., increased distress, suicidality, and substance use) that could arise during the treatment. While these concerns are present for MBCT with any group, as patients with PTSD often have concerns of immediate safety additional care needs to be taken in this crucial area.

The "content" adaptations we made to the 8-week MBCT protocol used with PTSD patients involved substituting psychoeducation about depression in Session 4 with psychoeducation geared toward PTSD and stress physiology. We shortened the length of the mindfulness meditation in session and at home from 45 min to 15–20 min, and increased attention to distress from trauma memories during in-session and at-home exercises. Throughout the group, we invited patient discussion of PTSD symptoms at specific times during the sessions, and in exercises like the "Unpleasant Event Calendar." We specifically invited patients to use a formal mindfulness exercise (the "3-Minute Breathing Space") as well as informal mindfulness practice when experiencing distressing situations that activated PTSD symptoms during the week. This was used as way to bring themselves more fully into the situation rather than to avoid it, and encourage them to respond in a manner reflecting as much balance as they could.

Establish Safety

Working to establish and communicate the physical safety of the space, and the emotional safety of what will go on in the group is an important early step, i.e., establishing a sense of literal and figurative "safety" in the room where the sessions occur, and within the in-session and at home exercises. In particular for exercises when members engaged in activities not "standard" for many group therapies, such as lying down, doing stretching exercises, or sitting silently, we let members know that the door to the room would be locked after the group begins, and members arriving late were invited to knock softly. As in other group treatments for PTSD, we endeavor to enhance feelings of emotional safety by sharing specific group guidelines on confidentiality, speaking in turn, etc. Many veterans were not interested in hearing other group members' "war stories," which they feared could elicit responses of distress, horror, and/or anger. Since the version of MBCT we utilized specifically did not include trauma processing, we reminded members that in this group we would not be discussing explicit memories of traumatic events, and invited them to keep the focus of group discussion on the present. As is standard in MBCT, in-session discussion was led be facilitators and focused first on the exercise just completed, then on members experiences doing the mindfulness exercises during the week. Only after these fundamental practices was there focus on other experiences of the week as these often include times when distress and PTSD symptoms arose for them. We asked members to share and discuss these experiences, but gently invited them to reframe these discussions into what was their sensory experience in their body, leading them to focus on what they noticed, etc., in the spirit of mindfulness-based work. If members had particularly difficult memories, nightmares, or trauma anniversaries, they were invited again to share their reactions to these memories, but gently advised that it was not necessary to share the specific content and narrative of the memories with the group, that this was not the focus of this group, but if they wished they could discuss with a group facilitator after the group.

Use Invitational Language and Egalitarian Stance

A common aspect of mindfulness-based work is the facilitator's effort to use "invitational" language when describing particular mindfulness exercises, and when asking members to engage in the exercise. We feel this is particularly important when working with traumatized people. All exercises were technically "optional," in that members were asked to use their gut and best judgment (or "intrinsic wisdom," as beautifully put by Kimbrough et al. [107]) in whether they would accept our invitation to do a particular exercise. We felt that the egalitarian stance and appropriate self-disclosure by the group facilitators is particularly useful with this population. Therapists engaged in all the exercises (including discussion of the Unpleasant Event calendar, etc.) and sincerely shared their experiences with the mindfulness exercises in session and with their practice throughout the week. Therapists presented themselves as concerned people who had experience in mindfulness and in helping people struggling with symptoms of PTSD, rather than experts who were going to "fix" them, or "teach them" about their PTSD symptoms. Therapist also present themselves as people who experience real-life hassles and fears, etc. in their own lives, who work daily with formal mindfulness practices, and who try to engage principles of mindfulness themselves when confronted with real-life challenging experiences. Therapists also acknowledged differences in first-hand knowledge and personal experiences between themselves and group members, and expressed their respect both for group member's

knowledge and experience, and their intrinsic wisdom that in many cases, probably helped them survive highly dangerous situations. It was our feeling that such a nonhierarchical, sincere, and egalitarian approach was greatly appreciated by many veteran group members, and helped with engagement and group cohesion. We also acknowledged that some of the exercises might even seem at times "a little odd" but asked members to give us the benefit of the doubt, and if they were "OK with this," even if it did push the limits of their comfort a bit.

Consider Shorter Mindfulness Exercises

Initially we did 20 min of in-session exercises, and recommended group members practice 20 min exercises at home 5 days a week, along with prepared audio materials of mindfulness of breath, body scans, and mindful movement tracks that had both 20 and 40 min versions. We also shortened the length of the mindfulness meditation in session and at home from 45 min to 15–20 min. We believe it is very important not to overwhelm the group members or ask them to strive for unrealistic goals that they would have trouble attaining. It should be noted that Carmody and Baer also find in MBSR, while the amount of time spent on mindfulness exercises is related to increase in mindfulness measures, most people do not report 45 min daily of sitting meditation practice at home, but rather report the average as closer to 15–20 min a session at home [108].

Be Prepared for Upsetting Reactions to Sitting Quietly

It is important for PTSD therapists engaged in MBCT to be prepared for upsetting reactions, intrusive trauma memories, and/or flashbacks that could occur in any therapy, including the sitting mindfulness practice, and in particular, the lying body scan. It has been a common concern among PTSD therapists who have not done mindfulness work with their patients that paradoxical "relaxation-induced anxiety" or the lessening of the experiential avoidance that occurs with mindfulness practice may trigger such reactions or flashbacks in group sessions or at home, and this will increase patient distress. This did not occur as often as we initially expected (in fact, only a small handful of times in the hundreds of hours of mindfulness group sessions we have engaged in with veterans). In each case, these reactions were able to be processed in the group discussion using standard cognitive therapy skills to address, normalize, and reframe these in a therapeutic manner, itself a form of de-catastophization. Recognition and normalization of the fact that it is possible that trauma memories or other forms of avoided cognitions or internal experiences may in fact arise during the mindfulness exercises can be a form of motivation and openness for "exposure."

Use Particular Care with the Body Scan

We did however, have two strong patient reactions to the body scan in the first two MBCT groups we ran. In both cases, the veterans complied with the invitation to lie down and did not express any distress until the end of the session, and then shared that they had felt overwhelmed and distressed, and this contributed to their later dropping out of the group. Therefore, we have taken additional care to express that lying down (and closing their eyes) during the body scan is optional, and that members can also do this sitting in session (we invited them to try this at home in a safe place lying down). We also gently checked in with group members during the scan, reminding them that if they were experiencing strong feelings or distress, to please use their own best judgment and open their eyes, move to a sitting posture, or whatever they felt was appropriate at that moment. It is interesting that many veterans expressed a great appreciation for the body scan, and in particular many would use the body scan (with or without the guided audio) when they were having difficulty sleeping and lying awake in bed. They reported it was very

helpful for "clearing their head" of intrusive worries and ruminations, and was helpful for getting to sleep. Although the body scan is intended as a mindfulness exercise (to "fall awake" in the words of Jon Kabatt-Zinn) we felt it was important to validate the experiences the veterans had, and to be pragmatic with any use of the exercises to be helpful in the veteran's lives (with the exception as discussed below of using breathing or body awareness as an explicit avoidant strategy)

Consider Using the "R-Word" ("Relaxation")

As is common in mindfulness-based interventions, we explained that mindfulness involved experiencing mental phenomenon, whether they are sensations, emotions, or cognitions, as they occur and as they are, always attending to the present moment, and adopting a nonjudgmental, open, even "curious" attitude. We discussed the difference between mindfulness and "relaxation," and that the objective of mindfulness was not necessarily to attempt to produce a "peaceful" or "relaxed" state that is different than what might be encountered in the present moment, but rather to engage with whatever is occurring. We recognize, and the group members commented on, the fact that engaging in mindfulness sometimes results in a more relaxed and supple state of mind. We felt it was helpful to patients to acknowledge that relaxation could provide a respite from being continually "amped up" especially as PTSD is associated with hypervigilance and heightened sympathetic nervous system drive. We did encourage patients to acknowledge and benefit from "relaxation" they gained from their mindfulness practice done on a regular/daily basis, and if they liked, to approach the mindfulness work as also being "relaxation" and "time for themselves." However, we also encouraged members not to use formal or informal mindfulness or breathing practice a way to distract themselves from the feelings they may experience and toward something else, or as an avoidant technique when distress or trauma memories occurred, but rather as an opportunity to take note of the nature of distressing images and feelings in as balanced a manner as one is capable of at the moment. We feel the "attitude" of the MBCT is overall quite consistent with that of exposure based therapies. Patients are consistently invited and encouraged to move toward experiences rather than to distract or avoid distressing, upsetting thoughts and feeling. If patients can also experience a benefit from relaxation that occurs during their practice, this is to be appreciated.

Psychoeducation About PTSD Symptoms, Stress Physiology, and Mindfulness Practice

There is somewhat of an ethos in the practical application of MBSR and MBCT to emphasize experience over narrative, "being" over "doing," and the first sessions of MBCT tend to focus on the actual experience of eating a raisin and encountering your body, as opposed to didactic presentations and psychoeducation. One of the appeals of mindfulness and its potential mechanisms of action is getting people "out of their heads," i.e., with discursive thought and didactic forms of activity, and "into their bodies" (or lives etc.) with more experiential, "being" forms of activity. In the interest of establishing greater feelings of safety and a positive expectancy that this therapy may be "OK for them," we considered moving some basic psychoeducation about PTSD symptoms, and common effects on patients and their families, as well as stress physiology to the first sessions of the group. We recognize that, the level of psychoeducation and "symptom normalization" will vary with the amount of previous treatment the PTSD patients in the group have already completed. In the initial MBCT groups we included in our pilot research protocol, most of the group members had extensive previous trauma focused treatment. We limited any modification to adapt MBCT to PTSD treatment, and kept the "psychoeducation" in session 4, and simply replaced information about depression symp-

toms from the "Territory of Depression" with PTSD symptoms. In subsequent group work in our clinic, a substantial number of veterans had not engaged in much previous treatment, and we added sessions to work with PTSD psychoeducation before introducing the Raisin exercise and the rest of the MBCT protocol). Note that Polusny et al. [109] took a similar approach to introduce psychoeducation in the first session.

Informal Mindfulness and the Three Minute Breathing Space with PTSD Symptoms

Both informal mindfulness and the 3-min Breathing Space are integral parts of the MBCT protocol for depression relapse prevention, and represent how patients can make use of and apply the skills they practice. They also cultivate informal exercises for changing and improving the way they respond to upsetting symptoms and engage in their lives; moving their mindfulness practice from "the cushion" and into "the real world" of the rest of their life. We focused on "translating" the experiences and attitudes the group members during the formal sitting mindfulness exercises into other times in their lives, and inviting them to "play with" having a more open, curious stance about things in their lives (e.g., in the "Pleasant Experiences Calendar" identifying pleasant moments even in the context of the pain and stress of PTSD). In MBCT for depression relapse prevention, the 3 min Breathing Space is trained first at several planned times during the day, and then also brought to bear when distressing, self-critical, or depressogenic cognitions arise. In the PTSD adaptation, we follow the general scheme of beginning use of the 3-min exercise during predetermined "neutral" times in the day, and then to also use it when experiencing trauma memories or other distressing symptoms. If this is too difficult, members are invited to try to engage in the 3-min Breathing after the experience of symptoms has begun to somewhat subside. In the case of PTSD, this can mean that in time and with effort, to be able to bring your sense of mindful enquiry, metacognition, openness to experience, and nonjudgmental quality even to the experience of PTSD experiences like intrusive fearful or horrific memories, feelings of fear or danger in the environment, feelings of shame and self-blame. The practice of mindfulness also provides a concrete example and way to see that any mental phenomenon has a beginning, a middle, and an end, and that whatever the particular thought or feeling is, it (usually) does not last forever, even if it feels like it will last forever when one is experiencing it. This attitude lends itself to an informal, in vivo "experiential exposure," and one's intrusive symptoms experiences can try to be seen as a phenomena. Group members are encouraged to use the 3-min BS and/or "informal mindfulness" as a way to encounter these frequent but highly unpleasant and often frightening experiences in a way that tries to see them in the present moment, as well as considering the current *context*. Patients are encouraged to use their awareness of sensation to orient themselves to their current context. In this way they can notice—*Where am I now? What is the social context? What is actually happening this moment?* They are encouraged to try, even when painful, to be a little "curious" about these intrusive memories and distress, notice what they can of the experience, rather than immediately try to do anything they can to distract and get themselves out of it. We believe that it is also important to communicate the standard message of exposure therapy, which is that memories and the feelings they arouse can be distressing, although in and of themselves they are not necessarily dangerous. This is of course much easier for the therapist to say than for a person with PTSD to necessarily do, but this message bears gently sharing (and repeating) throughout the group.

Evidence for MBCT for PTSD

There have been several meta-analyses of effects of mindfulness-based interventions on symptoms and problems often accompanying PTSD, which have documented medium effect sizes for mindfulness-based interventions for symptoms such as depression, chronic pain, and anxiety [41,

110–113]. There have also been are a large number of studies of MBSR in life-threatening diseases such as terminal cancer, meta-analyses again show medium to large effects sizes for relieving anxiety and depression and general improvement of psychological health [114, 115]. While cancer is clearly associated with life-threat, only a few studies of cancer have included specific measures of PTSD; one RCT of mainly female cancer patients found MBSR was acceptable to cancer patients and relatively high completion rate (>80 %), and was associated with a small to moderate (Cohen's $d=0.41$) decrease in PTSD avoidant symptoms [116]. A recent empirical review of "mind-body" interventions [117], report several studies of effects of yoga, yoga breathing (pranayama), and mantra meditation, as well as well as interventions that include techniques that share elements in common with mindfulness meditation to have effects to improve PTSD. Some of the earliest reports of "mind-body" group interventions with traumatized persons were with "Mind-Body Skills Groups," developed by James Gordon, which includes multiple components (biofeedback, drawings, autogenic training, guided imagery, breathing techniques, etc.) as well as a form of mindfulness meditation. A study of this intervention with adolescent survivors of war-related trauma in Kosovo was associated with decreased PTSD symptoms [118, 119] and in subsequent groups with traumatized adolescents in Gaza was also reported to be helpful.

Studies of MBCT and MBSR with Civilian Trauma and PTSD

Although as yet there have been only a handful of controlled studies, there is accumulating evidence that interventions that include explicit mindfulness meditation (MBSR and MBCT) appear to be acceptable to persons with trauma exposure and PTSD, and also lead to clinically meaningful improvement in PTSD symptoms. There is also a recent empirical review of mindfulness-based approaches for PTSD [120] but to our knowledge no meta-analyses have been completed as of yet. However, to date, only a few studies have included an active intervention comparison control group, and more studies have been done with using MBSR than MBCT. Several pilot studies have examined MBSR groups with persons (mainly women) with civilian trauma, some of whom had PTSD. The first report we are aware of with MBSR adapted for traumatized persons was with adult survivors of childhood sexual abuse [107], and was a well-conducted, uncontrolled pilot study with a pre-post design, and a 4 month follow-up. Since this was a pilot study with an unproven intervention for a high risk group, all of the participants were required to be enrolled in concurrent individual psychotherapy. A total of 27 people (24 women) were enrolled in three groups of MBSR (ranging in size from 7 to 11 group members); 15 of the 27 members met current criteria for PTSD (based upon self-report PCL-C) at intake. The standard MBSR format (8 weekly 2.5–3 h sessions, and one 5-h "retreat") was followed, but the authors reported some modifications to the way the group was taught (rather than the specific content of the MBSR sessions) that were influenced by MBCT and positive psychology: sensitive attention to language used to direct group activities, encouraging members to "titrate" their mindfulness experiences with present-moment experiences (e.g., emotional distress), and efforts to build on strengths, express gratitude, encouraging connections among group members and cultivation of self-compassion. The groups appeared to be well tolerated (85 % completion rate), and were associated with statistically significant reductions in symptoms of PTSD (PCL-C) and depression (BDI), and increases in mindfulness (MAAS)—the effects sizes were large for all of these effects (Cohen's $d > 1.0$). A subsequent study reported on a two and a half year follow-up with these participants, and found that the majority of the clinical gains were retained, and the participants rated their experiences with MBSR favorably [122], indicating significant long-term improvements in depression, PTSD, anxiety symptoms, and mindfulness scores (effect sizes (Cohen's d) ranged from 0.5 to 1.0).

Another uncontrolled pilot study conducted at about the same time [122] used MBSR groups for women with physical and psychological interpersonal abuse, and also found large decreases in total PTSD symptoms (also measured by self-report PCL-C) including improvements in all three symptoms clusters. Again the effect size was large (total PTSD symptoms $d = 1.54$, with effect sizes for clusters ranging from 0.77 to 1.28). Although this study was unpublished (a doctoral dissertation) the methods and measures appear of good quality. Another smaller uncontrolled pilot study of MBSR ($N = 10$) with persons with mixed forms of trauma exposure [123]. In this study of ten people, nine were female, six met current PTSD diagnosis, and seven had a history of childhood maltreatment. They also found large effect sizes for reduction in PTSD symptoms (as measured by PCL), depression (BDI), and self-blame/shame based cognitions, but also reported that two participants had a transient increase in PTSD symptoms. A recent small pilot study of a "mindfulness-based exercise" ("MBX") intervention in nurses was a randomized controlled trial (RCT) of MBX ($N = 11$) compared to a waitlist control ($N = 11$). This study also reported high completion rate (96 %) and large pre-post effect sizes in improvement in PTSD symptoms, which were also significant compared to the waitlist control group (between group $d = 1.42$) [124]. Another interesting pilot study utilized a telephone-delivered mindfulness intervention with $N = 11$ survivors of critical illnesses recruited in the intensive care unit (ICU) and provided as post-discharge follow-up [125]. The 6-week telephone intervention was developed by the authors based upon focus groups with ICU survivors and literature review, and included several common elements with MBSR/MBCT (breath mindfulness, body scan, mindful eating and movement) and loving-kindness meditation. Although the improvement in PTSD symptoms (self report PTSS) was not significant, the majority of patients showed a decrease in symptoms.

Studies of MBCT, MBSR, and Related Interventions with Military Veterans with Combat-Related PTSD Delivered by VA Mental Health Workers

We are aware of a number of major Veterans Administration (VA) health systems across the country that have been offering mindfulness-based approaches, including MBCT and MBSR, for a number of physical and mental health conditions, including combat PTSD. Some of these clinics have been using these modalities clinically for several years, as well as performing clinical trials and other research. The results of a small number of these studies have now been published, but it is also important to note that it appears there are many VA clinical centers using MBCT and/or MBSR with unpublished findings at the time of this book. One of the earliest studies published with a mindfulness-based intervention delivered to veterans with combat-related PTSD was with a telephone-delivered adaptation of MBSR at the Boston VA by Barbara Niles and colleagues, that included two 45 min face-to-face sessions and six 20-min weekly telephone session [126]. Of the PTSD patients in this study, 64% served in Vietnam, 30% in OEF or OIF, and 6% in other deployments. Patients were allowed to have concurrent psychiatric and psychotherapy care at the VA or elsewhere. Thirty-three male combat veterans were randomly assigned to the tele-MBSR or to a comparison telehealth psychoeducation treatment. Veterans in the MBSR-telemedicine adaptation reported high levels of satisfaction and high levels of engagement and at-home mindfulness practice. They also showed a significant decrease in PTSD symptoms and score on the Clinician Administered PTSD Scale (CAPS), considered the "gold-standard" PTSD assessment, with pre-post mindfulness Cohen's $d = 0.70$, and a between-groups $d = 1.25$ at the "post" assessment. However, the improvement in PTSD symptoms was not sustained at the 6-week post intervention follow-up. The authors concluded that while the brief MBSR telemedicine treatment was feasible and showed good patient engagement, it may not be of adequate intensity to sustain effects on PTSD symptoms in combat veterans.

David Kearney, Tracy Simpson, and colleagues at the VA Puget Sound Health Care System near Seattle have for several years offered MBSR classes for to veterans suffering from a range of mental health and somatic problems, including veterans with combat PTSD. They have recently published well-conducted pilot studies measuring PTSD symptoms with a "standard" MBSR group intervention (eight weekly 2–3 h sessions and a daylong "retreat," with 20–25 group members), both single group and an RCT comparing added MBSR to treatment as usual (TAU) [127, 128], as well as pilot studies of a loving-kindness meditation group intervention they have developed for PTSD [100, 129]. In an initial naturalistic longitudinal study of MBSR [127], they followed 92 veterans (70 male and 22 female) who participated in a hospital-wide "standard" MBSR class for 6 months and measured PTSD (PCL-C) and depression symptoms (PHQ-9), as well as mindfulness (FFMQ) and other self-report. Group members were referred by a VA provider for any somatic or mental health issue, or self-referred; no psychiatric assessments were conducted in the study, but 32 had PTSD and 54 had depression codes listed at some point in their electronic medical record. At the 6-month follow-up they found significant improvements in PTSD symptoms ($d = 0.64$), depression ($d = 0.70$), and other self-report measures. Furthermore, about half of the veterans had clinically significant improvements in PTSD symptoms. In a subsequent RCT of "standard" MBSR [128], combat veterans with PTSD were randomized to one of two conditions: either taking a "standard" MBSR class at the VA (including eight weekly sessions and a daylong "retreat"), or continuing "treatment as usual" (TAU). PTSD patients in each condition did not differ in psychiatric medications or concurrent psychotherapy during the study. Each MBSR group was conducted at the VA and contained about 20–30 male and female veterans, about 5–10 of whom were PTSD patients participating in the study, and the rest were veterans without PTSD who were referred to MBSR for various clinical indications. MBSR was associated with a significant, moderate within group (pre-post) effect in improvement in self-report measures of PTSD (PCL-C, $d = 0.63$) and depression ($d=0.65$); however, the improvement in PTSD symptoms was only about seven points on PCL-C, and between-groups effects were not statistically different than TAU. Nonetheless, this was a highly important study demonstrating the feasibility and acceptability of standard MBSR (with groups of 20–25 members) with patients with history of PTSD, and improvement in PTSD symptoms. There findings provide evidence that "standard" MBSR classes with 20–25 patients that are not focused on PTSD may be an acceptable and useful adjunctive treatment for PTSD patients.

An uncontrolled pilot group of MBSR with eight combat veterans (seven male Vietnam veterans and one female OIF veteran) recruited from the Veterans Administration Hospital in Madison, Wisconsin [130] also reported improvement in PTSD immediately following the group and at a 4 week post-intervention follow-up as measured by CAPS (average 9-point drop at post, and 15-point drop at follow-up). All the group members completed the group, and half of the group (4 of 8) had a "clinically meaningful" improvement in PTSD symptoms (previously defined as a 10 point or greater drop in CAPS [131]). The decreases in CAPS scores ranged from 0 to 32 points. This pilot also measured heart rate variability using 24 h Holter at home measurement, and reported that parasympathetic tone increased in all five of the veterans they measured. Although small and uncontrolled, this pilot used the "gold-standard" CAPS assessment, and suggested that small mindfulness groups are acceptable to PTSD patients, and may be associated with larger effects than larger groups.

In studies we have conducted at the VA Ann Arbor Health System, we investigated specifically adapting of MBCT for PTSD, and running small groups (5–8 members) of PTSD patients [132]. As described in the section above, we targeted didactic content and discussion to PTSD symptoms as well as mindfulness, and encouraged patients to use their mindfulness skills to encounter their patterns of responses to their PTSD symptoms. In our pilot study, we examined the effects of MBCT for PTSD with 37 combat veterans with chronic PTSD; the majority ($N=29$ or 78%) were Vietnam veterans, and

also some older (Korean war) and younger (Desert Storm) veterans. We compared 20 veterans with chronic PTSD who participated in a MBCT for PTSD group (four groups with 4–6 members each), with 17 veterans with chronic PTSD who engaged in other brief (6–8 weeks) active psychotherapy groups offered in our clinic during the same time period (psychoeducation (two groups with 5-6 members each) or imagery rehearsal therapy (IRT) for PTSD nightmare reduction (one group of 5 veterans)). The patients were all male, mean age was about 60 years old, and the time from trauma (~35 years), the portion with service connection for disability (~60%), alcohol dependence in sustained remission (~60%), currently taking psychiatric medications (~65%) and number of years in previous psychiatric treatment (~4 years) were not different between the groups. The veterans with chronic PTSD who completed the MBCT group showed a clinically meaningful improvement in PTSD symptoms and a 16 point drop in CAPS (effect size Hedge's g (corrected for small sample size) was $g=0.67$ in completer and $g=0.55$ intent to treat [ITT] analyses) from pre- to post-treatment. In contrast, the veterans in the TAU groups did not show any improvement in PTSD symptoms. The between group analyses showed significantly better response in the MBCT group; RM-ANOVA group x time interaction was significant ($p=0.001$), and the between group effects sizes comparing MBCT to the other brief groups were 1.0 in completer and 0.77 in ITT analyses, both significant. Furthermore, 73% of patients in MBCT showed clinically meaningful improvement, compared to 33% in TAU groups. These results suggested that the MBCT group therapy targeted for combat-related PTSD is acceptable and a potentially effective novel therapeutic approach for PTSD symptoms and trauma-related negative cognitions. The majority of veterans enrolled in the mindfulness group showed good engagement in the "in session" exercises, and were also compliant with daily mindfulness practice, in fact several reported an unexpectedly high level of engagement and compliance with home mindfulness practice.

There was a 25 % dropout rate of veterans discontinuing MBCT (all within the first 3 weeks), a dropout rate that was not different from the TAU groups and appears t with typical dropout rates in outpatient treatment studies of PTSD. However, it is important to note that two patients who dropped reported increased anxiety during the mindfulness exercises as a factor contributing to dropping the group. This suggests that great attention should be paid to "body-focused" exercises such as the body scan, as we discuss below.

We felt these findings are particularly noteworthy in light of the short duration of MBCT, and the chronicity of PTSD symptoms reported by our veterans (15–50 years). Interestingly, the mindfulness group appeared to reduce mainly the avoidant cluster symptoms, on CAPS, suggesting potential specificity of action here, which is consistent with the emphasis on reduced avoidance of unwanted emotions and experiences in mindfulness training. Given that one might expect avoidance symptoms to change first, a longer intervention or follow-up assessments may show greater impact on intrusive and hyperarousal symptoms, although such speculation requires further study. Additionally, consonant with an emphasis on mindful attention to positive experiences and nonjudgmental acceptance, the intervention led to a significant decrease in cognitions of self-blame and a trend toward decreased perception of the world as a dangerous place. We noted that future RCT studies with larger samples will be needed to determine whether mindfulness-based interventions also significantly reduce PTSD symptoms beyond the avoidance cluster. Additionally, the lack of follow-up assessment in this study limited our ability to determine additional symptom changes subsequent to treatment. Given the long-term protection from depression relapse afforded by MBCT, future studies of this type of intervention should assess PTSD outcomes at later follow-ups.

The largest study of MBCT or MBSR for PTSD to date in any patient population was done with military veterans at VA Minneapolis, an RCT of $N = 116$ veterans [109] randomized to either MBSR or a 9-week group version of PCT (PCGT). The MBSR groups were offered to veterans of any era, and the overall sample was primarily Vietnam veterans (74 %), along with 15 % Gulf War (Desert Storm) veterans, and 10 % who served in the recent conflicts in Afghanistan (known as Operation Enduring Freedom, OEF) and/or Iraq (known as Operation Iraqi Freedom, OIF). The study was well-randomized on most demographics, and veterans assigned to MBSR or PCGT did not differ in age, deployment, comorbid depression, psychiatric medications, forms of trauma, etc. The groups appeared to have a nonsignificant difference in PTSD severity at intake (mean CAPS score was 69.9 (15.5) in the MBSR vs 62.5 (16.9) in the PCGT sample). The MBSR intervention was adapted for PTSD; the first session included psychoeducation about PTSD and an orientation to the group, followed by seven more 2.5–3 h classes in which the usual MBSR protocol of body scan, raisin exercise, and sitting meditation were performed. The average group size was 6.4 veterans, ranging from 4 to 11 group members. Thus, the size of the groups were similar to that of MBCT, rather than the large group sizes (up to 25 members) frequently utilized in "stress-reduction" focused MBSR. Furthermore, the groups were composed of all combat PTSD patients, contained PTSD psychoeducation, and thus appeared to be focused to PTSD, similar to previously reported MBCT adaptations for depression, GAD, and PTSD. The study found that both MBSR and PCGT led to improvements in PTSD, as measured by PCL-C (which the authors considered the primary outcome) and CAPS (considered a secondary outcome), but found significant group × time interactions in reductions in PCL-C scores at post-treatment and 2 month follow-up, and in CAPS scores at 2 month follow-up but not at post-treatment, MBSR reduced CAPS scores from ~70 at intake, to ~56 at post, to ~50 at 2 month follow-up, compared to PCGT CAPS scores of ~63 intake, ~52 at post and ~51 at 2 month follow-up. This ~20 point improvement in CAPS score by MBSR is considered clinically significant, and appear to represent a similar or somewhat greater improvement in PTSD than found in the previous studies of MBCT and small group MBSR for combat PTSD [130, 132]. This study also found significant difference in increased mindfulness skills (FFMQ) and quality of life (WHOQOL) at the 2 month follow-up, but the improvements in depression (PHQ-9) were not different. They also did not find a difference in the number of patients obtaining a pre- to post-treatment clinically significant improvement in PCL-C, CAPS, or depression (PHQ-9), but did find a significantly greater portion of patients in MBSR (49 %) vs PCGT (28 %) showed a clinically significant response to treatment at the 2 month follow-up. However, this paper did not report the number/proportion of PTSD patients achieving remission of PTSD (i.e., no longer meeting diagnostic criteria for PTSD) at the post-treatment of 2 month follow-up.

Taken together, these early results with large group MBSR with mixed diagnosis members that is not focused on PTSD appears to be acceptable to veterans with PTSD, and may be associated with benefits to some, but the overall effect was not significant. Early results with MBCT adapted for PTSD, and with smaller group (4–11 patients) MBSR with all PTSD patients and focused on PTSD appear to have statistically significant improvement in PTSD symptoms (on average, 15–20 point reduction in CAPS), and approximately 50–70 % of PTSD patients had clinically meaningful improvement. However, while clinically significant, these reductions in CAPS from mindfulness group interventions do not appear to be as large as those for trauma-focused individual interventions (often averaging 30 point to even 50 point reductions in CAPS) or for recent reports of non-trauma focused effective interventions, e.g., IPT.

As we have discussed, it is possible that 8-week group MBCT by itself, even if focused on PTSD, while it may be very helpful and importantly, actively liked and engaged in by veterans with PTSD, simply may not be a sufficient therapeutic dose for most combat veterans with PTSD. As discussed, using MBCT as a preparation for more rigorous trauma-focused

therapies that clearly have large effect sizes but are declined by many, or as an adjunctive treatment for individual therapy may be an effective way that the benefits of MBCT may be utilized. It may also be possible to find ways to "combine" MBCT (or parts of the curriculum of MBCT) with other effective PTSD therapies, whether they are trauma-exposure focused, in vivo exposure focused, cognitive-behavioral emotion regulation skills focused, or personal relationship focused. We have been actively working with two of these possibilities. We developed a novel multi-modal group intervention for returning OEF/OIF veterans with PTSD which combines MBCT with PTSD psychoeducation and personal relationship skills, relaxation and chi-kung, self-compassion exercises, loving kindness, and "in vivo exposure" (i.e., exposure to avoided situations or activities), but no trauma exposure. We conducted an RCT of this 16-week intervention (which we call "Mindfulness-based Exposure Therapy") with OEF/OIF veterans who had declined trauma-focused treatment (PE). The mindfulness intervention appeared acceptable to OEF/OIF veteran with PTSD; veterans appeared highly engaged and reported they liked the mindfulness and loving-kindness exercises and also showed greater retention in the MBET than an active control group therapy. We have also been testing using mindfulness in a novel treatment package for complex and often treatment-refractory cases of combat PTSD with co-morbid persistent depressive disorder, which includes CBT for insomnia, CBASP, and trauma processing. Some of these complex patients do not respond, and most show residual PTSD symptoms. A group intervention based on MBCT was conducted as a relapse prevention component for veterans who had completed the treatment. The mindfulness group has shown some improvement in both nonresponders and in those with residual symptoms. Thus, we are encouraged and are engaging in further study of mindfulness and self-compassion interventions as a treatment extender for more complex polysymptomatic presentations, and as a relapse prevention method.

Practical Considerations of MBCT for PTSD, Including Patient Selection, Home Practice, Group Size, Format, Facilitator Training

PTSD can be associated with severe emotional and psychological symptoms, including severe distress and fear, anxiety, and anger. It can be also associated with substance abuse, depression, and suicidality, which lead to both considerable safety concerns, as well as challenges for conducting a group intervention. While we were interested in making the mindfulness groups available to as many veterans with PTSD as possible, and while mindfulness-based approaches have shown some acceptability in patients with psychotic disorders, suicidality, and substance-use disorders, in our studies exclusion criteria were current psychotic disorder, current suicidality, current expression of borderline or antisocial personality traits that would interfere with a group intervention, and current substance dependence or abuse that is not in treatment and/or that would cause a safety concern. We used these as exclusion because they would either have the potential to interfere with the group modality, could potentially be exacerbated by the interventions, and/or would require greater safety monitoring that could better be provided in an individual modality. We note that similar exclusion criteria were used by Kearney et al. [127].

We feel the group sizes common in MBCT (5–8 members) with two co-therapists is important for the group cohesion, feelings of safety, and for the ability to share and discuss PTSD symptoms, which patients often find difficult to talk about and often are accompanied with guilt, shame, and other strong emotions. We also feel having groups of all PTSD patients, and having the content and discussion of the discussion focusing on PTSD symptoms is very helpful for effectively working with PTSD symptoms, Although we have discussed evidence that larger (ca. 20–25 member) "standard" MBSR groups not focused on PTSD, with veterans with "mixed" diagnostic status are both acceptable to patients with PTSD and potentially lead to clinically meaningful improvements in PTSD and depression symptoms [127–129], we note that larger improvements in PTSD symptoms

have been reported with smaller group sizes using MBCT [132] and MBSR [109] specifically adapted for combat PTSD.

Another practical consideration regards the clinical training required for treating patients with PTSD, who often have specific needs, challenges, and safety concerns, and for whom having specific expertise and experience in PTSD treatment is important. Of course, in addition to this, while MBCT and MBSR techniques are becoming widely disseminated, they also require fairly specialized training and other considerable commitments beyond the initial training, including the commitment of a personal mindfulness practice and attendance in annual weeklong silent meditation retreats, etc. These are qualifications not usually required of VA psychologists, and may not be practical to expect. In our work, we took the approach to use two co-therapists in each group, a common practice in VA group therapies, at least one of whom had specific training and expertise in MBCT, and at least one of whom was a VA PTSD-trained psychologist. This model has the potential to take advantage of community resources of highly trained MBCT therapists, who could be "cross-trained" in working with PTSD patients in coordination with a VA PTSD therapist, and allow PTSD therapists who do not yet have training in mindfulness-based modalities to deepen their experience in preparation for more formal training in MBCT.

Summary/Conclusions

Several initial studies now report that mindfulness-based approaches including MBSR and MBCT are acceptable for trauma-exposed people and people suffering from PTSD, including military veteran with combat-related PTSD. Standard 8-week MBSR, with relatively large groups of 20–25 veterans, and not specifically focused on PTSD symptoms appear to be acceptable to PTSD patients and may be helpful for some veterans, but to date have not shown a clinically significant effect size. This suggests that standard MBSR may be a highly useful and convenient adjunctive or alternative treatment for combat veterans to improve emotional reactivity, especially those who are not appropriate for or refuse more intensive, trauma-focused treatments. While it is recommended that PTSD patients remain under psychiatric care of a PTSD clinic while taking the group, the MBSR teacher may not need to have specific competency in PTSD therapy.

Similarly, three recent studies of brief 8-week MBCT, and small group MBSR focused specifically on combat PTSD intervention appeared acceptable to veterans in a VA PTSD clinic, who demonstrated high levels of engagement, and were associated with a statistically significant improvement in PTSD symptoms. Here the average improvement in PTSD symptoms was in the clinically meaningful range (15–20 point reduction in CAPS), with 50–70 % of PTSD patient in the studies reported to date having clinically meaning improvement. However, one of the studies was an uncontrolled pilot. Thus, while the recent large RCT of small-group PTSD-focused MBSR has shown encouraging results, as yet more evidence is needed.

Furthermore, while the improvements in PTSD are "clinically meaningful" the actual reduction in PTSD symptoms from the mindfulness groups appears considerably smaller than that shown in individual trauma-focused therapy, and the portion of PTSD patients who lose their diagnosis following treatment has not been reported. The 8-week MBCT adapted for PTSD, while clearly liked and engaged in by veterans PTSD, may not be a sufficient therapeutic dose for severe combat PTSD, and thus at present appears MBCT is best thought of as a adjunctive therapy and/or a treatment extender, that may be able to be combined with effective trauma-focused on non-trauma focused interventions to improve emotional regulation and distress tolerance in this population, and thus improve treatment outcomes.

References

1. Kessler, RC, Berglund, P, Demler, O, Jin, R, Merikangas, KR, Walters, EE. Lifetime Prevalence and Age-of-Onset Distributions of DSM-IV Disorders in the National Comorbidity Survey Replication; Arch Gen Psychiatry. 2005; 62(6): 593–602. doi:10.1001/archpsyc.62.6.593.

2. Cabrera OA, Hoge CW, Bliese PD, Castro CA, Messer SC. Childhood adversity and combat as predictors of depression and post-traumatic stress in deployed troops. Am J Prev Med. 2007;33(2):77–82. doi:10.1016/j.amepre.2007.03.019.

3. Hoge CW, Castro CA, Messer SC, McGurk D, Cotting DI, Koffman RL. Combat duty in Iraq and Afghanistan, mental health problems, and barriers to care. N Engl J Med. 2004;351(1):13–22.

4. Hoge CW, Riviere LA, Wilk JE, Herrell RK, Weathers FW. The prevalence of post-traumatic stress disorder (PTSD) in US combat soldiers: a head-to-head comparison of DSM-5 versus DSM-IV-TR symptom criteria with the PTSD checklist. Lancet Psychiatry. 2014;1(4):269–77. doi:10.1016/S2215-0366(14)70235-4.

5. Kang HK, Natelson BH, Mahan CM, Lee KY, Murphy FM. Post-traumatic stress disorder and chronic fatigue syndrome-like illness among Gulf War veterans: a population-based survey of 30,000 veterans. Am J Epidemiol. 2003;157(2):141–8.

6. Kulka RA, Schlenger WE, Fairbanks JA, Hough RL, Jordan BK, Marmar CR, et al. Trauma and the Vietnam War generation: report of findings from the National Vietnam veterans readjustment study. New York, NY: Brunner Mazel; 1990.

7. Greenberg PE, Kessler RC, Birnbaum HG, Leong SA, Lowe SW, Berglund PA, et al. The economic burden of depression in the United States: how did it change between 1990 and 2000? J Clin Psychiatry. 2003;64(12):1465–75.

8. Kang HK, Mahan CM, Lee KY, Murphy FM, Simmens SJ, Young HA, et al. Evidence for a deployment-related Gulf War syndrome by factor analysis. Arch Environ Health. 2002;57(1):61–8.

9. Kessler RC, Sonnega A, Bromet E, Hughes M, Nelson CB. Posttraumatic stress disorder in the National Comorbidity Survey. Arch Gen Psychiatry. 1995;52(12):1048–60.

10. Boscarino JA. Posttraumatic stress disorder and mortality among U.S. Army veterans 30 years after military service. Ann Epidemiol. 2006;16(4):248–56. doi:10.1016/j.annepidem.2005.03.009.

11. Boscarino JA. A prospective study of PTSD and early-age heart disease mortality among Vietnam veterans: implications for surveillance and prevention. Psychosom Med. 2008;70(6):668–76. doi:10.1097/PSY.0b013e31817bccaf.

12. Boscarino JA. PTSD is a risk factor for cardiovascular disease: time for increased screening and clinical intervention. Prev Med. 2012;54(5):363–4. doi:10.1016/j.ypmed.2012.01.001. author reply 365.

13. Berger W, Mendlowicz MV, Marques-Portella C, Kinrys G, Fontenelle LF, Marmar CR, et al. Pharmacologic alternatives to antidepressants in post-traumatic stress disorder: a systematic review. Prog Neuropsychopharmacol Biol Psychiatry. 2009;33(2):169–80. doi:10.1016/j.pnpbp.2008.12.004.

14. Bradley R, Greene J, Russ E, Dutra L, Westen D. A multidimensional meta-analysis of psychotherapy for PTSD. Am J Psychiatry. 2005;162(2):214–27.

15. Steenkamp MM, Litz BT, Hoge CW, Marmar CR. Psychotherapy for military-related PTSD: a review of randomized clinical trials. JAMA. 2015;314(5):489–500. doi:10.1001/jama.2015.8370.

16. Medicine I o. Treatment of posttraumatic stress disorder: an assessment of the evidence. Washington, DC: National Academy of Sciences; 2007.

17. Steenkamp MM, Litz BT. One-size-fits-all approach to PTSD in the VA not supported by the evidence. Am Psychol. 2014;69(7):706–7. doi:10.1037/a0037360.

18. Chard KM, Ricksecker EG, Healy ET, Karlin BE, Resick PA. Dissemination and experience with cognitive processing therapy. J Rehabil Res Dev. 2012;49(5):667–78.

19. Eftekhari A, Crowley JJ, Ruzek JI, Garvert DW, Karlin BE, Rosen CS. Training in the implementation of prolonged exposure therapy: provider correlates of treatment outcome. J Trauma Stress. 2015;28(1):65–8. doi:10.1002/jts.21980.

20. Eftekhari A, Ruzek JI, Crowley JJ, Rosen CS, Greenbaum MA, Karlin BE. Effectiveness of national implementation of prolonged exposure therapy in Veterans Affairs care. JAMA Psychiatry. 2013;70(9):949–55. doi:10.1001/jamapsychiatry.2013.36.

21. Pomerantz AS, Kearney LK, Wray LO, Post EP, McCarthy JF. Mental health services in the medical home in the Department of Veterans Affairs: factors for successful integration. Psychol Serv. 2014; 11(3):243–53. doi:10.1037/a0036638.

22. Kehle-Forbes SM, Meis LA, Spoont MR, Polusny MA. Treatment initiation and dropout from prolonged exposure and cognitive processing therapy in a VA outpatient clinic. Psychol Trauma. 2016;8(1): 107–14. doi:10.1037/tra0000065.

23. Markowitz JC, Meehan KB, Petkova E, Zhao Y, Van Meter PE, Neria Y, et al. Treatment preferences of psychotherapy patients with chronic PTSD. J Clin Psychiatry. 2015. doi:10.4088/JCP.14m09640.

24. Forbes D, Lloyd D, Nixon RD, Elliott P, Varker T, Perry D, et al. A multisite randomized controlled effectiveness trial of cognitive processing therapy for military-related posttraumatic stress disorder. J Anxiety Disord. 2012;26(3):442–52. doi:10.1016/j.janxdis.2012.01.006.

25. Schnurr PP, Friedman MJ, Engel CC, Foa EB, Shea MT, Chow BK, et al. Cognitive behavioral therapy for posttraumatic stress disorder in women: a randomized controlled trial. JAMA. 2007;297(8):820–30. doi:10.1001/jama.297.8.820.

26. Suris A, Link-Malcolm J, Chard K, Ahn C, North C. A randomized clinical trial of cognitive processing therapy for veterans with PTSD related to military sexual trauma. J Trauma Stress. 2013;26(1): 28–37. doi:10.1002/jts.21765.

27. Jeffreys MD, Reinfeld C, Nair PV, Garcia HA, Mata-Galan E, Rentz TO. Evaluating treatment of posttraumatic stress disorder with cognitive processing therapy and prolonged exposure therapy in a VHA specialty clinic. J Anxiety Disord. 2014;28(1):108–14. doi:10.1016/j.janxdis.2013.04.010.

28. Tuerk PW, Yoder M, Grubaugh A, Myrick H, Hamner M, Acierno R. Prolonged exposure therapy for combat-related posttraumatic stress disorder: an examination of treatment effectiveness for veterans of the wars in Afghanistan and Iraq. J Anxiety Disord. 2011;25(3):397–403. doi:10.1016/j.janxdis. 2010.11.002.

29. Rothbaum BO, Astin MC, Marsteller F. Prolonged exposure versus eye movement desensitization and reprocessing (EMDR) for PTSD rape victims. J Trauma Stress. 2005;18(6):607–16.

30. Morris DJ. After PTSD, more trauma. New York Times, 18 Jan 2015, p. A18.

31. Editor. V.A.'s treatment of veterans' trauma. Letters to the Editoe. New York Times, 23 Jan 2015.

32. Frost ND, Laska KM, Wampold BE. The evidence for present-centered therapy as a treatment for posttraumatic stress disorder. J Trauma Stress. 2014;27(1):1–8. doi:10.1002/jts.21881.

33. Markowitz JC, Petkova E, Neria Y, Van Meter PE, Zhao Y, Hembree E, et al. Is exposure necessary? A randomized clinical trial of interpersonal psychotherapy for PTSD. Am J Psychiatry. 2015;172(5):430–40. doi:10.1176/appi.ajp.2014.14070908.

34. Becker CB, Zayfert C, Anderson E. A survey of psychologists' attitudes towards and utilization of exposure therapy for PTSD. Behav Res Ther. 2004;42(3):277–92. doi:10.1016/S0005-7967(03)00138-4.

35. Schnurr PP, Friedman MJ, Foy DW, Shea MT, Hsieh FY, Lavori PW, et al. Randomized trial of trauma-focused group therapy for posttraumatic stress disorder: results from a department of veterans affairs cooperative study. Arch Gen Psychiatry. 2003;60(5):481–9.

36. Resick PA, Schnicke MK. Cognitive processing therapy for sexual assault victims. J Consult Clin Psychol. 1992;60(5):748–56.

37. Ma SH, Teasdale JD. Mindfulness-based cognitive therapy for depression: replication and exploration of differential relapse prevention effects. J Consult Clin Psychol. 2004;72(1):31–40.

38. Teasdale JD, Segal ZV, Williams JM, Ridgeway VA, Soulsby JM, Lau MA. Prevention of relapse/recurrence in major depression by mindfulness-based cognitive therapy. J Consult Clin Psychol. 2000;68(4):615–23.

39. Bondolfi G, Jermann F, der Linden MV, Gex-Fabry M, Bizzini L, Rouget BW, et al. Depression relapse prophylaxis with mindfulness-based cognitive therapy: replication and extension in the Swiss health care system. J Affect Disord. 2010;122 (3):224–31.

40. Segal ZV, Bieling P, Young T, MacQueen G, Cooke R, Martin L, et al. Antidepressant monotherapy vs sequential pharmacotherapy and mindfulness-based cognitive therapy, or placebo, for relapse prophylaxis in recurrent depression. Arch Gen Psychiatry. 2010;67(12):1256–64.

41. Chiesa A, Serretti A. Mindfulness based cognitive therapy for psychiatric disorders: a systematic review and meta-analysis. Psychiatry Res. 2011;187(3):441–53.

42. Barnhofer T, Crane C, Hargus E, Amarasinghe M, Winder R, Williams JM. Mindfulness-based cognitive therapy as a treatment for chronic depression: a preliminary study. Behav Res Ther. 2009;47(5):366–73.
43. Eisendrath S, Chartier M, McLane M. Adapting mindfulness-based cognitive therapy for treatment-resistant depression: a clinical case study. Cogn Behav Pract. 2011;18(3):362–70. doi:10.1016/j.cbpra.2010.05.004.
44. Eisendrath SJ, Gillung E, Delucchi K, Mathalon DH, Yang TT, Satre DD, et al. A preliminary study: efficacy of mindfulness-based cognitive therapy versus sertraline as first-line treatments for major depressive disorder. Mindfulness (NY). 2015;6(3):475–82. doi:10.1007/s12671-014-0280-8.
45. Eisendrath SJ, Gillung EP, Delucchi KL, Chartier M, Mathalon DH, Sullivan JC, et al. Mindfulness-based cognitive therapy (MBCT) versus the health-enhancement program (HEP) for adults with treatment-resistant depression: a randomized control trial study protocol. BMC Complement Altern Med. 2014;14:95. doi:10.1186/1472-6882-14-95.
46. Manicavasgar V, Parker G, Perich T. Mindfulness-based cognitive therapy vs cognitive behaviour therapy as a treatment for non-melancholic depression. J Affect Disord. 2011;130(1-2):138–44.
47. Evans S, Ferrando S, Findler M, Stowell C, Smart C, Haglin D. Mindfulness-based cognitive therapy for generalized anxiety disorder. J Anxiety Disord. 2008;22(4):716–21.
48. Hoge EA, Bui E, Marques L, Metcalf CA, Morris LK, Robinaugh DJ, et al. Randomized controlled trial of mindfulness meditation for generalized anxiety disorder: effects on anxiety and stress reactivity. J Clin Psychiatry. 2013;74(8):786–92. doi:10.4088/JCP.12m08083.
49. Yook K, Lee SH, Ryu M, Kim KH, Choi TK, Suh SY, et al. Usefulness of mindfulness-based cognitive therapy for treating insomnia in patients with anxiety disorders: a pilot study. J Nerv Ment Dis. 2008;196(6):501–3.
50. Weber B, Jermann F, Gex-Fabry M, Nallet A, Bondolfi G, Aubry JM. Mindfulness-based cognitive therapy for bipolar disorder: a feasibility trial. Eur Psychiatry. 2010;25(6):334–7.
51. Hepburn SR, Crane C, Barnhofer T, Duggan DS, Fennell MJ, Williams JM. Mindfulness-based cognitive therapy may reduce thought suppression in previously suicidal participants: findings from a preliminary study. Br J Clin Psychol. 2009;48(Pt 2):209–15.
52. Williams JM, Duggan DS, Crane C, Fennell MJ. Mindfulness-based cognitive therapy for prevention of recurrence of suicidal behavior. J Clin Psychol. 2006;62(2):201–10. doi:10.1002/jclp.20223.
53. Sachse S, Keville S, Feigenbaum J. A feasibility study of mindfulness-based cognitive therapy for individuals with borderline personality disorder. Psychol Psychother. 2011;84(2):184–200.
54. Teasdale JD, Moore RG, Hayhurst H, Pope M, Williams S, Segal ZV. Metacognitive awareness and prevention of relapse in depression: empirical evidence. J Consult Clin Psychol. 2002;70(2):275–87.
55. Hempel, S, Taylor, SL, Marshall, NJ, Miake-Lye, IM, Beroes, J M, Shanman, R, Solloway, MR, Shekelle, PG. Evidence map of mindfulness. VA-ESP Project #05-226; 2014.
56. Allen NB, Chambers R, Knight W, Melbourne Academic Mindfulness Interest G. Mindfulness-based psychotherapies: a review of conceptual foundations, empirical evidence and practical considerations. Aust N Z J Psychiatry. 2006;40(4):285–94. doi:10.1111/j.1440-1614.2006.01794.x.
57. Baer R. Mindfulness training as a clinical intervention: a conceptual and empirical review. Clin Psychol Sci Pract. 2003;10(2):125–43.
58. Jankowski T, Holas P. Metacognitive model of mindfulness. Conscious Cogn. 2014;28:64–80. doi:10.1016/j.concog.2014.06.005.
59. Shapiro SL, Carlson LE, Astin JA, Freedman B. Mechanisms of mindfulness. J Clin Psychol. 2006;62(3):373–86.
60. Teasdale JD, Segal Z, Williams JM. How does cognitive therapy prevent depressive relapse and why should attentional control (mindfulness) training help? Behav Res Ther. 1995;33(1):25–39.
61. Wallace BA, Shapiro SL. Mental balance and well-being: building bridges between Buddhism and Western psychology. Am Psychol. 2006;61(7):690–701.
62. Chambers R, Gullone E, Allen NB. Mindful emotion regulation: an integrative review. Clin Psychol Rev. 2009;29(6):560–72. doi:10.1016/j.cpr.2009.06.005.
63. Marchand WR. Neural mechanisms of mindfulness and meditation: evidence from neuroimaging studies. World J Radiol. 2014;6(7):471–9. doi:10.4329/wjr.v6.i7.471.
64. Roemer L, Williston SK, Eustis EH, Orsillo SM. Mindfulness and acceptance-based behavioral therapies for anxiety disorders. Curr Psychiatry Rep. 2013;15(11):410. doi:10.1007/s11920-013-0410-3.
65. Tang YY, Holzel BK, Posner MI. The neuroscience of mindfulness meditation. Nat Rev Neurosci. 2015;16(4):213–25. doi:10.1038/nrn3916.
66. van der Velden AM, Kuyken W, Wattar U, Crane C, Pallesen KJ, Dahlgaard J, et al. A systematic review of mechanisms of change in mindfulness-based cognitive therapy in the treatment of recurrent major depressive disorder. Clin Psychol Rev. 2015;37:26–39. doi:10.1016/j.cpr.2015.02.001.
67. Eftekhari A, Stines LR, Zoellner LA. Do you need to talk about it? Prolonged exposure for the treatment of chronic PTSD. Behav Anal Today. 2006;7(1):70–83.
68. Rauch SA, Eftekhari A, Ruzek JI. Review of exposure therapy: a gold standard for PTSD treatment. J Rehabil Res Dev. 2012;49(5):679–87.
69. Bonanno GA. Loss, trauma, and human resilience: have we underestimated the human capacity to thrive after extremely aversive events? Am Psychol. 2004;59(1):20–8. doi:10.1037/0003-066X.59.1.20.

70. Breslau N. Psychiatric morbidity in adult survivors of childhood trauma. Semin Clin Neuropsychiatry. 2002;7(2):80–8.

71. Janoff-Bulman R. Shattered Assumptions. 1992; New York: Free Press.

72. Beck AT, Haigh EA. Advances in cognitive theory and therapy: the generic cognitive model. Annu Rev ClinPsychol.2014;10:1–24.doi:10.1146/annurev-clinpsy-032813-153734.

73. Holliday R, Link-Malcolm J, Morris EE, Surís A. Effects of cognitive processing therapy on PTSD-related negative cognitions in veterans with military sexual trauma. Mil Med. 2014;179(10):1077–82. doi: 10.7205/MILMED-D-13-00309.

74. Foa E, Hembree E, Rothbaum BO: Prolonged Exposure Therapy for PTSD: Emotional Processing of Traumatic Experiences (Treatments That Work) 1st Edition, Oxford, Oxford University Press, 2007.

75. Ringell S, Brandell JR. Trauma: Contemporary Directions in Theory, Practice, and Research. 2012; Thousand Oaks, CA: SAGE Publications, Inc.

76. Mowrer, OH. Two-factor learning theory: summary and comment. Psychological Review. 1939;58(5):1951, 350–354. http://dx.doi.org/10.1037/h0058956.

77. Foa EB, Kozak MJ. Emotional processing of fear: exposure to corrective information. Psychol Bull. 1986;99(1):20–35.

78. Keane TM, Zimering RT, Caddell JM. A behavioral formulation of posttraumatic stress disorder inVietnam veterans. the Behavior Therapist. 1985;8(1): 9–12.

79. Manzoni GM, Pagnini F, Castelnuovo G, Molinari E. Relaxation training for anxiety: a ten-years systematic review with meta-analysis. BMC Psychiatry. 2008;8:41.

80. Hickling EJ, Sison Jr GF, Vanderploeg RD. Treatment of posttraumatic stress disorder with relaxation and biofeedback training. Biofeedback Self Regul. 1986;11(2):125–34.

81. Follette VM, Palm KM, Rasmussen Hall ML. Acceptance, mindfulness, and trauma. In: SC. Hayes, VM. Follette, & M. Linehan, (Eds.)., *Mindfulness and acceptance: Expanding the cognitive behavioraltradition* 2004; New York: Guilford Press.

82. Hembree EA1, Foa EB. Posttraumatic stress disorder: Psychological factors and psychosocial interventions. J Clin Psychiatry. 2000;61 (Suppl 7):33–9.

83. Beck AT, Rush AJ, Shaw BF, Emery G. Cognitive therapy of depression. New York, NY: Guilford Press; 1979.

84. Safran JD, Segal ZV. Interpersonal process in cognitive therapy. New York, NY: Basic Books; 1990.

85. Fresco DM, Segal ZV, Buis T, Kennedy S. Relationship of posttreatment decentering and cognitive reactivity to relapse in major depression. J Consult Clin Psychol. 2007;75(3):447–55.

86. Kingston T, Dooley B, Bates A, Lawlor E, Malone K. Mindfulness-based cognitive therapy for residual depressive symptoms. Psychol Psychother. 2007;80(Pt 2):193–203.

87. Ramel W, Goldin PR, Carmona PE, McQuaid JR. The effects of mindfulness meditation on cognitive processes and affect in patients with past depression. Cogn Ther Res. 2004;28(4):433–55.

88. Segal ZV, Williams JMG, Teasdale JD. Mindfulness-based cognitive therapy for depression: a new approach to preventing relapse. New York, NY: Guilford Press; 2002.

89. El Leithy S, Brown GP, Robbins I. Counterfactual thinking and posttraumatic stress reactions. JAbnormPsychol.2006;115(3):629–35.doi:10.1037/0021-843X.115.3.629.

90. Gill IJ, Mullin S, Simpson J. Are metacognitive processes associated with posttraumatic stress symptom severity following acquired brain injury? Disabil Rehabil. 2015;37(8):692–700. doi:10.3109/0963828 8.2014.939774.

91. Lysaker PH, Dimaggio G, Wickett-Curtis A, Kukla M, Luedtke B, Vohs J, et al. Deficits in metacognitive capacity are related to subjective distress and heightened levels of hyperarousal symptoms in adults with posttraumatic stress disorder. J Trauma Dissociation. 2015;16(4):384 98. doi:10.1080/1529 9732.2015.1005331.

92. Roussis P, Wells A. Psychological factors predicting stress symptoms: metacognition, thought control, and varieties of worry. Anxiety Stress Coping. 2008; 21(3):213–25. doi:10.1080/10615800801889600.

93. Wells A, Sembi S. Metacognitive therapy for PTSD: a preliminary investigation of a new brief treatment. J Behav Ther Exp Psychiatry. 2004;35(4):307–18.

94. Kleim B, Ehlers A, Glucksman E. Early predictors of chronic post-traumatic stress disorder in assault survivors. Psychol Med. 2007;37(10):1457–67. doi:10.1017/S0033291707001006.

95. Seligowski AV, Lee DJ, Bardeen JR, Orcutt HK. Emotion regulation and posttraumatic stress symptoms: a meta-analysis. Cogn Behav Ther. 2015;44(2):87–102. doi:10 .1080/16506073.2014.980753.

96. Michalak J, Holz A, Teismann T. Rumination as a predictor of relapse in mindfulness-based cognitive therapy for depression. Psychol Psychother. 2011;84(2):230–6.

97. Hiraoka R, Meyer EC, Kimbrel NA, DeBeer BB, Gulliver SB, Morissette SB. Self-compassion as a prospective predictor of PTSD symptom severity among trauma-exposed U.S. Iraq and Afghanistan war veterans. J Trauma Stress. 2015;28(2):127–33. doi:10.1002/jts.21995.

98. Thompson BL, Waltz J. Self-compassion and PTSD symptom severity. J Trauma Stress. 2008;21(6):556–8. doi:10.1002/jts.20374.

99. Gu J, Strauss C, Bond R, Cavanagh K. How do mindfulness-based cognitive therapy and mindfulness-based stress reduction improve mental health and wellbeing? A systematic review and meta-analysis of mediation studies. Clin Psychol Rev. 2015;37:1–12. doi:10.1016/j.cpr.2015.01.006.

100. Kearney DJ, McManus C, Malte CA, Martinez ME, Felleman B, Simpson TL. Loving-kindness medita-

tion and the broaden-and-build theory of positive emotions among veterans with posttraumatic stress disorder. Med Care. 2014;52(12 Suppl 5):S32–8. doi:10.1097/MLR.0000000000000221.

101. Kearney DJ, Simpson TL. Broadening the approach to posttraumatic stress disorder and the consequences of trauma. JAMA. 2015;314(5):453–5. doi:10.1001/jama.2015.7522.

102. Jovanovic T, Kazama A, Bachevalier J, Davis M. Impaired safety signal learning may be a biomarker of PTSD. Neuropharmacology. 2012;62(2):695–704. doi:10.1016/j.neuropharm.2011.02.023.

103. Liberzon I, Sripada CS. The functional neuroanatomy of PTSD: a critical review. Prog Brain Res. 2008;167:151–69. doi:10.1016/S0079-6123(07)67011-3.

104. Garfinkel SN, Abelson JL, King AP, Sripada RK, Wang X, Gaines LM, et al. Impaired contextual modulation of memories in PTSD: an fMRI and psychophysiological study of extinction retention and fear renewal. J Neurosci. 2014;34(40):13435–43. doi:10.1523/JNEUROSCI.4287-13.2014.

105. Stuart S. Interpersonal Psychotherapy. American Psychiatric Press, Washington DC. 2013.

106. McCullough Jr., James P. Treatment for chronic depression: Cognitive behavioral analysis system of Psychotherapy (CBASP). Guilford Press, 2000. ISBN 1-57230-965-2

107. Kimbrough E, Magyari T, Langenberg P, Chesney M, Berman B. Mindfulness intervention for child abuse survivors. J Clin Psychol. 2010;66(1):17–33. doi:10.1002/jclp.20624.

108. Carmody J, Baer RA. Relationships between mindfulness practice and levels of mindfulness, medical and psychological symptoms and well-being in a mindfulness-based stress reduction program. J Behav Med. 2008;31(1):23–33.

109. Polusny MA, Erbes CR, Thuras P, Moran A, Lamberty GJ, Collins RC, et al. Mindfulness-based stress reduction for posttraumatic stress disorder among veterans: a randomized clinical trial. JAMA. 2015;314(5):456–65. doi:10.1001/jama.2015.8361.

110. Bandelow B, Reitt M, Rover C, Michaelis S, Gorlich Y, Wedekind D. Efficacy of treatments for anxiety disorders: a meta-analysis. Int Clin Psychopharmacol. 2015;30(4):183–92. doi:10.1097/YIC.0000000000000078.

111. Franca RD, Milbourn B. A meta-analysis of mindfulness based interventions (MBIs) show that MBIs are effective in reducing acute symptoms of depression but not anxiety. Aust Occup Ther J. 2015;62(2):147–8. doi:10.1111/1440-1630.12198.

112. Goyal M, Singh S, Sibinga EMS, Gould NF, Rowland-Seymour A, Sharma R, et al. Meditation programs for psychological stress and well-being. JAMA Intern Med. 2014;174(3):357–68.

113. Grossman P, Niemann L, Schmidt S, Walach H. Mindfulness-based stress reduction and health benefits: a meta-analysis. J Psychosom Res. 2004;57(1):35–43. doi:10.1016/S0022-3999(03)00573-7.

114. Huang HP, He M, Wang HY, Zhou M. A meta-analysis of the benefits of mindfulness-based stress

reduction (MBSR) on psychological function among breast cancer (BC) survivors. Breast Cancer. 2015. doi:10.1007/s12282-015-0604-0.

115. Piet J, Wurtzen H, Zachariae R. The effect of mindfulness-based therapy on symptoms of anxiety and depression in adult cancer patients and survivors: a systematic review and meta-analysis. J Consult Clin Psychol. 2012;80(6):1007–20. doi:10.1037/a0028329.

116. Branstrom R, Kvillemo P, Brandberg Y, Moskowitz JT. Self-report mindfulness as a mediator of psychological well-being in a stress reduction intervention for cancer patients – a randomized study. Ann Behav Med. 2010;39(2):151–61. doi:10.1007/s12160-010-9168-6.

117. Kim SH, Schneider SM, Kravitz L, Mermier C, Burge MR. Mind-body practices for posttraumatic stress disorder. J Investig Med. 2013;61(5):827–34.

118. Gordon JS, Staples JK, Blyta A, Bytyqi M. Treatment of posttraumatic stress disorder in postwar Kosovo high school students using mind-body skills groups: a pilot study. J Trauma Stress. 2004;17(2):143–7. doi:10.1023/B:JOTS.0000022620.13209.a0.

119. Gordon JS, Staples JK, Blyta A, Bytyqi M, Wilson AT. Treatment of posttraumatic stress disorder in postwar Kosovar adolescents using mind-body skills groups: a randomized controlled trial. J Clin Psychiatry. 2008;69(9):1469–76.

120. Banks K, Newman E, Saleem J. An overview of the research on mindfulness-based interventions for treating symptoms of posttraumatic stress disorder: a systematic review. J Clin Psychol. 2015;71(10):935–63.

121. Earley MD, Chesney MA, Frye J, Greene PA, Berman B, Kimbrough E. Mindfulness intervention for child abuse survivors: a 2.5-year follow-up. J Clin Psychol. 2014;70(10):933–41. doi:10.1002/jclp.22102.

122. Smith SA. Mindfulness-based stress reduction: an intervention to enhance the effectiveness of nurses' coping with work-related stress. Int J Nurs Knowl. 2014;25(2):119–30. doi:10.1111/2047-3095.12025.

123. Goldsmith RE, Gerhart JI, Chesney SA, Burns JW, Kleinman B, Hood MM. Mindfulness-based stress reduction for posttraumatic stress symptoms: building acceptance and decreasing shame. J Evid Based Complement Altern Med. 2014;19(4):227–34. doi:10.1177/2156587214533703.

124. Kim SH, Schneider SM, Bevans M, Kravitz L, Mermier C, Qualls C, et al. PTSD symptom reduction with mindfulness-based stretching and deep breathing exercise: randomized controlled clinical trial of efficacy. J Clin Endocrinol Metab. 2013;98(7):2984–92. doi:10.1210/jc.2012-3742.

125. Cox CE, Porter LS, Buck PJ, Hoffa M, Jones D, Walton B, et al. Development and preliminary evaluation of a telephone-based mindfulness training intervention for survivors of critical illness. Ann Am Thorac Soc. 2014;11(2):173–81. doi:10.1513/AnnalsATS.201308-283OC.

126. Niles BK-G, Ryngala DJ, Silberbogen K, Paysnick A, Wolf EJ. Comparing mindfulness and psychoeduca-

tion treatments for combat-related PTSD using a tele-health approach. Psychol Trauma. 2012;4(5):538–47.

127. Kearney DJ, McDermott K, Malte C, Martinez M, Simpson TL. Association of participation in a mindfulness program with measures of PTSD, depression and quality of life in a veteran sample. J Clin Psychol. 2012;68(1):101–16. doi:10.1002/jclp.20853.

128. Kearney DJ, McDermott K, Malte C, Martinez M, Simpson TL. Effects of participation in a mindfulness program for veterans with posttraumatic stress disorder: a randomized controlled pilot study. J Clin Psychol. 2013;69(1):14–27. doi:10.1002/jclp.21911.

129. Kearney DJ, Malte CA, McManus C, Martinez ME, Felleman B, Simpson TL. Loving-kindness meditation for posttraumatic stress disorder: a pilot study. J Trauma Stress. 2013;26(4):426–34. doi:10.1002/jts.21832.

130. Bhatnagar R, Phelps L, Rietz K, Juergens T, Russell D, Miller N, et al. The effects of mindfulness training on post-traumatic stress disorder symptoms and heart rate variability in combat veterans. J Altern Complement Med. 2013;19(11):860–1. doi:10.1089/acm.2012.0602.

131. Krystal JH, Rosenheck RA, Cramer JA, Vessicchio JC, Jones KM, Vertrees JE, Horney RA, Huang GD, Stock C. Veterans Affairs Cooperative Study No. 504 Group. Adjunctive risperidone treatment for antidepressant-resistantsymptoms of chronic military service-related PTSD: a randomized trial. JAMA. 2011;306(5):493–502. doi:10.1001/jama.2011.1080.

132. King AP, Erickson TM, Giardino ND, Favorite T, Rauch SA, Robinson E, et al. A pilot study of group mindfulness-based cognitive therapy (MBCT) for combat veterans with posttraumatic stress disorder (PTSD). Depress Anxiety. 2013;30(7):638–45. doi:10.1002/da.22104.

Mindfulness-Based Cognitive Therapy for Patients with Suicidal Ideation and Behavior

16

Thomas Forkmann, Tobias Teismann, and Johannes Michalak

Clinical Case Study

Martin was a 66-year-old teacher. Since he was 31, he experienced five episodes of Major Depression. Between episodes, he largely reached a state of normal functioning. The last episode began 6 years ago. It was the most severe episode he has ever experienced and it resulted in a 5-month inpatient treatment. During his inpatient stay, he attempted suicide after he completely lost hope of recovering from depression. He tried to cut his wrists. However, the lesion was not severe enough to result in bleeding to death.

During his depressive episodes, he excessively ruminates about being not acceptable to other people because of being a queer card, being too silent and interacting in an inappropriate way. He met the criteria for social anxiety disorder and this disorder persisted between depressive episodes. After Martin had left the clinic, he was still depressed and had not reached normal functioning. He contacted the outpatient clinic because he wanted to work on his social anxiety and on the persistent depressive symptoms. The individual therapy

T. Forkmann, Ph.D. (✉)
Institute of Medical Psychology and Medical Sociology, University Hospital of RWTH Aachen University, Aachen, Germany
e-mail: tforkmann@ukaachen.de

T. Teismann, Ph.D.
Department for Clinical Psychology and Psychotherapy, Ruhr-Universität Bochum, Germany, Bochum, Germany

J. Michalak, Ph.D.
Department of Psychology and Psychotherapy, Witten/Herdecke University, Witten/Herdecke, Germany

focused on these issues: social anxiety was treated with the cognitive approach of Clark and Wells [1] and depression with behavior activation and cognitive restructuring. Martin's condition improved significantly during the individual therapy and the social anxiety disorder and major depression completely remitted within 4 months. However, he was still concerned about the possible recurrence of his major depression and was particularly worried of getting into a suicidal crisis again. Thus, he joined a mindfulness-based cognitive therapy (MBCT) course to learn skills to prevent relapse into depression and to deal with possible suicidal ideations.

Martin was very impressed by the principle of mindfulness at the beginning of the course. He regularly practiced the body scan in the first 2 weeks of the program. In the first week, he felt that he could get in contact with his body, an experience that was new and refreshing for him. However, within the second week during the body scan, thought patterns came up that circled around the question "Am I doing it right?" When he realized that he drifted with his attention, the thought "I am a failure. I should try harder to stay in contact with my body." came up. During inquiry, he realized the harshness of this inner voice and that this harshness was very familiar to him and was often the starting point of a depressive spiraling down. Moreover, he realized that this quality of harshness was one of the core features of his suicidal ideation. So he was invited to be aware of this way of relating to himself and to try to bring a more gentle and self-caring tone into situations, in which he becomes aware of drifting.

In the third session, he reported that he realized how often this self-critical and demanding voice came up during the week and how much this voice drove his daily activities. Especially, this resulted in starting too many activities during the day and being much oppressed when he did not manage to handle his plans for the day. In session 4 he decided

© Springer International Publishing Switzerland 2016
S.J. Eisendrath (ed.), *Mindfulness-Based Cognitive Therapy*, DOI 10.1007/978-3-319-29866-5_16

to take a breathing space every time he started a new activity and to use this "psychological space" to decide if he is really prepared and willing to act or if he just feels compelled to act because of the self-critical and demanding inner voice.

During the next weeks, he reported that he gradually learned to relate differently with more self-compassion to slips during formal mindfulness practice and to everyday "shortcomings." Moreover, he gradually managed to act with more mindfulness in everyday life and to calm the self-critical voice. He said that it was very important to him to learn to start action with greater awareness and to step out of a kind of "driven mode" into a more deliberate and mindful mode of action.

Another important experience was the development of an action plan that can be used in the face of lowered mood. He realized that there were a huge number of small decisions between a first sign of low mood and a full-blown episode of major depression including strong suicidal ideation.

After the end of the 8-week program, Martin practiced the body-scan or sitting meditation on a daily base and used informal mindfulness practice regularly. He stayed well for 5 years up to now and said that the MBCT course was very important to him because it deeply changed and enriched his perspective on life and on himself.

The Problem of Suicidal Ideation and Behavior

Worldwide about one million people die by suicide each year, making it the 15th leading cause of death. It is estimated that for each adult who dies of suicide, there are likely to be more than 20 others with one or more suicide attempts [2]. Furthermore, adults are reported to have a lifetime prevalence of up to 33 % experiencing suicide ideation [3]. For many individuals suicide behavior and suicide ideation is episodic: As such, Gibb et al. [4] found a reattempt rate of 28 % within 10 years after an initial suicide attempt. Suicide ideation and behavior occurs most frequently in the context of a mental disorder [5], most prominently affective disorders: In a 40–44-year prospective follow-up study of 406 formerly hospitalized major mood disorder patients, Angst et al. [6] found that 14.5 % of the unipolar depressed patients completed suicide. Although suicide rates in depressed patients significantly

differ depending on treatment status (inpatient vs. outpatient), symptom severity and gender [7, 8], it is well established that about 40 % of individuals who died by suicide experienced depressive illness before their death [5]. Furthermore, 8.7 % of people suffering from Major Depressive Disorder (MDD) and 10.1 % of those suffering from dysthymia have attempted suicide during their lifetime [9]. However, because the vast majority of depressed patients do not attempt suicide or die by suicide, research has focused on discovering additional risk factors and mechanisms that predict suicidal ideation and behavior.

Generally, it seems plausible to assume that psychological treatments for depression not only ease depressed affect but also suicidal ideation, but this assumption has lately been called into question: Cuijpers and coworkers [10] found in a meta-analysis only three randomized controlled studies for adult depression in which suicidal ideation and behavior was used as a clearly specified outcome measure. The pooled results indicated very small and nonsignificant effects of psychotherapy for depression on suicidality, but there was not enough statistical power to consider this a true effect. Therefore, it seems necessary to investigate further the effects of different forms of therapy on suicide ideation and behavior, as well as to attempt to adopt treatments to the specific needs of this population. One treatment approach that has been advocated by Williams et al. [11] for preventing recurrent suicidal ideation and behavior is mindfulness-based cognitive therapy (MBCT).

Theoretical Rationale of MBCT for Suicidal Ideation and Behavior

Williams and colleagues [11–15] propose that suicidality is partly explicable by Teasdale's [16] *differential activation hypothesis*. The original theory states that during a person's learning history and particularly during episodes of depression, low mood becomes associated with patterns of negative thoughts and information processing (biases in memory, interpretations, and attitudes), body states, and behaviors. These elements may occur together in fairly loose association the first time a person experiences a period of low mood. If depression occurs again, however, the pattern starts to become established and learned associations build up between the moods, the thinking, and the bodily associations. Any return of the mood reactivates the pattern and an interlock configuration of dysphoric mood and negative thinking can be established that may result in an increasing risk of relapse and recurrence of depression [16]. Lau et al. [15] suggest that suicidal ideation arises as part of such patterns of thinking during early episodes and, during these episodes, an association is formed between depressed mood and suicidal ideation, such that future depression will activate suicidal ideas. Since suicidal ideation represents an extremely severe form of negative self-referent thinking ("I can never be forgiven for the mistakes I made," "I can't bear the pain any longer"), the authors suspect that it is particularly likely that suicidal ideation will become part of the depressive processing pattern. Williams et al. [12] furthermore propose that during such repeated activation, suicidal ideas become more elaborated and other negative moods (such as anger, shame) may also become associated with the suicidal ideation.

Taken together, risk of further suicide ideation and behavior should therefore arise from the ease with which these patterns of processing become reestablished in the face of negative affect or autobiographical material—a process called *cognitive reactivity*. Cognitive reactivity does not only refer to certain themes of thinking, but also to certain thought processes, such as ruminative thinking. Ruminative thinking, broadly defined as a style of repetitive thinking about one's problems or negative experiences that is partly intrusive and difficult to disengage from [17], has not only been shown to be associated with the amplification and maintenance of negative moods, as well as a decrease in positive thinking, motivation, problem-solving abilities, and interpersonal functioning [18] but is also positively related to suicide ideation and suicide attempts [19–21]. Williams and Swales [22] assume that over time these ruminative thinking processes become more relevant in triggering suicidal ideation and behavior than stressful events.

Evidence—in line with the differential activation hypothesis—stems from a study comparing formerly depressed patients with and without a history of suicide ideation, showing that previously suicidal patients exhibited significant decreases in their interpersonal problem-solving ability following induction of sad mood. In contrast, problem-solving performance in those without a history of suicidal ideation remained relatively unchanged [23]. Furthermore, Williams et al. [14] showed, that individuals who reported suicidal ideation when depressed in the past indicated higher hopelessness/suicidality scores in a measure of cognitive reactivity to low mood. Moreover, they found that greater hopelessness/suicidality reactivity was associated with greater decrease in positive future thinking after a negative mood induction. These studies suggest that small changes in mood may reinstate cognitive processes and deficits that are thought to contribute to escalation of suicidal crisis. Moreover, these findings suggest that people who have been suicidal may retain a latent vulnerability to suicidality, which becomes manifest when mood is low.

Because a reactivity pattern seen in previously suicidal patients may reflect rapid, automatic activation of the suicidal mode of mind, treatments addressing suicidal reactivity would be of great help to those with a vulnerability to suicidal ideation and behavior. As in the prevention of depressive relapse/recurrence, mindfulness may be useful in interrupting the automaticity of the activation process; increasing the individual's awareness of the activation may decrease the impact of the activation [22]. "This awareness facilitates a move from automatic to conscious processing and creates the space to make choices: Ah! What's going on here? What is this? Do I recognize this? Is it an old tape playing? Do I need to engage with it? Can't I just stay with it, notice what it does, and watch it as it passes and dissolves?" ([11], p. 5). Thus, participants are supported in developing a different relationship to their thoughts that would otherwise open the way to suicide ideation and behavior. Furthermore mindfulness helps inhibiting ruminative processes, by training the ability to maintain the focus of attention on the present moment. Moreover, training in mindfulness might increase the awareness for early cognitive, emotional, or bodily warning signs for the escalating process of negative mood and negative thinking patterns and might allow patients to step out of this process at an early stage. These mechanisms deem important in the prevention of suicide ideation and behavior.

Modifications of MBCT for Suicidal Ideation and Behavior

In most studies evaluating MBCT for patients with suicidal ideation and behavior, MBCT was delivered in its original form without any modifications. In addition, the research group of Mark Williams and colleagues, who investigated MBCT for patients with a history of suicidal ideation and behavior who are at high risk of suicidal relapse, utilized the original MBCT manual. However, greater emphasis has been put on patterns of thoughts and feelings that might be associated with suicidal planning, factors that maintain and exacerbate such patterns, and preparation of explicit action plans for suicidal crisis (see for example [24]). In conclusion of their own study results, Barnhofer et al. [25] suggested the incorporation of a psychoeducational component on the impact of suicidal imagery.

Recently, a combination of MBCT and the Safety Planning Intervention (SPI) was tested [26]. The SPI is a manualized one-session intervention aiming at designing a written safety plan that lists different strategies, contacts, and resources for use in crises or when rescue is needed [27]. The authors describe this preliminary intervention combination as a 9-week program, in which participants develop an individualized crisis plan, learn and practice mindfulness, and receive education on factors that maintain depression and suicidality. The intention of this program is to provide participants with new ways of dealing with difficult emotions and behaviors. The first session is offered individually and is dedicated to developing the individualized crisis plan. The remaining sessions, conducted in a group setting, focus on mindfulness and include some elements of cognitive therapy (i.e., psychoeducation and relapse prevention planning). Suicide risk assessments are conducted individually immediately before each group treatment session begins. In MBCT-S, less at home mindfulness-meditation practice is conducted (3 days a week) as compared to the standard MBCT protocol (6 days of inter-session practice a week). Instead, participants review their safety plan daily and monitor their suicidal cognitions and urges using a worksheet on a daily basis [28]. However, in the study by Chesin et al. [28], participants practiced voluntarily on 5 days per week on average, which is nearly the extent of practice usually asked from participants in MBCT protocols.

Evidence of MBCT for Suicidal Ideation and Behavior

Although the rationale for applying MBCT in the prevention and treatment of suicidality appears appealing, only limited empirical research has been conducted thus far addressing the question whether MBCT may exert significant effects on symptomatology in patients with suicidal ideation and behavior. A first *empirical* study on this issue was published by Kenny and Williams [29]. In a clinical audit 79 patients (32 of them reported suicidal ideation before treatment) participated in a MBCT program consisting of eight 2-h classes with around 1 h of daily homework. Ninety-four percent completed all classes. MBCT reduced depression as assessed via the Beck Depression Inventory (BDI) significantly. Mean BDI score dropped from 24.3 (SD = 9.8) prior to MBCT to 13.9 (SD = 9.7) after MBCT referring to an effect size of $d = 1.04$. MBCT showed a similar sized effect in the suicidal subgroup of the sample indicating that MBCT may reduce depression in both patients with and without suicidal symptoms [29]. Crane and colleagues [30] found similar results. In their study, individuals in recovery following an episode of suicidal depression were randomly assigned either to MBCT ($N=19$) or to a waitlist control group ($n=23$). Results indicated that in the MBCT but not in the waitlist control group, depressive symptoms were reduced. However, it has to be noted, that these studies did not evaluate the effect of MBCT *on suicidality*, but rather the effect on depression in a sample of patients with a history of suicidal ideation.

In a first randomized-controlled trial that *directly* examined the effect of MBCT on suicidality, Barnhofer and colleagues [25] randomly assigned 28 patients with chronic depression and a history of suicidality either to MBCT or to a treatment-as-usual (TAU) condition. The MBCT treatment followed the recommendations by Segal et al. [31] including some alterations concerning suicidality (crisis plans, cognitive components addressing suicidal cognitions and hopelessness). Results showed that MBCT reduced depression severity as assessed with the BDI significantly. Most importantly, MBCT also reduced suicidal ideation itself with an effect size of $d=0.48$. However, this effect was not significant, probably due to power restrictions caused by the limited sample size. Participants practiced on average 4.9 days out of the 6 days they were asked to practice. No adverse events were recorded during treatment time.

Two recent studies gave further evidence for the effectiveness of MBCT in reducing suicidality. These studies reported results of secondary analyses of randomized-controlled trials (primary results reported in [32, 33]) that reanalyzed the impact of MBCT on suicidality.

Forkmann et al. [34] found a significant reduction in suicidal ideation in an MBCT group ($n=64$), whereas no significant changes occurred in a wait-list control-group ($n=66$) when comparing baseline and post treatment scores of the suicide item from the self-rating form of the Dutch version of the Inventory of Depressive Symptoms. This effect was independent from the impact of changes in depression, rumination, and mindfulness skills. However, change in worry was a significant covariate of the specific reduction of suicidality in the MBCT group as compared to the control group.

In a prospective, bi-center, randomized controlled trial, Forkmann et al. [35] compared the effects of MBCT plus treatment-as-usual (TAU) and Cognitive Behavioral Analysis System of Psychotherapy (CBASP; group version) plus TAU on suicidal ideation to TAU alone. The sample consisted of 106 outpatients with chronic depression. The study revealed different results, depending on whether suicidal ideation was assessed via self-report (BDI) or via clinician ratings with the Hamilton Rating Scale for Depression (HAM-D; [36]). Whereas significant reduction of suicidal ideation emerged when assessed via clinician rating in the MBCT and CBASP group, but not in the TAU group, there was no significant effect of treatment on suicidal ideation when assessed via self-report. All effects were of small to medium size and independent of changes in depressive symptoms, mindfulness skills, and interpersonal problems.

Recently, Chesin and colleagues [28] published results of a pilot study on the feasibility, acceptability, safety, and preliminary effectiveness of the MBCT-S (described above). In a sample of 18 participants at high suicide risk and with a history of serious suicidal ideation within the past 6 months, they found significant reduction in suicidal ideation and depression between pre- and post-treatment assessments for treatment completers.

MBCT for the treatment of suicidality in children and youth is even sparser. In a community sample of sixth graders, Britton et al. [37] compared students randomly assigned to a mindfulness-based intervention (MBI) of up to 12 sessions including traditional meditation practices to students randomly assigned to an active control group, which consisted of a 6-week curriculum in ancient African history and the construction of a three-dimensional life-sized model of a Pharaoh's tomb. The participants in the MBI-group were significantly less likely to report suicidal thoughts or self-harm behavior than those in the control group at post-intervention assessments [37].

Mechanisms of Change of MBCT for Suicidal Ideation and Behavior

Evidence for the effectiveness of MBCT in reducing suicidality or preventing risk of future suicide is promising but highly inconclusive. Moreover, little is known so far about potential mechanisms of action that are responsible for positive treatment effects of MBCT on suicidal ideation and behavior. Luoma and Vilatte [38] argue that mindfulness reduces suicide risk because it targets experiential avoidance as a transdiagnostic process in suicidal clients. Experiential avoidance conceives a tendency to escape or avoid unwanted thoughts, emotions, memories, and sensations, even when doing so is useless, not beneficial or causes harm [39]. It has been shown that interventions that target at an increase in mindfulness are capable of reducing experiential avoidance. Reductions of experiential avoidance in turn may reduce many known predictors of suicidality, such as substance abuse, depression, anxiety, chronic pain, and psychotic symptoms [40]. Luoma and Vilatte [38] suspect that MBCT might have much of its effect through changes in experiential avoidance, although appropriate mediational analyses are lacking.

Another hypothetical mechanism of action linking MBCT to reductions in suicidality is change in overgeneral memory. Williams et al. [41] showed that MBCT reduces overgeneral autobiographical memory in formerly depressed patients. That means that MBCT facilitates the retrieval of specific autobiographical events, which in turn may add in improving problem-solving behavior among suicidal patients, which reduces the risk of a suicidal crisis.

Suicidal patients tend to suppress suicidal thoughts and intrusive mental images from awareness [42], in order to reduce pain and suffering. However, ironically, it has been shown that this tendency to suppress unwanted thoughts is associated with suicidal ideation and that longitudinally the suppression of suicidal thoughts predicts suicidal thinking over time, even while controlling for depression [42]. In a randomized-controlled trial, Hepburn et al. [43] found that MBCT reduces thought suppression in previously suicidal participants so that reduction of thought suppression may be a potentially important mechanism mediating the effects of MBCT on suicidality.

Tucker and colleagues [44] demonstrated that the positive relationship between neuroticism and suicidal ideation weakens at high levels of dispositional mindfulness and the negative relationship between extraversion and suicidal thinking is explicitly strong at low levels of mindfulness. Thus, mindfulness could be understood as a coping mechanism that helps individuals high in neuroticism and low in extraversion to deal with critical situations in a way that prevents or reduces the occurrence of suicidal thinking. However, these results should be deemed preliminary since they are limited to a healthy student sample and dispositional mindfulness [44].

Moreover, it can be speculated that self-compassion [45], a mediator of the effects of MBCT on depression [46], might also be a mechanism of the potentially beneficial effects of MBCT on suicidality. Self-compassion encompasses self-kindness (in contrast to self-criticism), common humanity (in contrast to feelings of isolation when faced with suffering) and mindfulness (in contrast to suppression or over-identification of feelings). Since episodes of suicidality are characterized by self-criticism, feelings of isolation and suppression or over-identification, self-compassion, which is fostered by MBCT [46], might be an antidote to the suicidal state of mind.

Forkmann et al. [34] found that their results were associated with reductions in worry, which is in line with prior investigations [11, 19]. Thus, they suggest, that MBCT may help people to distance themselves from worrying cognitions, which in turn may add to a reduction in suicidality [34]. Remarkably, it has to be noted that the recently published randomized-controlled trials found that changes in suicidality were largely independent from changes in rumination or mindfulness skills [34, 35]. Thus, additional research appears needed to clarify the exact role the various proposed variables play in mediating the effect of MBCT on suicidal ideation and behavior.

Practical Considerations of MBCT for Suicidal Ideation and Behavior

Generally, MBCT for patients at suicide risk or with a history of serious suicidal ideation/behavior appears feasible and acceptable. When treating suicidal patients the standard MBCT protocol can be slightly modified. Greater emphasis should be given to patterns of thoughts and feelings that might be associated with suicidal planning. Moreover, factors that maintain and exacerbate such patterns, and preparation of explicit action plans for suicidal crises can be developed. These issues can be addressed during the entire program when appropriate and might be explicitly deepened in session 6 and 7 that deal with cognitions and skillful action to care of ourselves.

In their pilot study on MBCT-S, a combination of MBCT and the safety plan intervention as described above, Chesin et al. [28] found MBCT-S to be feasible and safe for high suicide risk patients. Percentage of dropouts was low and general adherence was good. Ninety-three percent of all participants would recommend the MBCT-S to a friend in a similar position (Chesin et al. [28]).

Moreover, Williams et al. [11] formulated the following recommendations for the prevention of recurrence of suicidal behavior:

- For patients with a given suicidal risk it is important to ensure that they have a clear sense of whom they can contact in the case that a crisis is building and they need help and support over and above the classes.
- An increased emphasis should be given to externally focused mindfulness practices when the crisis is building up, so that patients overwhelmed by intense affect and powerful negative thoughts have an extended repertoire of grounding meditations that help them to focus on moment-by-moment awareness of the physical world around them.
- It seems to be advisable to explicitly introduce examples of suicidal cognitions into classes. By "inviting these (cognitive) monsters in to tea" we might see the monsters more clearly and

discover that they do not need to dominate our life and determine our actions to such a degree.

Most importantly, Williams and Swales [22] emphasize that MBCT should be used for depressed and suicidal patients while they are relatively well. However, for patients suffering from acute and severe suicidality "we would not recommend an approach solely based on mindfulness" ([22], p. 325).

Summary/Conclusions

MBCT for suicidal ideation and behavior is feasible and safe and can be applied easily with some slight modifications of the MBCT protocol. Although research on the direct effects of MBCT on suicidal ideation and behavior is limited, the available empirical studies suggest medium to large effects. More research is needed addressing the effect of MBCT on suicidal *behavior* since most studies focus on suicidal cognitions and urges only. Moreover, studies that investigate potential mediators of the effect of MBCT on suicidal ideation and behavior, ideally in a longitudinal design, are of great importance for a better understanding of the relevant mechanisms of action.

References

1. Clark DM, Wells A. A cognitive model of social phobia. In: Heimberg RG, Liebowitz MR, Hope DA, Schneier FR, editors. Social phobia: diagnosis, assessment, and treatment. New York, NY: Guilford Press; 1995. p. 41–68.
2. WHO. Preventing suicide: a global imperative. Geneva: WHO Press; 2014.
3. Nock MK, Borges G, Ono Y. Suicide: Global perspectives from the WHO Worlds Mental Health Surveys. Cambridge: Cambridge University Press; 2014.
4. Gibb S, Beautrais A, Fergusson D. Mortality and further suicidal behavior after an index suicide attempt: a 10-year study. Aust N Z J Psychiatry. 2005;39:95–100.
5. Arsenault-Lapierre G, Kim C, Turecki G. Psychiatric diagnoses in 3275 suicides: a meta-analysis. BMC Psychiatry. 2004;4:37.
6. Angst J, Angst F, Gerber-Werder R, Gamma A. Suicide in 406 mood-disorder patients with and

without long-term medications: a 40 to 44 years' follow-up. Arch Suicide Res. 2005;9:279–300.

7. Bostwick J, Pankratz S. Affective disorders and suicide risk: a reexamination. Am J Psychiatry. 2000; 157:1925–32.

8. Blair-West G, Mellsop G, Eyeson-Annan M. Downrating lifetime suicide risk in major depression. Acta Psychiatr Scand. 1997;95:259–63.

9. Bernal M, Haro JM, Bernert S, Brugha T, de Graaf R, Bruffaerts R, et al. Risk factors for suicidality in Europe: results from the ESEMED study. J Affect Disord. 2007;101:27–34.

10. Cuijpers P, de Beurs DP, van Spijker BA, Berking M, Andersson G, Kerkhof AJ. The effects of psychotherapy for adult depression on suicidality and hopelessness: a systematic review and meta-analysis. J Affect Disord. 2013;144:183–90.

11. Williams JM, Duggan DS, Crane C, Fennell MJ. Mindfulness-based cognitive therapy for prevention of recurrence of suicidal behavior. J Clin Psychol. 2006;62(2):201–10.

12. Williams JM, Crane C, Barnhofer T, Duggan D. Psychology and suicidal behavior: elaborating the entrapment model. In: Hawton K, editor. Prevention and treatment of suicidal behavior. Oxford: Oxford University Press; 2005. p. 71–89.

13. Williams JM, Crane C, Barnhofer T, Van der Does AJW, Segal ZS. Recurrence of suicidal ideation across depressive episodes. J Affect Disord. 2006;91: 189–94.

14. Williams JM, Van der Does AJW, Barnhofer T, Crane C, Segal ZS. Cognitive reactivity, suicidal ideation and future fluency: preliminary investigation of a differential activation theory of hopelessness/suicidality. Cogn Ther Res. 2008;32:83–104.

15. Lau MA, Segal ZS, Williams JM. Teasdales's differential activation hypothesis: implications for mechanisms of depressive relapse and suicidal behaviour. Behav Res Ther. 2004;42:1001–17.

16. Teasdale JD. Cognitive vulnerability to persistent depression. Cogn Emot. 1998;2:247–74.

17. Ehring T, Zetsche U, Weidacker K, Wahl K, Schönefeld S, Ehlers A. The Perseverative Thinking Questionnaire (PTQ): validation of a content-independent measure of repetitive negative thinking. J Behav Ther Exp Psychiatry. 2011;42:225–32.

18. Nolen-Hoeksema S, Wisco BE, Lyubomirsky S. Rethinking rumination. Perspect Psychol Sci. 2008; 3:400–24.

19. Kerkhof A, van Spijker BA. Worrying and rumination as proximal risk factors for suicidal behavior. In: O'Connor R, Platt S, Gordon J, editors. International Handbook of Suicide Prevention: Research, Policy and Practice. Oxford: John Wiley Sons, Ltd.; 2011. p. 199–209.

20. Morrison R, O'Connor RC. A systematic review of the relationship between rumination and suicidality. Suicide Life Threat Behav. 2008;38:523–38.

21. Teismann T, Forkmann T. Rumination, entrapment and suicide ideation: a mediational model. Clin Psychol Psychother. 2015. doi: 10.1002/cpp.1999. [Epub ahead of print].

22. Williams JM, Swales M. The use of mindfulness-based approaches for suicidal patients. Arch Suicide Res. 2004;8:315–29.

23. Williams JM, Barnhofer T, Crane C, Beck AT. Problem solving deteriorates following mood challenge in formerly depressed patients with a history of suicidal ideation. J Abnorm Psychol. 2005;114:421–31.

24. Williams JM, Crane C, Barnhofer T, Brennan K, Duggan DS, Fennell MJ, et al. Mindfulness-based cognitive therapy for preventing relapse in recurrent depression: a randomized dismantling trial. J Consult Clin Psychol. 2014;82(2):275–86.

25. Barnhofer T, Crane C, Hargus E, Amarasinghe M, Winder R, Williams J. Mindfulness-based cognitive therapy as a treatment for chronic depression: a preliminary study. Behav Res Ther. 2009;47:366–73.

26. Chesin MS, Chaudhury S, Stanley B. Psychotherapeutic treatment approaches for suicidal individuals. In: Cannon KE, Hudzik TJ, editors. Suicide: phenomenology and neurobiology. Heidelberg: Springer; 2014. p. 223–36.

27. Stanley B, Brown GK. Safety planning intervention: a brief intervention to mitigate suicide risk. Cogn Behav Pract. 2012;19(2):256–64.

28. Chesin MS, Sonmez CC, Benjamin-Phillips CA, Beeler B, Brodsky BS, Stanley B. Preliminary effectiveness of adjunct mindfulness-based cognitive therapy to prevent suicidal behavior in outpatients who are at elevated suicide risk. Mindfulness. 2015;6(6):1345–55. doi:10.1007/s12671-015-0405-8.

29. Kenny MA, Williams JM. Treatment-resistant depressed patients show a good response to mindfulness-based cognitive therapy. Behav Res Ther. 2007;45(3):617–25.

30. Crane C, Barnhofer T, Duggan DS, Hepburn S, Fennell MV, Williams JMG. Mindfulness-based cognitive therapy and self-discrepancy in recovered depressed patients with a history of depression and suicidality. Cogn Ther Res. 2008;32(6):775–87.

31. Segal ZV, Williams JMG, Teasdale JD. Mindfulness-based cognitive therapy for depression: a new approach to preventing relapse. New York: Guilford; 2002.

32. Geschwind N, Peeters F, Huibers M, van Os J, Wichers M. Efficacy of mindfulness-based cognitive therapy in relation to prior history of depression: randomised controlled trial. Br J Psychiatry. 2012;201:320–5.

33. Michalak J, Schultze M, Heidenreich T, Schramm E. A randomized controlled trial on the efficacy of mindfulness-based cognitive therapy and a group version of cognitive behavioral analysis system of psychotherapy for chronically depressed patients. J Consult Clin Psychol. 2015;83(5):951–63.

34. Forkmann T, Wichers M, Geschwind N, Peeters F, Van OJ, Mainz V, et al. Effects of mindfulness-based cognitive therapy on self-reported suicidal ideation: results from a randomised controlled trial in patients with residual depressive symptoms. Compr Psychiatry. 2014;55(8):1883–90.

35. Forkmann T, Brakemeier E-L, Teismann T, Schramm E, Michalak J. The effects of mindfulness-based cognitive therapy and cognitive-behavioral analysis system of psychotherapy on suicidal ideation in chronic depression. J Affect Disord. in press, doi:10.1016/j.jad.2016.01.047.

36. Hamilton M. Development of a rating scale for primary depressive illness. Br J Soc Clin Psychol. 1967;6(4):278–96.

37. Britton WB, Lepp NE, Niles HF, Rocha T, Fisher NE, Gold JS. A randomized controlled pilot trial of classroom-based mindfulness meditation compared to an active control condition in sixth-grade children. J Sch Psychol. 2014;52(3):263–78.

38. Luoma JB, Villatte JL. Mindfulness in the treatment of suicidal individuals. Cogn Behav Pract. 2012;19(2):265–76.

39. Hayes SC, Wilson KG, Gifford EV, Follette VM, Strosahl K. Experimental avoidance and behavioral disorders: a functional dimensional approach to diagnosis and treatment. J Consult Clin Psychol. 1996;64(6):1152–68.

40. Hayes SC, Luoma JB, Bond FW, Masuda A, Lillis J. Acceptance and commitment therapy: model, processes and outcomes. Behav Res Ther. 2006;44(1):1–25.

41. Williams J, Teasdale J, Segal Z, Soulsby J. Mindfulness-based cognitive therapy reduces overgeneral autobiographical memory in formerly depressed patients. J Abnorm Psychol. 2000;109(1):150–5.

42. Pettit JW, Temple SR, Norton PJ, Yaroslavsky I, Grover KE, Morgan ST, et al. Thought suppression and suicidal ideation: preliminary evidence in support of a robust association. Depress Anxiety. 2009;26(8):758–63.

43. Hepburn SR, Crane C, Barnhofer T, Duggan DS, Fennell MJ, Williams JM. Mindfulness-based cognitive therapy may reduce thought suppression in previously suicidal participants: findings from a preliminary study. Br J Clin Psychol. 2009;48(Pt 2):209–15.

44. Tucker RP, O'Keefe VM, Cole AB, Rhoades-Kerswill S, Hollingsworth DW, Helle AC, et al. Mindfulness tempers the impact of personality on suicidal ideation. Pers Individ Dif. 2014;68:229–33.

45. Neff KD. The development and validation of a scale to measure self-compassion. Self Identity. 2003;2:223–50.

46. Kuyken W, Watkins E, Holden E, White K, Taylor RS, Byford S, et al. How does mindfulness-based cognitive therapy work? Behav Res Ther. 2010;48:1105–12.

Mindfulness Intervention for Attention-Deficit/Hyperactivity Disorder: Theory and Action Mechanisms

17

Poppy L.A. Schoenberg

Charles, a 33-year-old with diagnosed primary ADHD-I, presented chronic inattention symptoms impairing organization and performance in his job, i.e., timekeeping, attention to details, losing pertinent information/objects, and following instructions/requests. Charles also displayed secondary impulsive symptoms detrimental to social and work settings, e.g., impulsivity during conversations displaying lack of social etiquette or empathy. Charles felt that his ADHD had a controlling influence in his life. It produced a lack in concentration and discipline making it difficult to put creative entrepreneurial ideas into any kind of conceptual or practical use, hindered opportunities for promotion at work, caused an inability to "connect" with others and strain within his primary relations. As such, Charles also suffered long-standing self-esteem issues. Following a period of partial remission, he requested to reduce (and potentially stop) psychotropic medication dosage due to several side effects of chronic use including migraines and insomnia. Charles' psychiatrist subsequently referred him to a mindfulness-based cognitive therapy (MBCT) program, an adapted protocol utilizing the Mindful Awareness Practises for ADHD presented by Zylowska et al. [1]. The adapted program involved gradual and flexible delivery of mindfulness practice alongside visual cues and heuristics comprising psychoeducational modules specifically tailored for ADHD. Charles found the mindfulness practise very difficult to carry out initially, particularly the formal sitting meditation, needing at least 10-min before being able to "find any calmness to be able to practise and keep up with the breath awareness." Progressively, he could remain mindful for increasingly longer intervals, and was more aware when he was distracted. Charles found observing how he "felt" in his body provided an accurate guide to his internal state and behavior, i.e., symptoms. This feeling was clearer and more centered than the "jittery" feeling he had when on psychotropic medication. In everyday life, Charles was able to persevere with tasks for longer periods, and refocus when he went off-task. Charles felt that he had more space to choose how to behave to a given situation, inhibiting (often problematic) automatic reactions. He became aware of being more attentive and able to listen to others for longer without interrupting, or losing the thread of a conversation. In turn, Charles was better able to connect with other people, increasing a sense of belonging and validation. Overall, Charles felt positive about himself, and more confident that he could redirect his symptoms, as opposed to the other way around.

Attention deficit/hyperactivity disorder (ADHD) is a neurobehavioral developmental disorder ensuing significant cognitive, emotional, social, and professional impairment. Its childhood onset has high persistence into adulthood, with an

P.L.A. Schoenberg, Ph.D. (✉)
Departments of Psychiatry and Cognitive
Neuroscience, Radboud University Medical Center,
Postbus 9010, Nijmegen 6500GL, The Netherlands
e-mail: poppy@science.ru.nl

estimated 2.5% adult worldwide prevalence [2]. The DSM defines three distinct subtypes/symptomatic clusters; inattention (ADHD-I), hyperactivity/impulsivity (ADHD-II), or combined type (ADHD-C). Subsequently, ADHD represents a complex disorder conceptualized as a multisystem condition with variable clinical expression based on degree of heterogeneity and dysfunction in pertinent neural systems, and epigenetic mechanisms. Adverse impacts to these processes thus account for phenotypic variation, observable in neurohormonal, neuroimaging, neurochemical, neurophysiological, and neuropsychological markers.

Pharmacological intervention represents mainstream treatment, principally comprising amphetamine-based, methylphenidate-based psychostimulants, non-stimulant selective norepinephrine re-uptake inhibitors, and non-stimulant selective alpha-2A adrenergic receptor agonists. Such medications primarily aim to alter neuromodulators of discrete transmitter networks within the brain. Because the neuromodulation is contrived, various contraindications, side effects, chemical/hormonal system imbalances leading to comorbid psychopathology and/or somatic problems, in addition to increased risk of medication addiction, to name a few considerations, emerge. Therefore, inducing similar neuromodulational change via less artificial bio-behavioral mechanisms presents a clinically cogent and ethical solution. Since the concept of ADHD represents a multisystem disorder with variation in pathology from relatively focal dysfunction to a large range of abnormalities organized along domains of neural systems and behavior; logically, treatment thus also requires a multisystem approach with flexibility and versatility to target multiple pathophysiological factors.

Mindfulness-based therapies for various medical and psychological conditions premise the following working pathways; (1) attention regulation; (2) somatic awareness; (3) emotion regulation; and (4) distance from a maladaptive self-perspective [3]. Theoretically, points (1)–(3) suggest high clinical relevance for attention deficits and related disorders, and as outlined later, for its mechanistic advantage for disorders underlined by dysfunctional fronto-limbic prefrontal (PFC)-amygdala

cortical networks. Specifically, mindfulness-based cognitive therapy (MBCT) is a form of sustained attention training incorporating psychoeducational units tailored for symptomatology. Preliminary studies demonstrate the efficacy of mindfulness for the treatment of adult ADHD, assessed using standardized clinical measures [4–6]. Whilst translational research into MBCT and cognate techniques are accumulating, empirical investigations and theory pertaining to neurodevelopmental disorders, including ADHD, remain marginal. This chapter offers an overview of the restricted extant research base concerning mindfulness interventions in the treatment of ADHD. An additional purpose of this chapter is to delineate the possible neural and psychological mechanisms involved. The research base regarding ADHD treatment with MBCT is limited, thus, several portions of this chapter aim to present germane theory connected to the possibilities of how mindfulness intervention could alleviate ADHD symptoms, supported by direct and indirect evidence. Interactions between the mindfulness technique and brain are introduced, providing a foundation for conjectures on brain-cognitive/behavioral mechanisms for ADHD.

Indirect Evidence: Theorizations in Directions for Mechanisms

Neurological/Anatomical Mechanism: Alterations in Brain Structure and Organization

Consistent principal findings regarding the neurobiological architecture of ADHD pertain to widespread cortical atrophy, altered gray and white matter morphology, in addition to impaired inter/intra-hemispheric connectivity. Whilst the involved cortical regions, neural systems, and clinical interplays of ADHD are convoluted, it is suggested that the pathophysiology of the disorder largely pertains to a cerebellar–prefrontal–striatal network [7]. The largest reductions in brain volume primarily allude to cerebellar structures, such as the posterior inferior vermis and splenium areas of the corpus callosum, compared to nonsignificant findings in non-splenium areas of the CC (see meta-analysis of Valera et al., [8]). Additionally, large volumetric differences between ADHD and control populations have been found in prefrontal and other frontal lobe areas. The prefrontal cortex (PFC), specifically the dorsolateral PFC (DLPFC) and fronto-orbital cortex (FOC), has high relevance to ADHD, due to their important roles in goal-directed operations (DLPFC) such as planning, organization, working memory, executive functioning, and the reward system (FOC).

Another important cortical region in terms of pathogenesis and function in ADHD is the anterior cingulate cortex (ACC), wherein reduced cortical thickness in this region has been associated with increased ADHD symptom severity, arising from dysregulation of the anterior attention network, i.e., rostral ACC/rACC [9]. Furthermore, the ACC is a key structure of the default-mode network/DMN [10], comprising other regions such as the precuneus, posterior cingulate cortex (PCC), and lateral parietal inferior gyri [11], wherein internally focused, stimuli-independent performance/task-specific processing is regulated by this system. The DMN component of the system interplays with the task-positive network (TPN), associated with moment-to-moment attention/processing for performance/task-specific functions. Evidence suggests ADHD adults and children [12, 13] display detrimentally prolonged DMN activity when task-specific processing, i.e., dominance of the TPN, is required, thus, interfering with the ability to perform attention/performance related tasks. Moreover, functional connectivity appears to be disrupted within the network at rest in ADHD [14], suggesting the ability to efficiently modulate DMN activity is hampered [15]. Prolonged mindfulness exposure has been associated with increased connectivity within the DMN system [16], in addition to between DMN structures and medial orbitofrontal regions interconnected to the limbic system, viscera-motor processing, and reward/pleasure pathways [17]. Enhanced connectivity of these regions with the DMN implicates increased processing capacity to disengage/engage the relevant networks (i.e., default/executive) via a salience network incorporating bottom-up visceral signals

alongside top-down cortical control [17]. Relevant to ADHD, diminished connectivity and regulation of this DMN/TPN interplay would entail inefficiency in disengaging-DMN/engaging-TPN activity to salient cues.

Peripherally connected research suggests that the haemodynamic brain correlates of the DMN are linked to specific temporal—(grossly) spatial electrocortical oscillations across differing frequencies reflecting an intrinsic baseline brain state [18, 19]. Due to the ubiquity of electrical oscillations within the brain, evidence supports the likelihood that the EEG-DMN connects to multiple frequencies, during eyes-closed and eyes-open resting-states [18]. Fronto-central distributed theta (4–7 Hz), bilateral distribution in posterior regions for alpha-1 (7.5–9.5 Hz) alpha-2 (10–12 Hz), and beta-1 (13–23 Hz), and prefrontal beta-2 (23–34 Hz) and gamma (35–45 Hz) distributions have been connected to EEG-DMN activity. Moreover, associations between blood oxygen level dependent (BOLD) fluctuations within DMN regions and cross-spectral electrocortical "signatures" present discrete functional significance [20]. Limited research examining mindfulness-induced changes to the DMN, gauged via EEG mean phase coherence (MPC), has shown increased α-activity and bilateralized decrease in functional connectivity; reduced right hemispheric theta compared to left hemispheric alpha and gamma MPC [21]. Putting these pieces together, MBCT presents a plausible mechanism to adaptively regulate the DMN/TPN interplay. This has been explored by a study currently under peer-review investigating EEG-DMN correlates in adult ADHD patients treated with 12-weeks MBCT versus wait-list controls [Schoenberg et al., currently unpublished]. In brief, beta-power increase was observed at rest, suggesting MBCT appeared to modulate the electro-cortical correlate viably connected to enhanced cortical alertness/activation and arousal of the DMN system, in turn, conceivably aiding the more efficient regulation of the DMN-TPN interplay within the disorder.

Returning to the neuroimaging evidence, remarkably structural and functional mindfulness-related changes in neuroanatomy have been observed. An uncontrolled non-randomized cross-sectional study presented increased gray matter density (cortical thickness) in prefrontal and parietal areas of the brain in meditators compared to non-meditators. Reported alterations were in structures pertinent to the pathophysiology of ADHD, such as regions associated with the dysregulation of attention, interoception, and sensory processing. Despite the methodological limitations of this first study [22], replicated findings of altered brain morphology have ensued (see review and meta-analysis, Fox et al., Tomasino et al., [23, 24]). Differing gray matter morphology have also been displayed in lower brain stem regions such as the medulla oblongata [26], a brain structure involved in connecting the central and autonomic nervous systems, and bridging lower brain regions with prefrontal regions. Such changes in brain structure are apparent at rest opposed to exclusively during meditation, highlighting the long-term effects on organic brain organization and function. Interestingly, gray matter density within the cerebellum, a subcortical region with the largest difference between (reduced levels in) ADHD versus controls, has been reported as higher in Tibetan Buddhist meditators practising a "pure" form of mindfulness compared to clinical interventions [25]. Although clearly accumulating, such neuroimaging data cannot infer causality, leading to the explanation that perhaps these various differences in cortical structure and organization between meditators and non-meditators reflects a predisposed alteration in brain morphology effecting meditators' drives, attention, and behaviors to engage in mindfulness (and other forms of meditation) initially. However, significantly increased gray matter density within the cerebellum, in addition to other less pertinent ADHD-related regions, has been observed during a longitudinal study investigating the effects of Mindfulness-Based Stress Reduction/MBSR [26]; wherein both MBCT and MBSR utilize the same mindfulness processes. Such data does not guarantee the translation of similar effects, or adaptive "recalibration," of these same altered cortical structures in ADHD. Albeit, they do provide plausible theoretical perspectives with regards to putative directions for future research

lines into the neuro-anatomical therapeutic pathways of mindfulness-based interventions in the treatment of ADHD and its sequelae.

White matter morphology and cortical connectivity also traverse both ADHD and mindfulness-based therapy outcomes. Significantly diminished deep frontal white matter in ADHD compared to controls may have pertinent implications, due to its involvement in cholinergic innervation to the brain. Altered cholinergic system activity asserts the primary neuromodulator involved in the combined ADHD-C subtype [27], thus, regulatory functions of attention, emotion, and goal-directed behavior. For example, frontal structural lesions in white matter disrupt cholinergic axonal projections originating in the basal forebrain, giving rise to significant cognitive complications [28, 29]. Likewise, attenuated fractional anisotropy of white matter tracts, reflecting impaired white matter fiber orientation and integrity [8, 30], have also, as with altered gray matter density, been found in cerebellar structures, and associated with increased severity of clinical (Conner's) inattention scores in ADHD [31]. Enhancement in white matter of meditators compared to non-meditators, particularly in regions associated with connectivity networks within the brain, such as the corpus callosum and superior longitudinal fasciculus, has been highlighted [23]. The latter structure pertains to bi-directional neuronal bundles that serve to connect the anterior and posterior regions of the cerebrum, detrimental to information transfer within various germane cognitive and affective operations, such as motor behavior control, focused spatial attention, and working memory.

Additionally, cortical connectivity has implications for sensory coding related to feedback interplays from higher-order cortical circuits towards the adaptive integration of sensory input with behavioral context [32]. Thus, enhancing connectivity within the cortex, via MBCT and related mindfulness interventions (as the indirect evidence suggests), may enact plausible mechanisms upon sensory-behavioral deficits in ADHD. For example, neuroimaging resting state data examining high versus low mindful breathing practise indicated those who engaged in mindfulness for longer exhibited increased connectivity within attentional networks [17].

Neuroendocrine/Physiologic Mechanisms: Chemical/Hormonal Pathways

Impact of the endocrinal system in the pathogenesis of ADHD has relatively recently entailed comprehensive research interest. As ADHD displays a multilayer disorder, the role of the endocrine system in neural circuitry development and interaction with associated physiological, affective, and behavioral systems appears clinically apt [33]. For example, neurosteroids, such as dehydroepiandrosterone sulfate (DHEA/DHEA-S), are principal substrates involved in mood, energy, aggression, and levels of activity [34], thus, have pertinent roles in goal-directed and self-regulation behaviors in ADHD.

One particular substrate of the endocrine system highly relevant to ADHD pertains to the hypothalamic–pituitary–thyroid (HPT) axis, involved in thyroid hormone production and regulation. Thyroid hormones are detrimental to human-fetal brain development [35], towards dendritic and axonal growth, synaptogenesis, neural migration, and the myelination of key neural networks and circuitry, particularly in hippocampal and prefrontal regions. Thus, enacting mechanisms involved in memory and attention operations. One measurement of the HPT-axis is thyroid stimulating hormone (TSH), found to be higher in children with ADHD compared to a highly prosocial group [36], where TSH levels have not shown any relationship to neurocognitive attention domains, rather have been linked to hyperactivity/impulsivity symptoms and dysregulation in mood within the disorder [37, 38]. Moreover, other hormonal mechanisms suggest elevated testosterone levels in ADHD, whereby gonadal hormones shape prenatal development of dopaminergic neural circuitry and pathways (connected to hyperactivity/impulsivity ADHD-II branch) in the pertinent cortical regions associated with ADHD morphology and functioning, namely the nucleus accumbens, striatum, and prefrontal cortex [33].

These findings are interesting considering a different technique of meditation (emphasizing focused concentration training) has highlighted long-term effects on hormonal changes in the human body, such as progressive decrease in serum TSH, growth hormone, and prolactin levels - peptide hormones largely associated with human immune system regulation [39]— further to lowering testosterone levels [40]. These previous studies offer peripheral evidence, in that, although it is not necessarily plausible to surmise findings from one meditation technique will translate to another, both the cited meditation technique and mindfulness train the process of "concentration" (being totally immersed in the "here and now" or on a fixed point), which may be the component that enacts neurochemical impact to the endocrine system via changes in cortico-subcortical projections and alterations in thyroid and steroid hormone concentrations.

An outstanding contention regarding the interplay between mindfulness and the neuroendocrine system concerns the hypothalamic–pituitary–adrenal (HPA) axis, regulated by limbic brain structures such as the amygdala, hippocampus, and hypothalamus and subsequent interaction with the adrenal (or suprarenal) glands. The HPA axis is central within the neuroendocrine system towards controlling emotional and bodily reactions to stress, general mood and emotions, and other bodily functions. Thus, potentially implicated in sensory- and emotion- regulation disturbances connected to hyperactive/impulsive ADHD subtype. One measure of HPA activity is the steroid hormone cortisol, wherein diminished levels have been noted in ADHD [41, 42] and weakly correlate with hyperactivity symptoms in children (6–17 years). Low cortisol levels indicate HPA-axis dysfunction, and may be associated with basal metabolic underarousal within the disorder, also evident within the cortical system, ensuing elevated thresholds to environmental cues and "over-compensatory" symptoms (i.e., increasing sensation from external stimuli/activity). Mindfulness has shown to "normalize" abnormal basal serum cortisol concentrations in post-traumatic stress disorder treatment [43], and the concentration meditation technique has shown to lower cortisol levels in healthy people [44]; in these cases cortisol modulation served to adaptively reduce physiological and emotional lability towards stressors. It remains to be determined, and presents an interesting avenue to explore, whether mindfulness treatment has potential scope to optimize/normalize discrete components of the HPT- and HPA-axes, and associated neuroendocrine system function in ADHD.

A further psychoneuroendocrinological avenue of potential interest pertains to mindfulness-related effects upon immune cell telomerase activity and structure (see reviews of Schutte and Malouff, [45]). Telomerase activity is an indicator of cellular variability and immune cell longevity, with high genetic heritability, and has been associated with the hyperactivity/impulsivity dimension in ADHD [46]. The concept that detrimental cellular effects and their interplay with adverse environmental exposure, can be mediated by mindfulness intervention poses a highly interesting epigenetic research avenue with regards to mindfulness mechanisms in the treatment of ADHD, particularly for behavioral problems arising from hyperactivity/impulsivity symptoms and related exacerbation in executive functioning. It remains to be determined what degree of specificity such a concept (and the currently limited empirical data) presents within ADHD.

Direct Evidence: Extant Progress on Mindfulness Intervention Mechanisms for ADHD

Neurotransmitter/Chemical Mechanisms: Mediated Synaptic Pathways

The brain is arguably the most complex system known to humankind. The average human brain consists of an estimated $2.0-5.0 \times 10^{11}$ cortical neurons arranged in intricate neural networks, which "communicate" via the process of neurotransmission fired by a conjectured 10^{14} synapses; roughly 2000–5000 "tagged" to each neuron. Electroencephalographic (EEG) recording amplifies the electrical activity generated by synaptic "firing" of large populations of neurons (neural networks) within the brain, thus constituting a peripheral measure of neurotransmission.

One etiological pathway of ADHD posits dysregulation in neurotransmitter systems. Moreover, diversification in neurotransmission levels can be linked to variation in clinical symptomatology. The complex neurochemical and neurotransmission interactions involved are intricate and beyond the scope of this chapter, thus to categorize, principal inattention subtype (ADHD-I) largely connects to altered norepinephrine levels (regulated by norepinephrine transporter genes), whilst hyperactivity subtype (ADHD-II) is largely associated with dopaminergic levels regulated by dopamine transporter genes [47, 48]. It is suggested that combined type (ADHD-C) patients may also be characterized by mutated choline transporter genes, in turn affecting acetylcholine neurotransmission levels [27]. Additionally, although less emphasized, impairments in the serotonergic system of ADHD patients can have adverse impact on emotion regulation within the disorder [49].

Psychopharmacological treatments for ADHD primarily target adrenomedullary neurohormones, in sum, by enhancing the availability of catecholamines in the synaptic cleft. The majority of medications target either the dopaminergic systems or norepinephrine systems, with a large portion of ADHD patients also taking anti-depressant medications aiming to focus on serotonin metabolism and alleviation of emotion regulation problems implied in professional-, social-aspects, and quality of life. Presently, the cholinergic system is largely ignored by psychopharmacological treatments, with no specific extant medications developed to target such neurotransmitters. Interestingly, a recent proposal by Potter et al. [50] has advocated the development of ADHD-specific interventions that target the nicotinic cholinergic system for its affective regulatory role in cortical connectivity and effects upon the adaptive regulation of the neural reward system.

Despite the centrality of dysregulation in neurohormonal homeostasis in ADHD, no presently published neurochemical studies have examined transmission level and change in the disorder following exposure to MBCT, potentially providing greater insight into the neural and clinical working mechanisms of the intervention. However, the investigation of various event-related potentials (ERPs) associated with sustained attention, performance monitoring, and inhibitory control, thus providing peripheral measurement of catecholaminergic functioning, have been examined in adult ADHD patients pre-to-post MBCT intervention [6]. Neurophysiological data were collected concomitant to a continuous performance task (CPT-X), wherein the ERN and Pe (error processing), NoGo-N2 (conflict monitoring), and No-P3 (inhibitory/motor control) ERPs were observed. The study highlighted MBCT-related modulation in ERPs underpinned by the adrenergic system (norepinephrine neurotransmission), namely the NoGo-P3, rather than dopaminergic system such as the ERN. Furthermore, enhanced NoGo-P3 amplitude indexing improved inhibitory and motor control were associated with alleviation in inattention symptoms, whilst increased Pe amplitudes reflecting improved error saliency/awareness correlated with amelioration in hyperactivity/impulsivity symptoms also supported by a positive correlation with the "act-with-awareness" mindfulness domain. Change in the Pe component of the error processing system also implied an improvement in emotional self-regulation of the affect-motivation-arousal matrix, a facet of ADHD symptomatology often overshadowed by more pressing attentional and executive deficits.

In sum, MBCT appears to enact comparable neurophysiological change connected to attention and self-regulation as pharmacology. However, the findings also allude to the potential scope of mindfulness-based interventions to engage both "top-down" neural pathways implicated in attention and executive control, in addition to "bottom-up" bio-behavioral and emotional self-regulatory neural pathways, wherein its primary target is to increase vigilance via innervation of the adrenergic system, opposed to increasing focused attention mechanisms related to the dopaminergic system.

Neurocognitive/Psychological Mechanisms: Modulated Brain Function

The majority of neurocognitive deficits in ADHD pertain to executive functions, such as planning, organization, performance monitoring, behavioral adjustment, working memory, and problem solving. The preceding sections have provided some information as to the neuro-anatomical/chemical/physiological basis of these "distal phenotypes." Mechanistically, executive functioning may be subsumed into three overarching components: (1) shifting between tasks or mental sets, (2) updating and monitoring of working memory representations, and (3) inhibition of prepotent responses [51], wherein all three units show disruption in ADHD.

Theories outlining multiple neurocognitive pathways connected to ADHD essentially propose that deficits in performance monitoring and subsequent behavioral control to environmental cues are likely fostered by insufficient signalling between the prefrontal cortex from subcortical and posterior systems. Thus, such models posit either dysregulation in the signalling of bottom-up mechanisms ensuing diminished capacity in context-template upgrading, such as to detect discrepancies between current and subsequent/expected outcomes. Alternatively, adaptive signalling in the presence of diminished top-down control mechanisms. ADHD represents a syndrome with discrete clinical subtypes, wherein a dual pathway concept proposes that deficits in attention and executive functioning are related to dysregulation in prefrontal–striatal circuits, whereas hyperactivity is connected to dysregulation of fronto-limbic system [52].

Available specific evidence illustrates that, aside from distinct potential attention training pathways, mindfulness-based techniques have modulating roles within the principal executive domains (outlined above). For example, actions upon aspects of performance monitoring, including mental "switching" capacity and its subsequent efficacy upon inhibitory control, have been found in adults with ADHD exposed to MBCT, not evident in a waitlist control group [6]. Not directly related to ADHD, although still pertinent, improvements in working memory capacity concomitant to diminished mind-wandering in those with high distractibility, have been reported [53].

Whilst the concept of attention training is paramount in the neurocognitive/psychological therapeutic pathway of MBCT for ADHD, executive functioning may also be an outcome of enhanced affective self-regulation. For example, a neurophysiological correlate of affective evaluation to error-making, usually attenuated in ADHD, increased pre-to-post MBCT, in turn improving inhibitory control. It could be reasoned that this process came about by elevation within the arousal-activation-motivation matrix [54], positively impacting self-regulation and engagement within a sustained attention cognitive task, ergo increasing task saliency. An aside, motivational salience towards stimuli has been connected to increased prefrontal norepinephrine levels [55]. Overall, empirical evidence suggests MBCT has the potential to target both top-down and bottom-up pathways concomitant to amelioration in the inattentive/executive functioning and hyperactivity/impulsivity symptom domains.

Considerations

The caution required when assimilating the regulatory effects of mindfulness-based intervention for psychiatric conditions is already well highlighted within the scientific community. Presently, mindfulness research is limited with regards to multifaceted methodological limitations, regarding experiment design issues and causality, generalizability of results across different mindfulness techniques and studied clinical populations, controlling for medication (especially applicable to ADHD), the need for standardization in mindfulness treatment programs especially adapted for ADHD, standardization in reporting such information, conscience of a purely objective opposed to an overly "pro-mindfulness" scientific stance, and so on (*other points covered here* [56]). Minimal comprehensive research has been conducted into possible "side effects" of mindfulness programs for the different disorders, and none into ADHD. Perhaps such information will be elucidated alongside more insightful neuro/clinical mechanistic understanding. A "dark" fringe movement within mindfulness research is forming [57, 58], spurred by the idea [59] that the psychiatric and psychotherapeutic fields still lack considerable illumination with regards to treatment interplays at micro and macro scales. Conversely, a large portion of detrimental effects reported via such practise may be from incorrect technique and not from standardized treatment programs such as MBCT. Moreover, the knowledge, effort, and skill development required to implement mindfulness correctly is rarely acknowledged in scientific reports. Despite these considerations, the fact remains that data advocating mindfulness treatment for various psychiatric disorders, and as outlined here, its pertinent applicability to ADHD, is exponentially accruing. Mindfulness is not a simple internal process; ergo, the associated outputs and interplays are unsurprisingly complex. Hence, the importance of mindfulness to be incorporated systematically into clinical treatment programs, such as MBCT, for its optimal impact for ADHD.

Synthesis

The etiological matrix of ADHD is convoluted and multileveled involving altered genetic and phenotypic interplays. Epigenetic factors impart early developmental/environmental stressors significantly affecting genetic mutations specific to attention disorders, thus altering phenotypic expression, cortical structure/function, synaptic development and plasticity. Based on the course of these factors, germane dysregulation in neurotransmitter systems/metabolism and cortical organization of pertinent neural circuitry, determine deficits in brain function pertaining to attention, motivation, cortical arousal, motor control, and executive functioning. The limited evidence base thus far infers that neuroanatomical alterations in brain structure and organization via mindfulness intervention may largely be implicated with attentional deficits. Furthermore, increased connectivity within and between viable cortical regions plausibly serves the efficient regulation of cortical-subcortical circuitry and networks, implicated in attention and executive function. Conversely, amelioration in the hyperactivity/impulsivity domain suggest optimization of pertinent neuro-endocrine/-hormonal regulatory mechanisms. In turn, neurochemical alteration to adrenergic system metabolism and activity ensues, associated with norepinephrine neurotransmission in ADHD. Less support is available for dopaminergic pathway clinical action. Mindfulness intervention for ADHD suggests scope to target sensory visceral "bottom-up" signalling concomitant to enhanced cortical control in "top-down" neural circuitry. These preliminary findings pertaining to mindfulness treatment in ADHD must be interpreted with caution. Albeit, direct and indirect evidence attests MBCT as a polymorphic clinical construct with the possibility to target concurrent pathways pertaining to ADHD, on neuro-anatomical, -chemical, -hormonal, -cognitive and -psychological dimensions.

References

1. Zylowska L, Smalley SL, Schwartz JM. Mindful awareness and ADHD. In: Fabrizio D, editor. Clinical handbook of mindfulness. New York, NY: Springer; 2009. p. 319–38.
2. Simon V, Czobbor P, Baliant S, Meszaros A, Bitter I. Prevalence and correlates of adult attention-deficit hyperactivity disorder: meta-analysis. Br J Psychiatry. 2009;194:204–11. doi:10.1192/bjp.bp.107.048827.
3. Hölzel BK, Lazar SW, Gard T, Schuman-Olivier Z, Vago DR, Ott U. How does mindfulness meditation work? Proposing mechanisms of action from a conceptual and neural perspective. Perspect Psychol Sci. 2011;6:537–59.
4. Zylowska L, Ackerman DL, Yang MH, Futrell JL, Horton NL, Hale TS, et al. Mindfulness meditation training in adults and adolescents with ADHD: a feasibility study. J Atten Disord. 2008;11:737–46. doi:10.1177/1087054707308502.
5. Mitchell JT, McIntyre EM, English JS, Dennis MF, Beckham JC, Kollins SH. A pilot trial of mindfulness meditation training for ADHD in adulthood: impact on core symptoms, executive functioning, and emotion dysregulation. J Atten Disord. 2015;2015:16 pages. doi:10.1177/1087054713513328.
6. Schoenberg PLA, Hepark S, Kan CC, Barendregt HP, Buitelaar JK, Speckens AEM. Effects of mindfulness-based cognitive therapy on neurophysiological correlates of performance monitoring in adult attention-deficit/hyperactivity disorder. Clin Neurophysiol. 2014;125:1407–16.
7. Giedd JN, Blumenthal J, Molloy E, Castellanos FX. Brain imaging of attention deficit/hyperactivity disorder. In: Wasserstein J, Wolf L, editors. Adult attention deficit disorder: brain mechanisms and life outcomes. Annals of the New York Academy Sciences, vol. 931. New York, NY: Academy of Sciences; 2001.
8. Valera EM, Faraone SV, Murray KE, Seidman LJ. Meta-analysis of structural imaging findings in attention-deficit/hyperactivity disorder. Biol Psychiatry. 2007;61:1361–9.
9. Bledsoe JC, Semrud-Clikeman M, Pilszka SR. Anterior cingulate cortex and symptom severity in attention-deficit/hyperactivity disorder. J Abnorm Psychol. 2013;122:558–65.
10. Raichle ME, MacLeod AM, Snyder AZ, Powers WJ, Gusnard DA, Shulman GL. A default mode of brain function. Proc Natl Acad Sci U S A. 2001;98:676–82.
11. Buckner RL, Andrews-Hanna J, Schachter D. The brain's default network: anatomy, function, and relevance to disease. Ann N Y Acad Sci. 2008;1124:1–38.
12. Cortese S, Kelly C, Chabernaud C, Proal E, Di Martino A, Milham MP, et al. Toward systems neuroscience of ADHD: a meta-analysis of 55 fMRI studies. Am J Psychiatry. 2012;169:1038–55.
13. Hart H, Radua J, Nakao T, Mataix-Cols D, Rubia K. Meta-analysis of functional magnetic resonance imaging studies of inhibition and attention in attention-deficit/hyperactivity disorder: exploring task-specific, stimulant medication, and age effects. Arch Gen Psychiatry. 2013;70:85–198.
14. Uddin LQ, Kelly AMC, Biswal BB, Margulies DS, Shehzad Z, Shaw D, et al. Network homogeneity reveals decreased integrity of default-mode network in ADHD. J Neurosci Methods. 2008;169:249–54.
15. Fair DA, Posner J, Nagel BJ, Bathula D, Dias TGC, Mills KL, et al. Atypical default network connectivity in youth with attention-deficit/hyperactivity disorder. Biol Psychiatry. 2010;68:1084–91.
16. Taylor VA, Daneault V, Grant J, Scavone G, Breton E, Roffe-Vidal S, et al. Impact of meditation training on the default mode network during restful state. Soc Cogn Affect Neurosci. 2013;8:4–14.

17. Hasenkamp W, Barsalou LW. Effects of meditation experience on functional connectivity of distributed brain networks. Front Hum Neurosci. 2012;6:38. doi:10.3389/fnhum.2012.00038.

18. Chen ACN, Feng W, Zhao H, Yin Y, Wang P. EEG default mode network in the human brain: spectral regional field powers. Neuroimage. 2008;41:561–74.

19. Mantini D, Perrucci MG, Del Gratta C, Romani GL, Corbetta M. Electrophysiological signatures of resting state networks in the human brain. Proc Natl Acad Sci U S A. 2007;104:13170–5.

20. Neuner I, Arrubla J, Werner CJ, Hitz K, Boers F, Kawohl W, et al. The default mode network and EEG regional spectral power: a simultaneous fMRI-EEG study. PLoS One. 2014;9, e88214. doi:10.1371/journal.pone.0088214.

21. Berkovich-Ohana A, Glicksohn J, Goldstein A. Studying the default mode and its mindfulness-induced changes using EEG functional connectivity. Soc Cogn Affect Neurosci. 2013. doi:10.1093/scan/nst153.

22. Lazar SW, Kerr CE, Wasserman RH, Gray JR, Greve DN, Treadway MT, et al. Meditation experience is associated with increased cortical thickness. Neuroreport. 2005;16:1893–7.

23. Fox KCR, Nijeboer S, Dixon ML, Floman JL, Ellamil M, Rumak SP, et al. Is meditation associated with altered brain structure? A systematic review and meta-analysis of morphometric neuroimaging in meditation practitioners. Neurosci Biobehav Rev. 2014;43:48–73.

24. Tomasino B, Chiesa A, Fabbro F. Disentangling the neural mechanisms involved in Hinduism- and Buddhism-related meditations. Brain Cogn. 2014;90:32–40.

25. Vestergaard-Poulsen P, van Beek M, Skewes J, Bjarkam CR, Stubberup M, Bertelsen J, et al. Long-term meditation is associated with increased gray matter density in the brain stem. Neuroreport. 2009;20:170–4.

26. Hölzel BK, Carmody J, Vangel M, Congleton C, Yerramsetti SM, Gard T, et al. Mindfulness practice leads to increases in regional brain gray matter density. Psychiatry Res. 2011;191:36–43.

27. English BA, Hahn MK, Gizer IR, Mazel-Robison M, Steele A, Kurnik DM, et al. Choline transporter gene variation is associated with attention-deficit hyperactivity disorder. J Neurodev Disord. 2009;1: 252–63.

28. Bohnen NI, Bogan CW, Müller MLTM. Frontal and periventricular brain white matter lesions and cortical deafferentation of cholinergic and other neuromodulatory axonal projections. Eur Neurol J. 2009;1:33–50.

29. Schmahmann JD, Smith EE, Eichler FS, Filley CM. Cerebral white matter: neuroanatomy, clinical neurology, and neurobehavioral correlates. Ann NY Acad Sci. 2008;1142:266–309.

30. Makris N, Papadimitriou GM, Worth AJ, Jenkins BG, Garrido L, Sorenson AG, et al. Diffusion tensor imaging. In: Davis KL, Charney D, Coyle JT, Nemeroff C, editors. Neuropsychopharmacology: the fifth generation of progress. New York, NY: American College of Neuropsychopharmacology. Lippincott Williams & Wilkins; 2002. p. 357–71.

31. Ashtari M, Kumra S, Bhaskar SL, Clarke T, Thaden E, Cervellione KL, et al. Attention-deficit/hyperactivity disorder: a preliminary diffusion tensor imaging study. Biol Psychiatry. 2005;57:448–55.

32. Harris KD, Mrsic-Flogel TD. Cortical connectivity and sensory coding. Nature. 2013;503:51–8.

33. Martel MM, Klump K, Nigg JT, Breedlove SM, Sisk CL. Potential hormonal mechanisms of attention-deficit/hyperactivity disorder and major depressive disorder: a new perspective. Horm Behav. 2009;55:465–79.

34. Wang L-J, Chen C-K. The potential role of neuroendocrine in patients with attention-deficit/hyperactivity disorder. In: Banerjee S, editor. Attention-deficit hyperactivity disorder in children and adolescents. Rijeka: InTech; 2013.

35. De Escobar GM, Obregon MJ, del Rey FE. Maternal thyroid hormones early in pregnancy and fetal brain development. Best practice and research. Clin Endocrinol Metab. 2004;18:225–48.

36. Al-Thwaini AN, Abdul-Wahid SSH, Jawad SQ. Level of thyroid stimulating hormone concentration in a sample of hyperactive versus pro-social school children in Iraqi city. Int J Pure Appl Biosci. 2014;2:118–23.

37. Hauser P, Soler R, Brucker-Davis F, Weintraub BD. Thyroid hormones correlate with symptoms of hyperactivity but not inattention in attention deficit hyperactivity disorder. Psychoneuroendocrinology. 1997;22:107–14.

38. Stein MA, Weiss RE. Thyroid function tests and neurocognitive functioning in children referred for attention deficit/hyperactivity disorder. Psychoneuroendocrinology. 2003;28:304–16.

39. Werner OR, Wallace RK, Charles B, Janssen G, Stryker T, Chalmers RA. Long-term endocrinologic changes in subjects practising the transcendental meditation and TM-Sidhi program. Psychosom Med. 1986;48:59–66.

40. MacLean CRK. Effects of the transcendental meditation program on adaptive mechanisms: changes in hormone levels and responses to stress after 4 months of practise. Psychoneuroendocrinology. 1997;22:277–95.

41. Isaksson J, Nilsson KW, Nyberg F, Hogmark A, Lindblad F. Cortisol levels in children with attention-deficit/hyperactivity disorder. J Psychiatr Res. 2012;46:1398–405. doi:10.1016/j.jpsychires.2012 .08.021.

42. Kariyawasam SH, Zaw F, Handley SL. Reduced salivary cortisol in children with comorbid attention deficit hyperactivity disorder and oppositional defiant disorder. Neuroendocrinol Lett. 2002;23:45–8.

43. Kim SH, Schneider SM, Bevans M, Kravitz L, Mermier C, Qualls C, et al. PTSD symptom reduction with mindfulness-based stretching and deep breathing exercise: randomized controlled clinical trial of efficacy. J Clin Endocrinol Metab. 2013;98:2984–92.

44. Rafael JI, Peran F, Martinez M, Roldan A, Poyatos R, Ruiz F, et al. ACTH and β-endorphin in transcendental meditation. Physiol Behav. 1998;64:311–5.

45. Schutte NS, Malouff JM. A meta-analytic review of the effects of mindfulness meditation on telomerase activity. Psychoneuroendocrinology. 2014;42:45–8.

46. Costa DS, Rosa DVF, Barros AGA, Romano-Silva MA, Malloy-Diniz LF, Mattos P, et al. Telomere length is highly inherited and associated with hyperactivity-impulsivity in children with attention deficit/hyperactivity disorder. Front Mol Neurosci. 2015;8:28. doi:10.3389/fnmol.2015.00028.

47. Kim CH, Hahn MK, Joung Y, Steele AH, Gizer I, Cohen BM, et al. A polymorphism in the norepinephrine transporter gene alters promoter activity and is associated with attention-deficit hyperactivity disorder. Proc Natl Acad Sci U S A. 2006;103:19164–9.

48. Mazei-Robison MS, Couch RS, Blakely RD. Sequence variation in the human dopamine transporter gene in children with attention deficit hyperactivity disorder. Neuropharmacology. 2005;49:724–36.

49. Nikolas M, Friderici K, Waldman I, Jernigan K, Nigg JT. Gene x environment interactions for ADHD: synergistic effect of 5HTTLPR genotype and youth appraisals of interparental conflict. Behav Brain Funct. 2010;6:23. doi:10.1186/1744-9081-6-23.

50. Potter AS, Schaubhut G, Shipman M. Targeting the nicotinic cholinergic system to treat attention-deficit/hyperactivity disorder: rationale and progress to date. CNS Drugs. 2014;28:1103–13.

51. Miyake A, Friedman NP, Emerson MJ, Witzki AH, Howerter A, Wager TD. The united and diversity of executive functions and their contributions to complex "frontal lobe: tasks: a latent variable analysis. Cogn Psychol. 2000;41:49–100.

52. Sonuga-Barke EJ. The dual pathway model of AD/HD: an elaboration of neuro-developmental characteristics. Neurosci Biobehav Rev. 2003;27:593–604.

53. Mrazek MD, Franklin MS, Phillips DT, Baird B, Schooler JW. Mindfulness training improves working memory capacity and GRE performance while reducing mind wandering. Psychol Sci. 2013;24:776–81.

54. Barkley RA. Behavioral inhibition, sustained attention, and executive functions: constructing a unifying theory of ADHD. Psychol Bull. 1997;121:65–94.

55. Ventura R, Latagliata EC, Morrone C, La Mela I, Puglisi-Allegra S. Prefrontal norepinephrine determines attribution of "high" motivational salience. PLoS One. 2008;3, e3044.

56. Tang YY, Posner MI. Tools of the trade: theory and method in mindfulness neuroscience. Soc Cogn Affect Neurosci. 2013;8:118–20.

57. Britton W, Lindahl J, and colleagues. http://cheetahhouse.org. Accessed 31 July 2015.

58. Compson J. Meditation, trauma and suffering in silence: raising questions about how meditation is taught and practiced in western contexts in light of a contemporary trauma resiliency model. ConBuddh. 2014. doi:10.1080/14639947.2014.935264.

59. Dimidjian S, Hollon SD. How would we know if psychotherapy were harmful? Am Psychol. 2010; 65:21–33.

Mindfulness-Based Cognitive Therapy and Caregivers of Cancer Survivors

18

Andrew W. Wood, Jessica Gonzalez, and Sejal M. Barden

Introduction

The use of mindfulness-based cognitive therapy (MBCT) is vast, as illustrated throughout this book. The use of MBCT and its related therapies has extended into medical settings, which is appropriate as mindfulness-based stress reduction (MBSR), from which MBCT was based, originated in a medical setting [1, 2]. However, a caregiving population has not been explicitly highlighted in MBCT literature. Existing on the periphery of formalized medical care, informal caregivers experience significant burden in providing care for others (e.g., family and friends). We believe that informal caregivers, specifically those of cancer survivors, would greatly benefit from MBCT treatment as a way to relieve burden and to

transition into a "being mode" while providing care. The purpose of this chapter is to introduce the application of MBCT for caregivers of cancer survivors. In this chapter, we detail the rationale for using MBCT with caregivers of cancer survivors, highlighting how MBCT could meet the needs of caregivers of cancer survivors, and how to adapt the current MBCT format [3] to a group of those providing care for cancer survivors. Recommendations based on various clinical concerns, questions for reflection, and resources are also included at the conclusion of this chapter.

Caregiver Concerns

In a 2015 survey, National Alliance for Caregiving (NAC) and American Association for Retired People (AARP) [4] surveyed 1248 informal caregivers in the USA; results estimated that 43.5 million people in the USA have served as informal caregivers to adults within the last year, identifying cancer as one of the five reasons they were providing care. Formal caregivers are paid professionals such as nurses or government employees that receive payment to assist in the daily needs of people who are physically or mentally ill. Informal caregivers are often unpaid family members or friends who are assisting in the care of family members who are physically or mentally ill, resulting in 83 % of overall caregivers [5]. For the purposes of this chapter, the term caregiver indicates informal caregivers,

A.W. Wood, Ph.D. (✉)
School of Applied Psychology, Counseling, and Family Therapy, Clinical Mental Health Counseling, Antioch University, 2326 Sixth Ave., Seattle, WA 98121, USA
e-mail: awood5@antioch.edu

J. Gonzalez, Ph.D.
College of Health and Human Science, School of Education Counseling and Career Development, Colorado State University, 1588 Campus Delivery, Fort Collins, CO 80523-1588, USA

S.M. Barden, Ph.D.
Child, Family and Community Sciences, College of Education, University of Central Florida, 12494 University Boulevard, Orlando, FL 32816, USA

© Springer International Publishing Switzerland 2016
S.J. Eisendrath (ed.), *Mindfulness-Based Cognitive Therapy*, DOI 10.1007/978-3-319-29866-5_18

unless otherwise stated. Thirty-eight percent of caregivers report having emotional stress and 20% report having physical strain from their caregiving responsibilities [4]. Furthermore, caregivers of cancer survivors experience unique features while providing care.

Despite advances in early detection of cancer and treatment, a cancer diagnosis persists as a life stressor for cancer patients and their caregivers. The American Cancer Society [6] reports that cancer is the second most common cause of death, with an average of 1600 deaths per day in the USA. Family members are often the primary caregivers of cancer survivors and often overlook their own needs, placing emphasis on the needs of their loved ones. Results from a 2013 longitudinal study investigating the most common unmet needs reported by cancer caregivers were (1) fear of a cancer diagnosis returning; (2) reducing stress in the person they are providing care for; and (3) increased understanding of the cancer experience for whom they are providing care [7]. Thus, caregivers identify their primary responsibilities as caring for another individual and tend to put aside their self-care needs, influencing their quality of life.

Quality of life is the overall sense of well-being individuals have in various aspects of their lives and is a common variable measured to understand the effect of cancer on one's life. Informal caregivers' quality of life can be positively or negatively impacted by caregiver burden [8]. While some caregivers report experiencing positive changes such as finding personal meaning through caregiving [9] more commonly reported symptoms or effects include heightened experiences of dysphoria, fatigue, and depression [10, 11]. The activities of providing care for another individual can contribute to caregiver fatigue. Fatigue, or burnout, is a frequently disabling symptom [10, 12] experienced by caregivers [13]. Contributions to caregiver fatigue include caregivers' lack of social support [14] and economic stressors (e.g., taking time off from paying jobs to provide on average of 21 h or more per week of care) [4]. Untreated caregiver fatigue can lead to impairment in daily functioning [13, 15], anxiety [16], and depression [17].

Informal caregivers are the primary support system for the person they are providing care for, yet often do not have a support system of their own. Lack of perceived social support can negatively impact caregivers' ability to cope with daily stressors [14] and can increase the likelihood of fatigue, anxiety, burden of care, and overall quality of life [4, 18]. Conversely, informal caregivers who have a perceived social support may have decreased symptoms of caregiver burden. Ownsworth et al. [19] assessed cancer caregivers for factors that may moderate caregiver psychological well-being and found that psychological well-being was associated with satisfaction in social support and resources. In a study with caregivers of individuals with intellectual disabilities, results indicated that symptoms of depression and anxiety decreased while positive social interactions increased after the intervention [20]. Similarly, results from a review of 30 quantitative and quasi-experimental controlled trialed studies on the effectiveness of support groups for caregivers of patients suffering from dementia indicated that support groups are benef icial for caregivers [21].

Caregivers experience both positive and negative aspects of caregiving [22]. Although interventions can be used to focus on strength-based coping [23], it may be necessary for many caregivers to alleviate mental health symptoms directly to improve the quality of life of caregivers and those for whom they care [24]. MBCT may be an intervention that can aid caregivers in their own lives and in providing care for cancer survivors.

Theoretical Rationale of MBCT for Caregivers

Addressing the broad array of burdens that caregivers face during the MBCT sessions allows caregivers to share with other group members in a safe environment, a task that is difficult for caregivers, especially for those that have been caring for extended periods of time [25]. The needs that cancer survivors have such as transportation to medical appointments or frailty due to medical treatment form one type of caregiver burden. Caregivers may also experience psychological distress from watching those who they provide care for suffer through their disease and treatments.

MBCT is an intervention that can be used in group form that encourages informal caregivers to discuss their caregiver burden experiences and increase coping mechanisms to decrease symptoms of depression and anxiety. Further, because a group format is commonly used with MBCT, caregivers can see the strain that other caregivers face and can build a group that promotes hope, universality, catharsis, and other curative factors that groups provide [26]. Further, MBCT can be helpful because it focuses on a set of skills to impart to members to help them increase their well-being, regardless of a major psychiatric diagnosis or overarching symptoms (e.g., anxiety). Due to the burden that caregivers face, focusing on thoughts and feelings relating to guilt, anger, and sadness should be a primary concern for MBCT practitioners [3, 11]. Recognizing thoughts and feelings as they occur can help caregivers accept them as unique and decrease instances of rumination during their day-to-day care activities.

Additional reasons that MBCT may be helpful with caregivers of cancer survivors are the fear of recurrence in cancer and the focus on destabilizing this mindset in MBCT. A fear of recurrence is common in cancer survivors and their caregivers [27]. However, a main focus of MBCT is to recognize recurring thoughts and meet them with acceptance rather than challenge or delving into usual thought patterns. As Teasdale and colleagues [28] found, MBCT was helpful in working with individuals to break from recurrent depressive episodes. Part of the reasoning for MBCT's effectiveness is a focus on breaking from ruminating thoughts into acceptance of initial thoughts before a snowball effect occurs [3]. Similarly, with a fear of recurrence, the ruminating thoughts about the possibility of a cancer coming back, while being realistic concerns, can be met with acceptance rather than rumination, possibly causing an increased well-being in caregivers of cancer survivors.

Another benefit of using MBCT with caregivers is the brevity of the intervention. MBCT is provided in a group format, which is presented in 2-h group sessions for 8 weeks [3]. Group members are encouraged to practice mindful exercises and homework related to cognitive processes between sessions (e.g., noticing positive, negative, and activating events leading to thoughts). Group members are only in sessions for a short amount of time, so a focus of MBCT is to help group members utilize the lessons learned from the MBCT group sessions outside of class in their everyday life to prevent relapse of negative emotions [3, 28]. The brevity of MBCT can also be helpful in that caregivers already devote a great deal of time to providing care [4], and thus a short treatment would provide less of a burden in conjunction with their caregiving duties. Also, if planned effectively by a cancer treatment center or hospital, the group could take place during the treatment of cancer survivors, limiting the travel time and costs associated with receiving the MBCT intervention. In addition to the stated rationale to use MBCT with caregivers of cancer survivors, there is evidence that its putative mechanisms of change may be effective in this population.

Mechanisms of Change

The processes by which MBCT can be effective with caregivers of cancer survivors are multifaceted. As stated previously, informal caregivers provide care for family members or friends. This caregiving relationship alters the relationship between caregivers and cancer survivors. In order to accommodate a changing relationship and impending caregiver burden, MBCT can work to bring awareness to feelings of anxiety, stress, or depression due to caregiving and help caregivers to appropriately process their feelings.

To support these purported mechanisms of change, the current evidence for the use of MBCT with caregivers of cancer survivors will be discussed. Some of the support for the use of MBCT is derived from mindfulness and similar therapeutic approaches used with caregivers, as well as evidence for MBCT's use to combat issues that caregivers can face. Recently, there has been a surge of empirical evidence that supports the efficacy of MBCT with a variety of individuals [29–31].

Empirical Support of MBCT for Caregivers of Cancer Survivors

A review of empirical support for MBCT must be qualified in that there is only limited evidence for its use with caregivers of cancer survivors. Thus, it is necessary to investigate the components of MBCT and related treatments to understand how MBCT can be effective with this population. We provide a short review of empirical evidence supporting the use of mindfulness with caregivers, MBSR with caregivers, and finally MBCT with caregivers.

In a review of mindfulness studies, Keng et al. [32] found that mindfulness practice provides an overall increase in well-being and emotional reactivity, as well as a reduction of psychological symptoms (e.g., symptoms of anxiety). In more recent research, Paller and colleagues [33] found that a mindfulness program developed for caregivers of individuals with Alzheimer's disease experienced increased quality of life and fewer depressive symptoms after the course. Kögler and colleagues [34] found that mindfulness was a predictor of less psychological distress, increased meaning in life, and increased quality of life in caregivers of individuals receiving palliative care. Furthermore, Lunksy et al. [35] developed a mindfulness-based coping with stress group for caregivers of individuals with developmental disabilities, ranging from children to adults. Lunksy and colleagues found that caregivers reported lower stress after the intervention. Further evidence for using MBCT with caregivers of cancer survivors can be found in evidence that supports the use of MBSR with caregivers. Further evidence for suggesting that MBCT may be useful with caregivers of cancer survivors can be found in evidence supporting the use of MBSR.

Mindfulness-based stress reduction interventions, from which MBCT is based, have been found to be effective in numerous caregiving settings. Li et al. [36] conducted a systematic review of literature on MBSR's use with family caregivers. Li and colleagues found that MBSR had an overall positive influence on the health and well-being of caregivers with no reported side effects or complaints. In particular, Hou and colleagues [37] studied family caregivers of individuals with chronic illnesses that experienced caregiver strain and found that MBSR, versus a self-help control group, decreased depressive symptoms, improved anxiety symptoms, and increased in self-efficacy. Similarly, Whitebird and colleagues [38] investigated the use of MBSR with family caregivers of individuals with dementia. Compared to a group of individuals in a caregiver education and support intervention, the MBSR group was more effective in reducing stress, reducing depression symptoms, and increasing overall mental health for caregivers. It should be noted in Whitebird and colleagues' [36] study that the caregiver education and support intervention group also had increases in mental health, leading to an inference that a more supportive group format like MBCT may be even more effective for this population than MBSR. Lengacher and colleagues [39] found that in a study of advanced-stage cancer survivors and their caregivers that MBSR was helpful in increasing quality of life for caregivers, but that increase was not statistically significant over time. Caregivers had lower levels of cortisol and interleukin-6 levels after the MBSR program, which indicated lower stress. Finally, an MBSR intervention was used with a group of lung cancer survivors and their partners, many with caregiving responsibilities, in a pilot study conducted by van den Hurk et al. [40]. Although lung cancer survivors did not experience significant changes, their partners experienced significant decreases in caregiver burden.

Although there is evidence for mindfulness strategies and MBSR programs in treating caregivers and caregivers of cancer survivors, very few studies exist examining MBCT and how it can help caregivers. Norouzi et al. [41] investigated the use of MBCT with women caregivers of individuals with dementia. Norouzi and colleagues found that MBCT was effective in decreasing depression and caregiver burden at 2-month follow-up. Additionally, current research supports the use of MBCT when working with caregivers of persons with dementia [42]. Oken and colleagues [42] conducted a study on the efficacy of mindfulness, with results indicating that both mindfulness and MBCT interventions decreased caregiver stress when compared to control group participants that received only respite care, supporting the use of these interventions when working with caregivers.

Modifications of MBCT for Caregivers

Using MBCT with caregivers allows practitioners to use a manualized treatment [3]. Along with brevity in care, relying on manualized treatments is appealing to managed care providers and can also help counselors to better adapt their practices [43]. In using mindfulness-based cognitive therapy for depression as a guide, along with the suggestions in the next section for tailoring the practice to caregivers of adults with cancer, practitioners can guide themselves in providing treatment to alleviate the burden caregivers experience. In order to meet the needs of caregivers of cancer survivors, the MBCT curriculum [3] has been modified. The modifications detailed pertain mostly to the unique concerns that caregivers face while providing care. The modifications enhance and inform the content to be more applicable to caregivers of cancer survivors. In short, the modifications to the MBCT curriculum include a focus on how caregiving relationships can be both the cause of emotional distress and the solution to emotional distress, sometimes simultaneously. This can be explored by using caregiving relationships in positive ways (e.g., planning mindfulness days with those for whom they provide care). Further, because there is rarely respite in caregiving relationships, group leaders should focus on helping members to learn how to conduct mindfulness practices while immersed in providing care, rather than having time outside of caregiving duties to practice mindfulness. Thus, adding role-playing will give

caregivers a chance to practice immediately with others after the group. Other general modifications pertain to the health of cancer survivors (e.g., terminal or nonterminal illnesses), other cancer-specific concerns (e.g., recurrence of cancer), and caregiver concerns (e.g., relationship with cancer survivor).

Throughout the chapter we have discussed the role caregivers have, the burden that being a caregiver can have on individuals, and how MBCT can be effective in treating caregivers of cancer survivors. A case study will be provided to illustrate how to use a modified form of MBCT with a group of informal caregivers that can be adapted to meet their needs in a therapeutic environment to provide better care for cancer survivors. The application of MBCT to this population is a fairly straightforward process. Although MBCT can be applied to individuals (e.g., [44]), we have chosen to illustrate the original group format [3] as cancer treatment centers can see a variety of types of cancer caregivers who would have an ability to meet on a weekly basis while cancer survivors receive treatment.

Case Study

Although the use of MBCT with groups allows for groups of around 12 individuals [3], for illustrative purposes, the case study for this chapter consists of a group of four caregivers of cancer survivors. Each individual has a specific set of issues based on various factors including location of cancer (e.g., breast or prostate), type of treatment (e.g., surgery or radiation), age, cultural background, and role in relationships (e.g., husband/wife or child). However, caregivers face many similar concerns, regardless of illness.

The 8-week group consists of four informal caregivers: Brenda, a 56-year-old African-American female providing care for her husband with prostate cancer; Randy, a 60-year-old Hispanic male providing care for his wife with breast cancer; Leah, a 24-year-old White female providing care for her fiancé with testicular cancer; and Michelle, a 40-year-old African-American female providing care for her father with metastatic cancer. Brenda, Randy, and Leah's partners are currently receiving treatment or are in recovery for treatment at the facility and Michelle's father received treatment previously. The members of the group joined an MBCT group to help cope with caregiving demands, focusing on relieving caregiver burden and regulating their own emotions while being caregivers. Notably characteristics of the group include Michelle's care as her father is facing metastatic cancer that originated in the colon and is receiving palliative care, where a focus is on reducing symptoms to improve the quality of life for individuals with terminal diseases [45–47], as well as Leah's younger age (reflective of diagnostic trends for testicular cancer), and the older age of Brenda and Randy.

During the first session, the MBCT group leader discusses the members' reasons for coming to the group. Brenda comments that providing care for her husband is causing a strain on their relationship through her helping him to cope with weakness from his treatments, embarrassment from helping him with daily needs (e.g., managing a colostomy), and a financial strain from having to drive him to treatments each day of the work-week for multiple months. Randy notes that providing care for his wife is a burden due to trying to meet her emotional needs after her double mastectomy, which causes him to become angry with increasing haste. Leah states that she is having trouble dealing with the anger her fiancé has over his diagnosis and treatment in their relationship, as well as a strain in providing care for him almost constantly due to his weakened state during chemotherapy treatment. Michelle concludes the discussion saying that she is scared of the possibility of her father's death and sadness due to seeing her father in a terminal state while still trying to provide competent care.

Session One

The first MBCT session sets the proverbial stage for the entirety of the intervention [3]. Goals of the first MBCT session include

practitioners assessing for the burden and pressure that group members face in providing care. Group members are told that individuals often drift into doing modes, that is, not being mindful of the actions they are participating in. Due to the demands of caregiving, it is important for practitioners to validate and be empathetic to the variety of tasks and jobs that can cause group members to be overwhelmed with when providing care; drifting into doing modes is natural and happens to most people. To encourage someone to focus on paying attention to the individual tasks and thoughts they are having may be different from their traditional behavior. As such, asking group members to donate their full attention to themselves can be overwhelming because they are used to focusing a majority of their concerns and time to the cancer survivor. Thus, it is important to have an idea of the types of care and tasks that each group member is involved in during the first session (as mentioned previously). It is also important for group members to state their intention and goal of participating in the group (e.g., better personal quality of life or providing better care) and assess what each member hopes to get from the group.

Group leaders should be aware of the types of caregiving that group members provide, whether it is before, during, or after treatment, or if it is palliative. Because their needs are different as caregivers, the barriers to participating in mindfulness practices may differ as well. Thus, the education of what MBCT entails and gauging members' readiness to participate in the group is important.

Session Two

In the second MBCT session, group members are encouraged to process the previous week's group and homework; group leaders explain connections between thoughts and feelings; and more mindfulness practices are introduced. Segal and colleagues [3] note that during the second session, group members often bring up difficulties they have had in applying mindfulness practices at home. In providing MBCT for caregivers, it is possible to experience resistance from group members that did not accomplish homework due to being too busy dealing with caregiving tasks [48]. Complaints of not finding time to practice mindfulness activities or general issues with the mindfulness practices (e.g., mind wandering or frustration) can occur during the second session and can be discussed in the group [3]. Feelings of guilt can arise in group members from doing mindfulness practices during the group rather than actively providing care and may present as group member resistance [49]. In this case, it would be important for practitioners to demonstrate empathy and aid in group members reiterating the purpose for the group taking place and what caregivers can gain from participating in the group. Group members may also be instructed to make a positive experiences calendar [3], listing activities they have done in the past week with individuals they provide care for that have generated feelings of happiness. Group members may continue to exhibit resistance as daily distress or feelings of being overwhelmed by caregiving responsibilities can contribute to having difficulty characterizing positive experiences. However, encouraging group members to keep positive experiences calendars may help them to find moments of positivity in their lives.

Group members like Randy or Leah may easily dismiss practice, as the care they provide can be emotionally draining. Similarly, someone like Michelle may dismiss practice as unimportant in light of her father's impending death. It is important for practitioners to also encourage the positive aspects of caregiving and the relationships that caregivers have. Putting an emphasis on how self-care can yield better caring may encourage members to participate, so that the group can be seen as a way to provide better care, making the group seem more selfless.

Session Three

In the third MBCT session, group members are encouraged to increase practice of active mindfulness such as mindful stretching and hearing exercises (e.g., focusing on sounds). It is during this session that increased awareness of thoughts and feelings is incorporated along with bodily sensations from previous sessions. Practitioners can take precautions in encouraging group members to focus on thoughts or emotions if they cause adverse reactions (e.g., remembering traumatic events). Focusing on thoughts or feelings related to being a caregiver could increase group members' feelings of frustration or joy involved with providing care; therefore practitioners should allow for adequate time to process negative thoughts and feelings so that they will be able to provide sufficient care after the MBCT session. Similar to the second MBCT group, group members are encouraged to construct an unpleasant experiences calendar similar to the positive experiences calendar. Finally, group members are taught the three-minute breathing space [3] which allows for more immediate mindfulness practices outside of the longer practices that have been learned so far in the course, and it also helps to set up the lessons later in the course. The "three-minute breathing space" is a short mindfulness practice that is used to help group members become aware of thoughts, feelings, and bodily sensations at that particular time. This brief mindfulness activity helps group members to become aware of thoughts, feelings, and bodily sensations in the first minute, focus on the feeling of their breath in the second minute, and then focus on the feeling of their body as a whole in the third minute, thus increasing a mindful awareness of group members in a short period of time.

The "three-minute breathing space" can be especially helpful for the group members if previous practices have been successful. In the midst of caregiving duties, the "three-minute breathing space" can be a short time to refocus and take a break from duties. For example, Brenda can take time from providing care for her husband and helping him with treatment effects (e.g., colostomy) and notice her passing thoughts, rather than being attributed to her husband or their relationship. The practice can be a short personal time and relief from caregiver burden.

Session Four

The fourth MBCT session focuses on understanding the group members' aversion to thoughts and emotions [3]. Challenges specific to group members include understanding how aversion to thoughts and feelings is triggered by the person for whom they provide care. Thoughts or feelings that contribute to aversion are related to other individuals or events that they can become disconnected from. However, caregiving group members' thoughts or feelings that can trigger aversion are often related to individuals they provide care for. Group members may be in a constant state of aversion, therefore increasing challenge of recognizing aversion. Patience during this session is helpful in helping group members to recognize aversion and returning to focus on the thoughts and emotions that cause aversion. Automatic negative thoughts are also explored in the fourth MBCT session. Practitioners are encouraged to process the halfway point of the group and note progress that has been made thus far.

The state of aversion that the group members are in could be due to emotions elicited through providing care for cancer survivors. In this session, it may be difficult to separate the person from the burden, as the caregiving relationship has mixed the two concepts. Thus, understanding and recognizing aversion can mean that group members focus on unpleasant experiences rather than discounting them and focusing on their need to be caregivers. The caregivers in the case study can care deeply for the person they provide care for; thus it may be hard for them to associate negative thoughts or feelings (e.g., resentment) to their partners or parents. Aversion then becomes a quick fix to their thoughts and emotions related to providing care, but understanding aversion may provide a long-term solution.

Session Five

In the fifth MBCT session, group members discuss allowing their thoughts and emotions to exist as they are, rather than applying aversion techniques or being judgmental of their thoughts or emotions [3]. The use of the phrase, turning toward, is applicable for group members that are caregivers, as they start to understand that the thoughts they have can be triggered by the individuals they are providing care for. Group members' awareness of thoughts that are causing negative emotions triggered by the person they are providing care for can be difficult. Practitioners can focus on the application of becoming aware of thoughts as they are having them while the individual who triggered the thought is in the room. Thus, we suggest other practices such as role-playing or other related techniques be integrated into MBCT sessions in order for the group members to learn how to become aware of their thoughts as they are happening while still being able to provide care in an effective way.

Group leaders can guide Leah through a role play exercise of being a caregiver and Randy can role-play the person receiving care in a relatable situation to caregivers, such as taking their family member to a doctor's appointment. Then, practitioners can encourage other group members to provide feedback for the caregiver of how they reacted to the person receiving care. This role play can be applied to various caregiving relationships (e.g., romantic or familial).

Session Six

The sixth MBCT session focuses on thoughts being free of emotion [3]. This session focuses on the nonjudgmental portion of MBCT, treating thoughts as completely separate from emotions. This session is difficult as many individuals learn that thoughts and emotions are connected to one another. In this session, practitioners help group members to nonjudgmentally accept thoughts as unique experiences, rather than tied to any specific emotion. It is also emphasized in this session that negative moods are passing events that should not be attributed to a larger theme, but sole negative moods. Continued practice from the fifth MBCT session is encouraged, along with more mindfulness practices, in order to help group members identify as many thoughts as they can and practice accepting those thoughts. It is also encouraged between the sixth and seventh MBCT sessions to plan a day of mindfulness. A day of mindfulness can be difficult for caregivers, as many of their tasks are routinized [48]. Therefore, in adapting the day of mindfulness for caregivers' schedules, it may be more realistic to encourage them to plan a half-day. Group members can also be encouraged to practice their everyday care tasks in a mindful way in order to increase awareness of thoughts and feelings as they occur.

Thus, in the mindfulness day, caregivers can be encouraged to plan the day with their partner or parents in order for both to benefit from the day [50]. Michelle and her father can plan a mindfulness day that could also possibly lead to a relief of physical or emotional pain during his palliative care. During the mindfulness day, the lessons can be applied even if both individuals do not participate in the mindfulness day, with Randy providing emotional care in a mindful way regardless of the activities of his wife.

Session Seven

The purpose of the seventh MBCT session is to increase activity in recognizing negative thoughts and feelings before or as they occur [3]. In the seventh MBCT session, group members are encouraged to acquire an understanding of when their moods start to lower or the triggers that cause their moods to lower. Group members are then given the time and space to think of positive or pleasurable activities to engage in in order to raise their moods. Similar to the second MBCT session, this session can be difficult for group members as they have to plan positive and pleasurable activities, rather than just providing care. Practitioners can encourage group members to revisit the rationales stated during the first session as to why the group members are using the MBCT group. On the other hand, the positive and pleasurable

activities could be related to giving care, which provides group members with a positive outlet while still providing care. Group members can list positive or pleasurable activities they can engage in with the individual they provide care for, whether it is going for a walk or playing board games.

This session can be a relief to those who find it difficult to provide care and who are overwhelmed by providing care. Brenda, in the midst of driving to and from work and treatment appointments, can be overwhelmed by the negative experiences of caregiving. Hopefully by this point in the group, she is learning to approach thoughts with acceptance and awareness, rather than an "auto-pilot" mode. Brenda can plan enjoyable activities while in route to the cancer treatment center with her husband to help encourage positive experiences in providing care.

Session Eight

The final MBCT session focuses on maintaining the lessons learned in previous sessions and expanding on those lessons [3]. A review of the course and termination activities can take place during the eighth MBCT session in order to help group members retain information gained from the group. Relapse prevention is important during this session as well. A unique struggle that caregivers can face when leaving the MBCT group is that the individual they care for can get worse over time and possibly put them back into the thought patterns that they previously held. Group members can exchange contact information with someone in the group they related to in order to maintain connections and have an outlet to vent to. Thus, relapse prevention and possible follow-up sessions are important in maintaining progress in dealing with negative thoughts and emotions while maintaining healthy stress levels and providing effective care. Group members can also be provided with additional resources, such as the MBCT guide developed for clients, The Mindful Way Through Depression [51].

Practical Considerations of MBCT for Caregivers

While the efficacy of MBCT for caregivers seems promising, practitioners are encouraged to consider factors such as role responsibilities, client selection, group size, facilitator training, cultural relevance, and spiritual backgrounds of caregivers. Given that many caregivers provide full-time care for their family members [52], accommodations need to be made to provide some caregiving relief or services during group sessions. We suggest providing MBCT to caregivers in conjunction with adult day-care services or treatment centers to provide MBCT to caregivers and services for those they care for. Practitioners are encouraged to partner with local hospitals or adult day-care services to enable caregivers to more readily accept help due to a temporarily lessened burden [53]. Cultural and spiritual needs of the caregivers should also be considered.

Exploring caregivers' cultural and spiritual needs throughout MBCT interventions will allow practitioners to increase awareness of their group members' needs. Cultural considerations include understanding caregivers' roles in the family and their personal beliefs and values about health. Another consideration to be aware of in providing MBCT is religious or spiritual considerations. As mindfulness practices originated in Buddhist philosophies [54], it is important to ensure that group members feel comfortable engaging in practices that originate from a religion or spiritual practice that is possibly different from their own. For guidance in providing care for those with a variety of cultural or religious and spiritual backgrounds, counselors are encouraged to consult the *Multicultural and Social Justice Counseling Competencies* [55] or the *Association for Spiritual, Ethical, and Religious Values in Counseling Spiritual Competencies* [56].

In addition to cultural concerns surrounding MBCT, there are a variety of logistical concerns for the group. The group size is a concern when many caregivers may be interested in joining a group. Segal and colleagues [3] state that a 12-person group is appropriate for MBCT groups; however, depending on the severity of burden, a smaller group may be necessary. Also, the developers of MBCT [3] believe that practitioners should be well versed in their own mindfulness practices and should experience an MBCT group themselves as group members. Training is available through the Mindfulness-Based Professional Training Institute (www.mbpti.org) to receive teacher qualification in MBCT.

Although an MBCT group can be helpful for individuals with a variety of problems, there are guidelines for screening that should be followed [57]. MBCT is a type of therapy that encourages group members to be self-guided between and after sessions. Caregivers looking for directive and/or long-term therapies can be referred to practitioners that meet those specific needs. Further, serious mental disorders that are not currently controlled (e.g., actively suicidal or individuals experiencing psychotic symptoms) can pose a problem for groups. Caregivers that have serious mental health concerns should seek more intensive individual therapy or specialized group therapies. To ensure a productive group process, it will be helpful to screen out disruptive group members before beginning a group, and refer them to other practitioners accordingly. In addition, as demonstrated in this chapter, it would be helpful to have a group with one type of caregiver (e.g., cancer survivors) rather than a larger variety of caregivers (e.g., parents of children with autism). Formal caregivers and informal caregivers should be kept separate, as both possibly come from different backgrounds in providing care (e.g., formal caregivers have established coursework and training in providing care).

Finally, the adaptation of MBCT for caregivers of cancer survivors is a theoretical application. Empirical research on the subject does not currently exist. Although research is under way, we can infer that MBCT will be a beneficial treatment through the application of MBSR and other mindfulness therapies for caregivers, and for caregivers of cancer survivors specifically. Further, wide-scale research will need to be conducted in order to support its efficaciousness, but it is a theoretically sound application given adjustments to the MBCT curriculum.

Conclusion

Caregiver burden negatively influences physical and mental health leading to sleep disturbances, psychological distress, lowered immune system, and financial distress [24]. Caregivers' levels of distress can also decrease the level of quality care provided to patients [58, 59]. Utilizing psychological interventions such as psychoeducation, counseling, or skill training has been shown to decrease symptoms of distress, though these interventions are rarely implemented [60]. Potential barriers in implementing effective psychological interventions for caregivers include lack of resources, lack of awareness of caregivers' needs, or limited education of health care professionals on how to implement interventions.

MBCT may be an effective intervention for informal caregivers of cancer patients that can help overcome these barriers, offering a step-by-step integrated intervention of psychoeducation, skill training, and counseling. As demonstrated in the case study, numerous changes were made in order to adapt the MBCT curriculum to caregivers of cancer survivors. Modifications included looking at how caregiving relationships can cause both strain and benefit for caregivers; focusing on helping group members learn how to conduct mindfulness practices while immersed in providing care; and including cancer-specific concerns and caregiver concerns in the curriculum. In sum, by adapting current MBCT lessons and activities [3] for caregivers of cancer survivors, practitioners can use an empirically supported, manualized, and time-sensitive treatment to decrease caregiver burden and increase caregiver quality of life.

Resources

The following resources provide informational and further resources concerning caregiving, cancer, and related issues.

Family Caregiver Alliance: https://www.caregiver.org
American Cancer Society: https://www.cancer.org
National Cancer Institute: https://www.cancer.gov

American Psychosocial Oncology Society: https://www.apos-society.org

Reflection Questions

1. What challenges may group leaders face when conducting an MBCT group for caregivers? What are some techniques group leaders can use to reduce challenges?
2. What are the benefits and challenges of having an MBCT group in a cancer care facility or hospital?
3. How would an MBCT group look different for formal caregivers (e.g., nursing staff or other treatment specialists)? What accommodations would need to be made for this group vs. informal caregivers?
4. Based on the cultural backgrounds on the group members of the case study, what considerations or alterations to MBCT would need to be made in order to run a culturally sensitive group?
5. What are some ways group leaders can adapt MBCT groups to accommodate the needs of group members from different cultural or socioeconomic backgrounds?

References

1. Kabat-Zinn J. Full-catastrophe living: Using the wisdom of your body and mind to face stress, pain, and illness. Revth ed. New York, NY: Bantam; 2013.
2. Smith JE, Richardson J, Hoffman C, Pilkington K. Mindfulness-based stress reduction as supportive therapy in cancer care: systematic review. J Adv Nurs. 2005;52:315–37.
3. Segal ZV, Williams JMG, Teasdale JD. Mindfulness-based cognitive therapy for depression: a new approach to preventing relapse. 2nd ed. New York, NY: The Guilford Press; 2013.
4. National Alliance for Caregiving & Association of American Retired Persons. Caregiving in the U.S.; 2015. http://www.caregiving.org/caregiving 2015/
5. Family Caregiver Alliance. Selected caregiver statistics. Fact Sheet: Selected Caregiver Statistics. 2005. http://www.caregiver.org
6. American Cancer Society. Cancer facts and figures 2012. Cancer. 2013. http://www.cancer.org

7. Girgis A, Lambert S, McElduff P, Bonevski B, Lecathelinais C, Boyes A, et al. Some things change, some things stay the same: a longitudinal analysis of cancer caregivers' unmet supportive care needs. Psychooncology. 2013;22(7):1557–64.

8. Bevans M, Sternberg EM. Caregiving burden, stress, and health effects among family caregivers of adult cancer patients. JAMA. 2012;307:398–403.

9. Hansen T, Slagsvold B, Ingebretsen R. The strains and gains of caregiving: an examination of the effects of providing personal care to a parent on a range of indicators of psychological well-being. Soc Indic Res. 2013;114(2):323–43. doi:10.1007/s11205-012-0148-z.

10. Clark MM, Atherton PJ, Lapid MI, Rausch SM, Frost MH, Cheville AL, et al. Caregivers of patients with cancer fatigue: a high level of symptom burden. Am J Hosp Palliat Care. 2014;31(2):121–5. doi:10.1177/1049909113479153.

11. Kim Y. Emotional and cognitive consequences of adult attachment: the mediating effect of the self. Pers Individ Dif. 2005;39:913–23.

12. Lawrence DP, Kupelnick B, Miller K, Devine D, Lau J. Evidence report on the occurrence, assessment, and treatment of fatigue in cancer patients. J Natl Cancer Inst. 2004;32:40–50.

13. Chiu YC, Lee YN, Wang PC, Chang TH, Li CL, Hsu WC, et al. Family caregivers sleep disturbance and its associations with multilevel stressors when caring for patients with dementia. Aging Ment Health. 2014; 18:92–101.

14. Hasson-Ohayon I, Goldzweig G, Braun M, Galinsky D. Women with advanced breast cancer and their spouses: diversity of support and psychological distress. Psychooncology. 2010;19(11):1195–204.

15. Kotronoulas G, Wengstrom Y, Kearney N. Sleep patterns and sleep-impairing factors of persons providing informal care for people with cancer a critical review of the literature. Cancer Nurs. 2012;36:1–15.

16. Cooper C, Balamurali T, Livingston G. A systematic review of the prevalence and covariates of anxiety in caregivers of people with dementia (English). Int Psychogeriatr. 2006;19(2):175–95.

17. Lambert S, Girgis A, Lecathelinais C, Stacey F. Walking a mile in their shoes: anxiety and depression among partners and caregivers of cancer survivors at 6 and 12 months post-diagnosis. Support Care Cancer. 2012;21:75–85.

18. Gaston-Johansson F, Lachica E, Fall-Dickson J, Kennedy M. Psychological distress, fatigue, burden of care, and quality of life in primary caregivers of patients with breast cancer undergoing autologous bone marrow transplantation. Oncol Nurs Forum. 2004;31(6):1161–9.

19. Ownsworth T, Henderson L, Chambers SK. Social support buffers the impact of functional impairments on caregiver psychological well-being in the context of brain tumor and other cancers. Psychooncology. 2010;19(10):1116–22.

20. Wei Y, Chu H, Chen C, Hsueh Y, Chang Y, Chang L, Chou K. Support groups for caregivers of intellectually disabled family members: Effects on physical

psychological health and social support. J Clin Nur 2012;21(11–12).

21. Chien L, Chu H, Guo J, Liao Y, Chang L, Chen C, Chou K. Caregiver support groups in patients with dementia: A meta-analysis. International Journal of Geriatric Psychiatry 2011;26(10):1089–1098.

22. Schulz R, Sherwood PR. Physical and mental health effects of family caregiving. Am J Nurs. 2008;108(9 Suppl):23–7.

23. Peacock S, Forbes D, Markle-Reid M, Hawranik P, Morgan D, Jansen L, et al. The positive aspects of the caregiving journey with dementia: using a strengths-based perspective to reveal opportunities. J Appl Gerontol. 2010;29:640–59.

24. Northouse L, Williams A, Given B, McCorkle R. Psychosocial care for family caregivers of patients with cancer. J Clin Oncol. 2012;30:1227–34.

25. Phillips AC, Gallagher S, Hunt K, Der G, Carroll D. Symptoms of depression in non-routine caregivers: the role of caregiver strain and burden. Br J Clin Psychol. 2009;48:335–46.

26. Yalom ID, Leszcz M. The theory and practice of group psychotherapy. New York, NY: Basic Books; 2005.

27. Simard S, Thewes B, Humphris G, Dixon M, Hayden C, Mireskandari S, et al. Fear of cancer recurrence in adult cancer survivors: a systematic review of quantitative studies. J Cancer Surviv. 2013;7:300–22.

28. Teasdale JD, Segal ZV, Williams JMG, Ridgeway VA, Soulsby JM, Lau MA. Prevention of relapse/recurrence in major depression by mindfulness-based cognitive therapy. J Consult Clin Psychol. 2000;68:615–23.

29. Geschwind N, Peeters F, Drukker M, van Os J, Wichers M. Mindfulness training increases momentary positive emotions and reward experience in adults vulnerable to depression: a randomized controlled trial. J Consult Clin Psychol. 2011;79(5): 618–28.

30. Haydicky J, Shecter C, Wiener J, Ducharme JM. Evaluation of MBCT for adolescents with ADHD and their parents: impact on individual and family functioning. J Child Fam Stud. 2013;24(1):76–94. doi:10.1007/s10826-013-9815-1.

31. Kaviani H, Hatami N, Javaheri F. The impact of mindfulness-based cognitive therapy (MBCT) on mental health and quality of life in a sub-clinically depressed population. Arch Psychiatry Psychother. 2012;1:21–8.

32. Keng S, Smoski MJ, Robins CJ. Effects of mindfulness on psychological health: a review of empirical studies. Clin Psychol Rev. 2011;31:1041–56.

33. Paller KA, Creery JD, Florczak SM, Weintraub S, Mesulam M, Reber PJ, et al. Benefits of mindfulness training for patients with progressive cognitive decline and their caregivers. Am J Alzheimers Dis Other Demen. 2015;30:257–67.

34. Kögler M, Brandstätter M, Borasio GD, Fensterer V, Küchenhoff H, Fegg MJ. Mindfulness in informal caregivers of palliative patients. Palliat Support Care. 2013;13:11–8.

35. Lunksy Y, Robinson S, Reid M, Palucka AM. Development of a mindfulness-based coping with stress group for parents of adolescents and adults with developmental disabilities. Mindfulness. 2015. Advance online publication. doi:10.1007/s12671-015-0404-9

36. Li G, Yuan H, Zhang W. The effects of mindfulness-based stress reduction for family caregivers: systematic review. Arch Psychiatr Nurs. 2015. Advance online publication. doi:10.1016/j.apnu. 2015.08.014

37. Hou RJ, Wong SY, Yip BH, Hung ATF, Lo HH, Chan PHS, et al. The effects of mindfulness-based stress reduction program on the mental health of family caregivers: a randomized controlled trial. Psychother Psychosom. 2014;83:45–53.

38. Whitebird RR, Kreitzer M, Crain AL, Lewis BA, Hanson LR, Enstad CJ. Mindfulness-based stress reduction for family caregivers: a randomized controlled trial. Gerontologist. 2013;53:676–86.

39. Lengacher CA, Kip KE, Barta M, Post-White J, Jacobsen PB, Groer M, et al. A pilot study evaluating the effect of mindfulness-based stress reduction on psychological status, physical status, salivary cortisol, and interleukin-6 among advanced-stage cancer patients and their caregivers. J Holist Nurs. 2012; 30(3):170–85.

40. van den Hurk M, Schellekens J, Molema J, Speckens AE, van der Drift MA. Mindfulness-based stress reduction for lung cancer patients and their partners: results of a mixed methods pilot study. Palliat Med. 2015;29.652–60.

41. Norouzi M, Golzari M, Sohrabi F. Effectiveness of mindfulness based cognitive therapy on the quality of life, depression and burden of demented women caregivers. Zahedan J Res Med Sci. 2014;16(9):5–11.

42. Oken BS, Fonareva I, Haas M, Wahbeh H, Lane JB, Zajdel D, et al. Pilot controlled trial of mindfulness meditation and education for dementia caregivers. J Altern Complement Med. 2010;16:1031–8.

43. Mitchell CG. Patient satisfaction with standard interventions in a managed care context. Res Soc Work Practice. 2001;11:473–484.

44. Tovote KA, Fleer J, Snippe E, Peeters AC, Emmelkamp PM, Sanderman R, et al. Individual mindfulness-based cognitive therapy and cognitive behavior therapy for treating depressive symptoms in patients with diabetes: results of a randomized controlled trial. Diabetes Care. 2014;37:2427–34.

45. Harding R, Higginson IJ. What is the best way to help caregivers in cancer and palliative care? A systematic literature review of interventions and their effectiveness. Palliat Med. 2003;17:63–74.

46. Lorenz KA, Lynn J, Dy S, Shugarman LR, Wilkinson A, Mularski RA, et al. Evidence for improving palliative care at the end of life: a systematic review. Ann Intern Med. 2008;148:147–59.

47. Sampson C, Finlay I, Byrne A, Snow V, Nelson A. The practice of palliative care from the perspective of patients and carers. BMJ Support Palliative Care. 2014. Advanced online publication.

48. Parkenham KI. Caregiving tasks in caring for an adult with mental illness and associations with adjustment outcomes. Int J Behav Med. 2012;19(2):186–98.

49. Spillers RL, Wellisch DK, Kim Y, Matthews BA, Baker F. Family caregivers and guilt in the context of cancer care. Psychosomatics. 2008;49(6):511–9.

50. Smith EL, Jones FW, Holttum S, Griffiths K. The process of engaging in mindfulness-based cognitive therapy as a partnership: a grounded theory study. Mindfulness. 2015;6:455–66.

51. Williams JMG, Teasdale JD, Segal ZV, Kabat-Zinn J. The mindful way through depression: Freeing yourself from chronic unhappiness. New York, NY: The Guilford Press; 2007.

52. Yabroff K, Kim Y. Time costs associated with informal caregiving for cancer survivors. Cancer. 2009;115(18):4362–73.

53. Zarit HS, Kim K, Femia EE, Almeida DM, Savla J, Molenaar PCM. Effects of adult day care on daily stress of caregivers: a within-person approach. J Gerontol B Psychol Sci Soc Sci. 2011;66B(5):538–46.

54. Maex E. The Buddhist roots of mindfulness training: a practitioners view. ConBuddh. 2011;12:165–75.

55. Ratts MJ, Singh AA, Nassar-McMillan S, Butler SK, McCullough JR. Multicultural and social justice counseling competencies. 2015. http://www.multiculturalcounseling.org/index.php?option=com_content&view=article&id=205:amcd-endorses-multicultural-and-social-justice-counseling-competencies&catid=1:latest&Itemid=123

56. Association for Spiritual, Ethical, and Religious Values in Counseling. Competencies for addressing spiritual and religious issues in counseling. Alexandria, VA: Author; 2009.

57. Gladding ST. Groups: A counseling specialty (6th ed.). Upper Saddle River, NJ: Pearson. 2011.

58. Pinquart M, Sörensen S. Differences between caregivers and noncaregivers in psychological health and physical health: a meta-analysis. Psychol Aging. 2003;18:250–67.

59. Smith G, Williamson G, Miller L, Schulz R. Depression and quality of informal care: a longitudinal investigation of caregiving stressors. Psychol Aging. 2011; 26(3):584–91.

60. Northouse L, Katapodi M, Song L, Zhang L, Mood D. Interventions with family caregivers of cancer patients meta-analysis of randomized trials. CA Cancer J Clin. 2010;60(5):317–39.

Mindfulness-Based Interventions as School-Based Mental Health Promoting Programs

Katleen Van der Gucht, Peter Kuppens,
Edel Maex, and Filip Raes

Approximately 20 % of adolescents around the world experience mental health problems, most commonly depression or anxiety [1]. Prevalence is high, especially among girls, and appears to be on the increase (e.g., [2, 3]). When also taking subthreshold depression and anxiety into account approximately half of European adolescents meet the criteria [4]. Given the high prevalence of youth mental health problems there is a critical need for effective low-threshold evidence-based mental health promoting programs.

Adolescence can be seen as a period of heightened vulnerability and as the point at which much of the disease burden from mental disorders later in life emerges [5, 6]. It is a period marked by increases in emotionality, greater sensitivity to social interactions, and greater reward seeking and concomitant risk taking behavior [7]. It is also a transitional stage characterized by changes in development of adaptive attentional, emotional, and behavioral regulation and, thus, might be seen as a critical time window to deliver effective mental health promoting interventions. Neurobiological research has shown that during adolescence connections among brain regions increase and communication between the prefrontal cortex (PFC) and other cortical and subcortical regions become more efficient enabling better regulation of thought, emotion, and action [6]. Brain regions, particularly plastic during this period (such as certain regions in the PFC, the hippocampus) are also highly vulnerable to stress and negative life events, which might partly explain the increased risk of developing mental illness [8]. From the neurodevelopmental perspective the heightened brain plasticity might also be seen as a critical window to introduce interventions that actively support the development of brain regions involved in adaptive emotion and cognition regulation [9]. As poor emotion regulation is seen as a core feature of many mental (depression, anxiety [10]) and behavioral problems (self-injury, eating disorders [11], substance abuse [12], aggression [13]) in adolescents, actively supporting these brain regions involved in adaptive emotion regulation might be very helpful.

As it is also important to focus not just on treatment, but also on preventative efforts to decrease the risk of later adult disorders

K. Van der Gucht, Ph.D. (✉) • P. Kuppens, Ph.D.
• F. Raes, Ph.D.
Faculty of Psychology and Educational Sciences,
University of Leuven,
Tiensestraat 102, 3000 Leuven, Belgium
e-mail: katleen.vandergucht@kuleuven.be

E. Maex, M.D.
Ziekenhuis Netwerk Antwerpen,
Leopoldstraat 26, 2000 Antwerpen, Belgium

© Springer International Publishing Switzerland 2016
S.J. Eisendrath (ed.), *Mindfulness-Based Cognitive Therapy*, DOI 10.1007/978-3-319-29866-5_19

[14] and to diminish the intergenerational transmission of risk for anxiety and depression [2], low threshold, universal approaches, offered to a whole population might have the most potential.[1]

Schools provide an excellent opportunity to implement community-wide prevention programs. Especially schools with a high percentage of disadvantaged youth might benefit from this kind of interventions, as these adolescents are often exposed to a range of economic, family and community stressors that place them at higher risk for psychological distress and mental health impairment [15].

Universal school-based programs may also reduce the stigma surrounding mental health treatment. Stigma still is a common reason why adolescents do not seek and receive mental health treatment [16], so universal school-based programs may help to normalize participation in behavioral interventions, especially when the intervention is not laden with the stigma of mental illness in the common perception. Universal school-based programs might also be seen as cost-effective alternatives to afterschool-programs and do not face the substantial costs associated with screening needed to deliver the selectively offered targeted interventions. They can be made available to all students including those currently deemed at lower risk but whose risk profile changes later.

So what is needed is programs that can be easily utilized by a large number of students, that are easy to implement, highly efficient and that are inexpensive (see also ref. [17]). The program should focus on training self-regulatory skills based on alterations in basic cognitive and emotional processes and may effect neural systems, psychological functions and behavioral outcomes. Self-regulatory skills that can enable young people to successfully cope with the challenges they will face in their future life.

Is There Evidence That Mindfulness Based Interventions (MBIs) Can Fulfill These Needs in Adolescent Populations?

Solid evidence is emerging that MBIs tick all these boxes. MBIs have proven to be efficacious and effective for youth, both in clinical (e.g., depression [18]; mixed mental health disorders [19, 20]) and nonclinical samples (in a school context; e.g., [21, 22]). Reviews show that MBIs can be successfully used with children and adolescents in different settings (e.g., [23–26]). A recent meta-analysis of 20 studies (published before July 2011) with participants under 18 years of age and using programs with mindfulness as the chief component found small to moderate omnibus effect sizes (0.15–0.31), larger effect sizes were found for psychological symptoms compared to other dependent variable types (0.37 versus 0.21) and for studies drawn from clinical samples (0.50 versus 0.20) [27]. A more recent meta-analysis including only randomized controlled trials (15 studies published until January 2014) using MBIs or Acceptance and commitment therapy (ACT) for children or adolescents found interventions based on MBSR and MBCT to be effective for stress, anxiety and depression, other MBIs were only effective improving anxiety and stress but not depression [28]. Overall, the positive findings are consistent with those reported in adult populations. Reported effect sizes for psychological problems (0.25–0.50) are only slightly smaller than those shown in meta-analyses of studies in adults samples (0.30–0.60) (e.g., [29]). However, many of the studies with adolescents so far appear to have substantial methodological shortcomings and there is a great variability in study design. There is also a lack of uniformity in program content. Studies have predominantly been outcome-based to understand the efficacy and effectiveness of the programs, with less focus on the possible working mechanisms.

The ability to effectively regulate one's emotions and cognitions during stressful experiences is viewed as foundational for well-being, academic performance, and positive adjustment

---

[1] There is an ongoing debate about delivering universal versus targeted interventions into schools based on both ethical and scientific arguments (e.g., [58–60]).

throughout the lifespan [30, 31] and serves as a protective factor against the emergence of symptoms of many mental disorders and behavioral problems [32–34]. And indeed, both cognitive and emotional reactivity are acknowledged as critical mechanisms in the proposed theoretical models of mindfulness [35, 36]. Empirical studies with adults show that MBIs may reduce symptoms of stress, anxiety and depression by both targeting processes that are known as vulnerability factors (cognitive and emotional reactivity, rumination, worry) for mental disorders and processes that are known as resilience factors (mindfulness skills, self-compassion) [37]. Although mindfulness interventions do not have any explicit instruction for changing the nature of thinking, or emotional reactivity, it has been shown to diminish the habitual tendency to emotionally (over-)react and ruminate [38]. For example, in a population of economically disadvantaged people we found evidence for a reduction in cognitive reactivity and overgeneralization and an improvement in mindfulness skills [39].

Not unimportantly, there is evidence that the effects of MBI are also attributable to increased mindfulness skills instead of more generic intervention factors. Findings from recent studies focusing on changes during a MBI confirm an impact on affect, cognition, and distress through the day-to-day development of mindfulness skills [40–42].

Also findings from neuroimaging studies imply that mindfulness reduces emotional reactivity by attenuating limbic responses to emotional triggers via specific top-down modulation processes localized at prefrontal areas [43, 44]. Based on evidence from adult fMRI research Sanger and Dorjee [45] suggest that mindfulness practice could encourage connections between the relevant prefrontal structures in adolescents, stabilizing arousal and reducing harmful risk-taking. In this context Sanger and Dorjee [46] refer to mindfulness based training as a potential helpful intervention, particularly as it can be sustainably implemented in schools [45].

Back from the viewpoint of adolescence, the first experimental and correlational studies with youth focusing on emotion and cognition regulation show preliminary findings suggesting that mindfulness can be seen as an important skill improving both emotion and cognition regulation. A study on acute experimental pain among adolescents showed ameliorated pain responses among adolescents with a regular meditation practice and these effects were mediated by reduced catastrophizing [46]. In a recent study with clinically depressed youth greater dispositional mindfulness predicted greater recovery from these symptoms and a greater tendency to use mindfulness as an emotion regulation strategy was associated with positive mental health outcomes and better quality of life [47]. Pearson et al. [48] found a sharp contrast in emotional functioning between subgroups of college students distinguished based on their mindfulness scores. Both the high mindfulness group (scoring high on all facets of mindfulness) and the nonjudgmental aware group (scoring high on nonjudging and acting with awareness but low on observing) had the most adaptive emotional outcomes (lower depressive symptoms, anxiety symptoms, affective lability, and distress intolerance). Since the largest subgroup in the sample of college students was the low mindfulness group (>57 %) the authors suggest that mindfulness-based interventions could have a meaningful impact in this population [48]. In a cross-sectional study Peters et al. [49] found that mindfulness may lead to reduced aggression in students via lower levels of anger rumination [49].

Concluding, based on theoretical and empirical research there are strong arguments to invest in future research further exploring the potential benefits of mindfulness for adolescents.

Already recognizing potential benefits of mindfulness, the cultivation of mindfulness in classrooms has gained enormous popularity [50] and a recently started large-scale trial, which will involve nearly six thousand students in schools across the UK, will assess effectiveness of teaching mindfulness in schools (http://www.oxford-mindfulness.org/learn/myriad/).

Many different intervention formats have emerged and variability is large in program content and length [51]. In a recent review a comprehensive description of the emergent programs for adolescents is provided [52].

Practical Considerations and Guidelines

To use mindfulness interventions in a school context, some practical considerations come into play. We here propose some key recommendations based on our own experience in schools [22] and recently published studies on school trials.

The *structure of the program* should be designed to be easily integrated into the school curriculum. The format should be adjusted, shorter sessions which fit in the time window of a class hour, in order to enlarge feasibility. The sessions can be spread over weeks or even one to several years.

The *content of the program* should capture the core components originating from adult programs (MBSR/MBCT) such as awareness of physical sensations, awareness of thoughts and emotions, mindful movement, loving kindness practice. As it is more challenging for adolescents to focus attention on a single activity for longer periods of time the formal exercises should be shorter and more repetitious. Exercises as body scan, mindful movement, loving kindness practice should be adapted to the world and language of the age group. Adolescents are also more likely to be engaged in frequent informal exercises throughout the day, as they incorporate these exercises in many of their daily activities (e.g., mindful listening to music); therefore, a great deal of attention should be given to informal mindful exercises. The core components are necessary to help students to regulate their attention and become aware of their experience. Practicing these core elements students learn to recognize and understand the nature of their thoughts and feelings (recognizing the transience of thoughts and emotions as temporary states). They learn to relate to these thoughts and feelings in a different way (letting go of maladaptive cognitions and not holding on to or identifying with negative thoughts). They become aware of the whole range of pleasant, unpleasant and neutral experiences with an attitude of non-judgment and acceptance of that experience and compassionate [53].

The *delivery* should become self-sustaining. For most of the peer-reviewed studies on MBIs in secondary schools the program was delivered by professional trainers (e.g., [21, 22, 54]). More self-sustaining alternatives exist as well, including training delivered by school teachers [55], or schools could work with Web-based interventions or audio audio-guided mindful awareness training programs [56]. As mindful awareness can be practiced in many different ways, mindful exercises can be combined with the core teachings of many disciplines such as art, science, religion, literature.

Given the influx of different paradigms and approaches, there is a strong need to explore facilitators and barriers in effective implementation. So far there is a broad range of translational techniques and a lack of uniformity in program content and implementation. Implementation should not be limited to brief interventions and researchers and mindfulness trainers need to work together when attuning the mindfulness programs. Therefore, future studies should not only apply a robust trial design but also clearly specify how the practices are adapted to be age appropriate. Clear descriptions of specific instructions are needed and manuals that provide such details should be made available. Not only should future studies focus on short-term outcomes but prospective cohort studies for instance in people at risk for health problems are recommended to study long term effects. Special attention should be payed to the importance of participant-specific variables (such as age, gender, and personality traits) to find out what works for whom.

Conclusion

At present, empirical evidence on the effectiveness of MBIs for adolescents is available, growing. Variability in study design and program content is large and studies focusing on processes and working mechanisms are still scarce. Mindfulness research conducted with adults and research (theoretical, empirical, neurobiological) focusing on psychological and emotional flexibility does provide a substantial theoretical rationale to further investigate the potential of MBIs as a mental training for enhancing mental well-being in adolescents. Based on the findings discussed here it is conceivable that mindfulness may have positive effects on transdiagnostic problems and health-related behavior. However, the speed at which the development of mindfulness-based programs in a school context is being assimilated leads to concerns. Concerns about whether the preliminary evidence justifies the growing popularity and about the authenticity of the approaches. Therefore, in the future, trainers and researchers should work together and focus on uniformity in program content, robust trial designs measuring participant-specific and long-term effects. Outcomes should be measured using multiple methods including neuroscience, behavioral science, physical health, if possible measured in real life, and behavioral outcomes should be rated by students, parents, and teachers. Also economic analyses indicating the potential financial benefits of such interventions are important.

If found to be effective, as could be expected based on both theoretical considerations and preliminary empirical results, mindfulness meditation may be an important factor in the developmental trajectory of our youth.

As Arthur Zajonc says: "The true goal of meditation is to achieve a way of directly experiencing the world and ourselves that is not imprisoned or distorted by mental habits or emotional desires. When free of these, we are opened to a richer exploration of reality that presents to us new insights into self and world" [57].

References

1. United Nations Publication. Mental Health Matters. Social inclusion of youth with mental health condition. New York: United Nations. 2014; http://www.un.org/esa/socdev/documents/youth/youth-mental-health.pdf.
2. Collishaw S, Maughan B, Natarajan L, Pickles A. Trends in adolescent emotional problems in England: a comparison of two national cohorts twenty years apart. J Child Psychol Psychiatry. 2010;51(8):885–94. doi:10.1111/j.1469-7610.2010.02252.x.
3. Patton GC, Coffey C, Romaniuk H, Mackinnon A, Carlin JB, Degenhardt L, et al. The prognosis of common mental disorders in adolescents: a 14-year prospective cohort study. Lancet. 2014;383(9926):1404–11. doi:10.1016/s0140-6736(13)62116-9.
4. Balazs J, Miklosi M, Kereszteny A, Hoven CW, Carli V, Wasserman C, et al. Adolescent subthreshold-depression and anxiety: psychopathology, functional impairment and increased suicide risk. J Child Psychol Psychiatry. 2013;54(6):670–7. doi:10.1111/jcpp.12016.
5. Gore FM, Bloem PJN, Patton GC. Global burden of disease in young people aged 10–24 years: a systematic analysis. Lancet. 2011;378(9790):486.
6. Paus T, Keshavan M, Giedd JN. OPINION why do many psychiatric disorders emerge during adolescence? Nat Rev Neurosci. 2008;9(12):947–57. doi:10.1038/nrn2513.
7. Allen NB, Sheeber LB. The importance of affective development for the emergence of depressive disorder during adolescence. In: Allen NB, Sheeber LB, editors. Adolescent emotional development and the emergence of depressive disorders. Cambridge: Cambridge University Press; 2008. p. 1–10.
8. Andersen SL, Teicher MH. Stress, sensitive periods and maturational events in adolescent depression. Trends Neurosci. 2008;31(4):183–91. doi:10.1016/j.tins.2008.01.004.
9. Spear LP. Adolescent neurodevelopment. J Adolesc Health. 2013;52(2):S7–13. doi:10.1016/j.jadohealth.2012.05.006.
10. Kullik A, Petermann F. The role of emotion regulation for the genesis of anxiety disorders in childhood and adolescence. Zeitschr Psychiatr Psychol Psychother. 2012;60(3):165–73. doi:10.1024/1661-4747/a000113.
11. Fischer S, Munsch S. Self-regulation in eating disorders and obesity – implications for the treatment. Verhaltenstherapie. 2012;22(3):158–64. doi:10.1159/000341540.
12. Siegel JP. Emotional regulation in adolescent substance use disorders: rethinking risk. J Child Adolesc Subst Abuse. 2015;24(2):67–79. doi:10.1080/1067828x.2012.761169.
13. Roell J, Koglin U, Petermann F. Emotion regulation and childhood aggression: longitudinal associations. Child Psychiatry Hum Dev. 2012;43(6):909–23. doi:10.1007/s10578-012-0303-4.
14. Kessler RC, Angermeyer M, Anthony JC, de Graaf R, Demyttenaere K, Gasquet I, et al. Lifetime prevalence and age-of-onset distributions of mental disorders in the World Health Organization's World Mental Health Survey Initiative. World Psychiatry. 2007;6(3):168–76.
15. Thapar A, Collishaw S, Pine DS, Thapar AK. Depression in adolescence. Lancet. 2012;379(9820):1056–67. doi:10.1016/s0140-6736(11)60871-4.
16. Bulanda JJ, Bruhn C, Byro-Johnson T, Zentmyer M. Addressing mental health stigma among young adolescents: evaluation of a youth-led approach. Health Soc Work. 2014;39(2):73–80. doi:10.1093/hsw/hlu008.

17. Shochet I, Montague R, Smith C, Dadds M. A qualitative investigation of adolescents' perceived mechanisms of change from a universal school-based depression prevention program. Int J Environ Res Public Health. 2014;11(5):5541–54.

18. Ames CS, Richardson J, Payne S, Smith P, Leigh E. Innovations in practice: mindfulness-based cognitive therapy for depression in adolescents. Child Adolesc Ment Health. 2014;19(1):74–8. doi:10.1111/camh.12034.

19. Biegel GM, Brown KW, Shapiro SL, Schubert CA. Mindfulness-based stress reduction for the treatment of adolescent psychiatric outpatients: a randomized clinical trial. J Consult Clin Psychol. 2009;77(5):855–66. doi:10.1037/a0016241.

20. Tan L, Martin G. Taming the adolescent mind: a randomised controlled trial examining clinical efficacy of an adolescent mindfulness-based group programme. Child Adolesc Ment Health. 2015;20(1):49–55. doi:10.1111/camh.12057.

21. Kuyken W, Weare K, Ukoumunne OC, Vicary R, Motton N, Burnett R, et al. Effectiveness of the mindfulness in schools programme: non-randomised controlled feasibility study. Br J Psychiatry. 2013;203(2):126–31. doi:10.1192/bjp.bp.113.126649.

22. Raes F, Griffith JW, Van der Gucht K, Williams JMG. School-based prevention and reduction of depression in adolescents: a cluster-randomized controlled trial of a mindfulness group program. Mindfulness. 2014;5(5):477–86. doi:10.1007/s12671-013-0202-1.

23. Burke CA. Mindfulness-based approaches with children and adolescents: a preliminary review of current research in an emergent field. J Child Fam Stud. 2010;19(2):133–44. doi:10.1007/s10826-009-9282-x.

24. Harnett PH, Dawe S. The contribution of mindfulness-based therapies for children and families and proposed conceptual integration. Child Adolesc Ment Health. 2012;17(4):195–208. doi:10.1111/j.1475-3588.2011.00643.x.

25. Zack S, Saekow J, Kelly M, Radke A. Mindfulness based interventions for youth. J Ration Emot Cogn Behav Ther. 2014;32(1):44–56. doi:10.1007/s10942-014-0179-2.

26. Zenner C, Herrnleben-Kurz S, Walach H. Mindfulness-based interventions in schools—a systematic review and meta-analysis. Front Psychol. 2014;5:603. doi:10.3389/fpsyg.2014.00603.

27. Zoogman S, Goldberg SB, Hoyt WT, Miller L. Mindfulness interventions with youth: a meta-analysis. Mindfulness. 2015;6(2):290–302. doi:10.1007/s12671-013-0260-4.

28. Kallapiran K, Koo S, Kirubakaran R, Hancock K. Effectiveness of mindfulness in improving mental health symptoms of children and adolescents: a meta-analysis. Child Adolesc Ment Health. 2015;20(4):182–94.

29. Khoury B, Lecomte T, Fortin G, Masse M, Therien P, Bouchard V, et al. Mindfulness-based therapy: a comprehensive meta-analysis. Clin Psychol Rev. 2013;33(6):763–71. doi:10.1016/j.cpr.2013.05.005.

30. Eisenberg N, Spinrad TL, Eggum ND. Emotion-related self-regulation and its relation to children's maladjustment. Annu Rev Clin Psychol. 2010;6:495–525.

31. Kashdan TB, Rottenberg J. Psychological flexibility as a fundamental aspect of health. Clin Psychol Rev. 2010;30(7):865–78.

32. Aldao A, Nolen-Hoeksema S, Schweizer S. Emotion-regulation strategies across psychopathology: a meta-analytic review. Clin Psychol Rev. 2010;30(2):217–37. doi:10.1016/j.cpr.2009.11.004.

33. Berking M, Wupperman P. Emotion regulation and mental health: recent findings, current challenges, and future directions. Curr Opin Psychiatry. 2012;25(2):128–34. doi:10.1097/YCO.0b013e3283503669.

34. Gross JJ. Emotion regulation: taking stock and moving forward. Emotion. 2013;13(3):359–65. doi:10.1037/a0032135.

35. Roemer L, Williston SK, Rollins LG. Mindfulness and emotion regulation. Curr Opin Psychol. 2015;3:52–7.

36. van der Velden AM, Kuyken W, Wattar U, Crane C, Pallesen KJ, Dahlgaard J, et al. A systematic review of mechanisms of change in mindfulness-based cognitive therapy in the treatment of recurrent major depressive disorder. Clin Psychol Rev. 2015;37:26–39. doi:10.1016/j.cpr.2015.02.001.

37. Gu J, Strauss C, Bond R, Cavanagh K. How do mindfulness-based cognitive therapy and mindfulness-based stress reduction improve mental health and wellbeing? A systematic review and meta-analysis of mediation studies. Clin Psychol Rev. 2015;37:1–12.

38. Teasdale JD, Chaskalson M. How does mindfulness transform suffering? In: Williams JMG, Kabat-Zinn J, editors. Mindfulness – diverse perspectives on its meaning, origins and applications. London: Routledge, Taylor & Francis Group; 2013. p. 89–124.

39. Van der Gucht K, Takano K, Van Broeck N, Raes F. A mindfulness-based intervention for economically disadvantaged people: effects on symptoms of stress, anxiety and depression, and on cognitive reactivity and overgeneralization. Mindfulness. 2014;6(5):1042–52. doi:10.1007/s12671-014-0353-8.

40. Garland EL, Geschwind N, Peeters F, Wichers M. Mindfulness training promotes upward spirals of positive affect and cognition: multilevel and autoregressive latent trajectory modeling analyses. Front Psychol. 2015;6:15. doi:10.3389/fpsyg.2015.00015.

41. Kiken LG, Garland EL, Bluth K, Palsson OS, Gaylord SA. From a state to a trait: trajectories of state mindfulness in meditation during intervention predict changes in trait mindfulness. Pers Individ Dif. 2015;81:41–6. doi:10.1016/j.paid.2014.12.044.

42. Snippe E, Nyklicek I, Schroevers MJ, Bos EH. The temporal order of change in daily mindfulness and affect during mindfulness-based stress reduction. J Couns Psychol. 2015;62(2):106–14. doi:10.1037/cou0000057.

43. Gard T, Holzel BK, Sack AT, Hempel H, Lazar SW, Vaitl D, et al. Pain attenuation through mindfulness is associated with decreased cognitive control and increased sensory processing in the brain. Cereb Cortex. 2012;22(11):2692–702. doi:10.1093/cercor/bhr352.

44. Murakami H, Katsunuma R, Oba K, Terasawa Y, Motomura Y, Mishima K, et al. Neural networks for mindfulness and emotion suppression. PLoS One. 2015;10(6):e0128005. doi:10.1371/journal.pone.0128005.

45. Sanger KL, Dorjee D. Mindfulness training for adolescents: a neurodevelopmental perspective on investigating modifications in attention and emotion regulation using event-related brain potentials. Cogn Affect Behav Neurosci. 2015;15(3):696–711.

46. Petter M, McGrath PJ, Chambers CT, Dick BD. The effects of mindful attention and state mindfulness on acute experimental pain among adolescents. J Pediatr Psychol. 2014;39(5):521–31. doi:10.1093/jpepsy/jsu007.

47. Chambers R, Gullone E, Hassed C, Knight W, Garvin T, Allen N. Mindful emotion regulation predicts recovery in depressed youth. Mindfulness. 2015; 6(3):523–34. doi:10.1007/s12671-014-0284-4.

48. Pearson MR, Lawless AK, Brown DB, Bravo AJ. Mindfulness and emotional outcomes: identifying subgroups of college students using latent profile analysis. Pers Individ Dif. 2015;76:33–8. doi:10.1016/j.paid.2014.11.009.

49. Peters JR, Smart LM, Eisenlohr-Moul TA, Geiger PJ, Smith GT, Baer RA. Anger rumination as a mediator of the relationship between mindfulness and aggression: the utility of a multidimensional mindfulness model. J Clin Psychol. 2015;71(9):871–84.

50. Shapiro SL, Lyons KE, Miller RC, Butler B, Vieten C, Zelazo PD. Contemplation in the classroom: a new direction for improving childhood education. Edu Psychol Rev. 2015;27(1):1–30. doi:10.1007/s10648-014-9265-3.

51. Shonin E, Van Gordon W, Griffiths MD. Mindfulness-based interventions: towards mindful clinical integration. Front Psychol. 2013;4:194. doi:10.3389/fpsyg.2013.00194.

52. Tan L. A critical review of adolescent mindfulness-based programmes. Clin Child Psychol Psychiatry. 2015;pii:1359104515577486.

53. Kabat-Zinn J. Wherever you go there you are: mindfulness meditation in everyday life. New York, NY: Hyperion; 1994.

54. Huppert FA, Johnson DM. A controlled trial of mindfulness training in schools: the importance of practice for an impact on well-being. J Posit Psychol. 2010; 5(4):264–74. doi:10.1080/17439761003794148.

55. Atkinson M, Wade T. Mindfulness-based prevention for eating disorders: a school-based cluster randomised controlled study. Int J Eat Disord. 2015;48(7):1024–37.

56. Bakosh LS, Snow RM, Tobias JM, Houlihan JL, Barbosa-Leiker C. Mindful learning: an innovative mindful awareness intervention improves elementary school students' quarterly grades. Mindfulness. 2015. doi:10.007/s12671-015-0387-6.

57. Zajonc A. Meditation as contemplative inquiry. Great Barrington, MA: Lindisfarne Books; 2010.

58. Fazel M, Hoagwood K, Stephan S, Ford T. Mental health interventions in schools in high-income countries. Lancet Psychiatry. 2014;1(5):377–87.

59. Robinson J, Cox G, Malone A, Williamson M, Baldwin G, Fletcher K, et al. A systematic review of school-based interventions aimed at preventing, treating, and responding to suicide-related behavior in young people. Crisis. 2015;34(3):164–82.

60. Sandler I, Wolchik SA, Cruden G, Mahrer NE, Ahn S, Brincks A, et al. Overview of meta-analyses of the prevention of mental health, substance use and conduct problems. Annu Rev Clin Psychol. 2014;10:243.

Index